Taste of Home
DIABETES
COOKBOOK

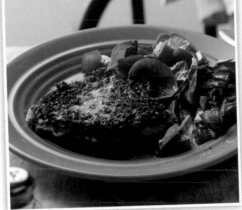

TASTE OF HOME BOOKS • RDA ENTHUSIAST BRANDS, LLC • MILWAUKEE, WI

Taste of Home

EDITORIAL

Vice President, Content Operations: Kerri Balliet
Creative Director: Howard Greenberg

Managing Editor, Print & Digital Books: Mark Hagen
Associate Creative Director: Edwin Robles Jr.

Editor: Christine Rukavena
Contributing Editor: Rachael Liska
Art Director: Raeann Thompson
Graphic Designer: Courtney Lovetere
Layout Designers: Catherine Fletcher, Dalma Vogt
Copy Chief: Deb Warlaumont Mulvey
Copy Editors: Dulcie Shoener (senior), Ronald Kovach, Chris McLaughlin, Ellie Piper
Contributing Copy Editor: Amy Rabideau Silvers
Editorial Services Manager: Kelly Madison-Liebe
Editorial Production Coordinator: Jill Banks

Content Director: Julie Blume Benedict
Food Editors: James Schend; Peggy Woodward, RDN
Recipe Editors: Sue Ryon (lead), Irene Yeh

Culinary Director: Sarah Thompson
Test Cooks: Nicholas Iverson (lead), Matthew Hass
Food Stylists: Kathryn Conrad (lead), Lauren Knoelke, Shannon Roum
Kitchen Operations Manager: Bethany Van Jacobson
Culinary Assistant: Aria C. Thornton
Food Buyer: Maria Petrella

Photography Director: Stephanie Marchese
Photographers: Dan Roberts, Jim Wieland
Photographer/Set Stylist: Grace Natoli Sheldon
Set Stylists: Melissa Franco (lead), Stacey Genaw, Dee Dee Schaefer

Business Architect, Publishing Technologies: Amanda Harmatys
Business Analysts, Publishing Technologies: Dena Ahlers, Kate Unger
Junior Business Analyst, Publishing Technologies: Shannon Stroud

Editorial Business Manager: Kristy Martin
Editorial Business Associate: Andrea Meiers
Rights & Permissions Assistant: Jill Godsey

BUSINESS

Publisher: Donna Lindskog
Strategic Partnerships Manager, Taste of Home Live: Jamie Piette Andrzejewski

TRUSTED MEDIA BRANDS, INC.

President & Chief Executive Officer: Bonnie Kintzer
Chief Financial Officer: Dean Durbin
Chief Marketing Officer: C. Alec Casey
Chief Revenue Officer: Richard Sutton
Chief Digital Officer: Vince Errico
Senior Vice President, Global HR & Communications: Phyllis E. Gebhardt, SPHR; SHRM-SCP
General Counsel: Mark Sirota
Vice President, Product Marketing: Brian Kennedy
Vice President, Consumer Acquisition: Heather Plant
Vice President, Operations: Michael Garzone
Vice President, Consumer Marketing Planning: Jim Woods
Vice President, Digital Product & Technology: Nick Contardo
Vice President, Digital Content & Audience Development: Kari Hodes
Vice President, Financial Planning & Analysis: William Houston

For other *Taste of Home* books and products,
visit **tasteofhome.com**

International Standard Book Number: 978-1-61765-683-5
Library of Congress Control Number: 2017935182

Cover Photographer: Jim Wieland
Set Stylist: Stacey Genaw
Food Stylist: Kathryn Conrad

Pictured on cover: Chocolate-Topped Strawberry Cheesecake, page 307
Pictured on back cover: (from left) Shrimp-Slaw Pitas, page 206; Cheesy Spinach-Stuffed Shells, page 237; English Muffin Egg Sandwich, page 29
Pictured on spine: Quick Hawaiian Pizza, page 198
Pictured on title page: Parmesan Pork Chops with Spinach Salad, page 192
Pictured below left: Garden Vegetable Beef Soup, page 62

Printed in China.
5 7 9 10 8 6

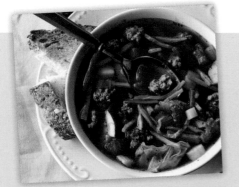

GET SOCIAL WITH US!

 LIKE US
facebook.com/
tasteofhome

PIN US
pinterest.com/
taste_of_home

To find a recipe
tasteofhome.com

FOLLOW US
@tasteofhome

  TWEET US
twitter.com/
tasteofhome

To submit a recipe
tasteofhome.com/submit

To find out about other
Taste of Home products
shoptasteofhome.com

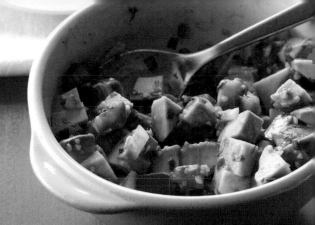

Contents

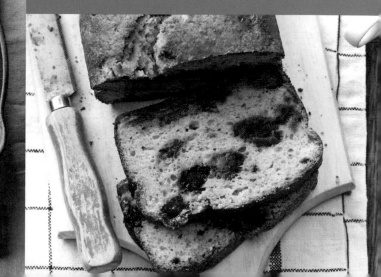

Understanding Diabetes

What is it?

Our bodies require insulin **to help get glucose into our cells** for energy. When you have diabetes, your body is either **not producing enough insulin to feed your cells** or **cells are resisting the insulin.** When this happens, the level of glucose rises in the blood, leading to a variety of dangerous consequences.

Type 1 diabetes occurs when the body's immune system destroys the cells in the pancreas that produce insulin. That's why people with Type 1 diabetes take insulin shots or use an insulin pump.

Type 2 diabetes occurs when your cells begin to resist the insulin produced by your pancreas. Healthy eating, physical activity and regular blood glucose testing are the main therapies for Type 2 diabetes.

Left untreated, high blood glucose can cause nerve damage, kidney or eye problems, heart disease and stroke, so it's important to talk to your doctor about whether you should be actively checking your blood glucose levels.

The key to successfully managing diabetes is to control blood sugar while getting the right amount of nutrients. And that starts with a healthy diet. Each of the 397 recipes in this book offers Nutrition Facts and Diabetic Exchanges, so you can choose the best recipes for you and your family.

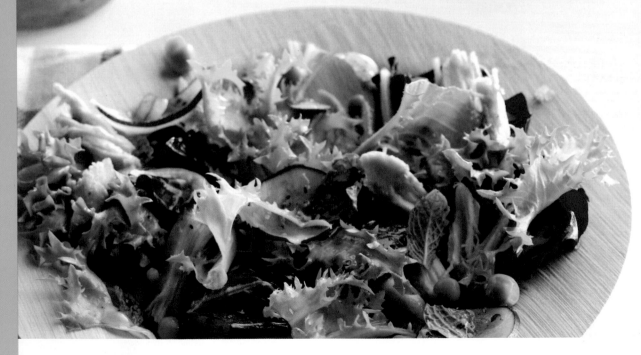

Three Myths Worth Busting

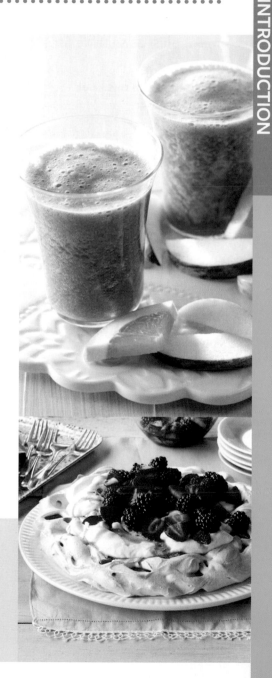

1 People with diabetes **have to eat different meals** and snacks from the rest of the family.
MYTH
It's true that family members with diabetes have to watch what they eat, but there's no need to cook separate dishes. Everyone will benefit from eating more leafy greens, high-fiber foods and lean proteins.

2 People with diabetes **can't eat sweets** or desserts.
MYTH
Almost everyone has a hankering for something sweet from time to time. A good way to deal with a food craving is to enjoy a little taste. Having a small portion on special occasions will prevent you from feeling deprived so you can keep focusing on healthful foods.

3 People with diabetes **shouldn't eat starchy foods.**
MYTH
Everyone needs carbohydrates for energy. Whole grains and starchy vegetables like potatoes, yams, peas and corn can be included in meals and snacks, but portion size is key. According to the American Diabetes Association, a good place to start is to aim for 45-60 grams of carbohydrate per meal or 3-4 servings per day of carbohydrate-containing foods. Depending on your needs and how you manage your diabetes, you may need to adjust this amount. Your health care team can help you determine suitable portions.

Quick Facts from the American Diabetes Association
- Twenty-nine million Americans have Type 2 diabetes and about 86 million have prediabetes—and the number is rising.
- Type 2 diabetes accounts for 90 to 95 percent of all cases of diabetes.
- Eating well and losing even a few pounds can reduce the risk of diabetes and other health problems.

How This Book Can Help

All the recipes in **Diabetes Cookbook** have been reviewed and approved by a registered dietitian nutritionist as suitable for someone with diabetes to consider including in meal plans.

The recipes in this book can help you:

- Incorporate more fruits, vegetables and whole grains into meals
- Prepare flavorful meals with just a few higher-fat, higher-sodium foods
- Eat healthy foods most of the time, while savoring an occasional indulgence

Smart Choices

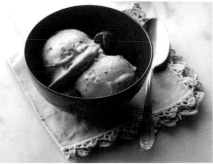

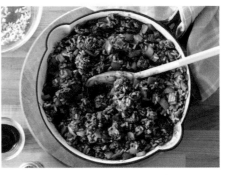

Milwaukee's **Melissa Hansen** uses the natural sweetness of raspberries and ripe bananas in **RASPBERRY-BANANA SOFT SERVE.** Her recipe uses less than 1 teaspoon of maple syrup per serving, compared to the 4-6 teaspoons of sugar you'd find in traditional ice cream. **P. 304**

Stay powered up all day with Texas home cook **Joan Hallford's** flavorful recipe for **MOM'S SPANISH RICE.** The dish stars satisfying ground beef and brown rice, while zesty peppers, tomatoes, and onion work in a full cup of veggies (2 vegetable exchanges) per serving. **P. 97**

Healthy Makeover Tips

Use these tricks to make over your own favorite recipes. See how quickly the savings add up!

	ORIGINAL	SUBSTITUTE	SAVE (per serving)
Spaghetti	1 pound Italian turkey sausage; *4 servings*	• ½ pound Italian turkey sausage • ½ pound lean ground turkey • 1 teaspoon Italian seasoning	200 mg sodium
Tacos	1 pound lean ground beef; *4 servings*	• ½ pound lean ground beef • 1 can black beans (rinsed and drained)	5 g fat (2 g saturated fat) (and add 4 g fiber)
Chili	2 cans tomatoes and 1 can tomato sauce; *8 servings*	• no-salt-added versions in the same amounts	400 mg sodium
Cream Soup	2 cups half-and-half cream; *8 servings*	• 2 cups reduced-fat evaporated milk	30 calories, 5 g fat (4 g saturated fat)
Pancakes	4 tablespoons melted butter; *8 servings*	• 2 tablespoons melted butter • 2 tablespoons canola oil	2 g saturated fat
Brunch Bake	12 large eggs; *8 servings*	• 4 large eggs • 2 cups egg substitute	42 calories, 5 g fat (2 g saturated fat)
Quick Breads	1 cup each chocolate chips and chopped pecans; *12 servings*	• ½ cup each in the bread • 1 tablespoon each sprinkled on top	57 calories, 5 g fat
Cupcakes	1 cup canola oil; *24 servings*	• ½ cup canola oil • ½ cup applesauce	36 calories, 5 g fat

About Our Nutrition Info

Diabetic Exchanges
A helpful tool in making smart food choices is the food-exchange system, which organizes foods into several groups—generally starches, fruits, vegetables, milk, meat and protein-based substitutes and fats. The idea behind the exchange system is that every item within a given category is nutritionally equivalent to every other item in the same category, providing roughly the same amount of carbohydrate, fat, protein and calories.

While Diabetic Exchanges are designed for people with diabetes, they can also be valuable for anyone trying to control calories, reduce fat and eat a balanced diet. Diabetic Exchanges are assigned to recipes in accordance with guidelines from the American Diabetes Association and the Academy of Nutrition and Dietetics.

Ranges of Exchanges
Some exchange lists are subdivided into groups that specify exchanges of, say, lean meats and substitutes (separate from high-fat meats), or fat-free milk products (separate from the whole-milk products). Foods within each category are nutritionally equivalent in the exchange system.

Total Sugars
We've added total sugars to our nutrition facts information. For example: 294 cal., 12g fat (2g sat. fat), 64mg chol., 218mg sodium, 20g carb. (13g sugars, 3g fiber), 24g pro.

Note: This number represents added sugars plus naturally occurring sugars, like what you see in the Nutrition Facts label on packaged foods.

Special Indicators
To help you find dishes to suit your needs, we clearly mark recipes with these helpful icons:

FAST FIX ▶ Table-ready in just 30 minutes or less

⑤INGREDIENTS Recipes made with 5 or fewer ingredients

SLOW COOKER 🍲 Set it and forget it

COMMON DIABETIC EXCHANGES

STARCHES
- 1 slice bread
- ½ cup cooked lentils
- ⅓ cup cooked pasta
- ½ cup corn
- 1 small potato

VEGETABLES
- ½ cup cooked carrots
- ½ cup cooked green beans
- 1 cup raw radishes
- 1 cup raw salad greens
- 1 large tomato

FRUITS
- 1 small banana
- ½ large pear
- 17 small grapes
- 2 tablespoons raisins
- ½ cup fruit cocktail

FAT-FREE AND LOW-FAT MILKS
- 1 cup skim or 1% milk
- 1 cup plain nonfat yogurt
- ⅔ cup low-fat fruit-flavored yogurt
- ⅔ cup evaporated nonfat milk
- 1 cup low-fat buttermilk

LEAN MEATS AND SUBSTITUTES
- 1 ounce skinless chicken breast
- 1 ounce canned tuna (in water or oil, drained)
- 1 ounce cheese with 3 grams of fat or less per ounce
- ¼ cup low-fat cottage cheese
- 2 egg whites

FATS
- 1 teaspoon oil
- 1 teaspoon stick butter
- 1½ teaspoons peanut butter
- 1 tablespoon reduced-fat margarine spread
- 1 tablespoon reduced-fat mayonnaise
- 6 almonds
- 4½ teaspoons reduced-fat cream cheese

How We Calculate Nutrition Facts

The **Diabetes Cookbook** provides a variety of recipes that fit into a healthy lifestyle.

- Whenever a choice of ingredients is given (such as ½ cup sour cream or plain yogurt), the first ingredient is used in our calculations.
- When a range is given for an ingredient, we calculate using the first amount.
- Only the amount of a marinade absorbed is calculated.
- Optional ingredients are not included in our calculations.

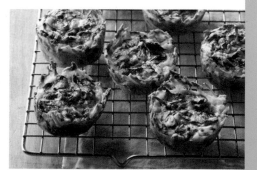

Pump Up Your Exercise Routine

Physical activity is one of the most effective ways to manage diabetes because it can shave off excess weight, and even a small loss can lead to improved glucose control. Exercise is almost like insulin in its ability to bring down blood sugar and boost insulin sensitivity. It also improves blood circulation, protects your heart by decreasing blood pressure and improving cholesterol, relieves stress, builds confidence and makes you feel good!

Before starting an exercise program, consult your doctor for recommendations tailored to your level of fitness and appropriate for your health. Walking is one of the best exercises to try if you're just getting started. It's easy, fun and free! Aim for 30 minutes of light to moderate activity five times a week, or 20 minutes of vigorous activity three times a week.

Get Moving!

In a landmark Harvard study of some 40,000 women over the age of 45, those who walked as little as one hour a week—even at a stroll—were half as likely to have coronary heart disease as those who rarely walked for exercise. Walking is easier with good form, so follow these easy tips for proper posture to start your path to healthier tomorrows!

HEAD
Imagine a string attached to the top of your head, pulling it straight toward the sky. Keep your chin lifted and your ears in line with your shoulders.

SHOULDERS
Keep them relaxed, down and slightly back. If they start hunching up toward your ears, take a deep breath and drop them back again.

ARMS
Elbows should be bent at about 90-degree angles, hands slightly cupped. Relax your arms and pump them forward and back as you walk; they should not crisscross in front of you. Walking with light hand weights can help build muscle and burn calories, but too much weight will strain the elbows and shoulders.

CHEST
Yoga practitioners sometimes refer to the breastbone area as your "heart light." Keep your heart light lifted and shining straight ahead.

ABDOMINALS
Pull your belly button toward your spine as if you were zipping up a snug pair of jeans. Keep those abs firm and tight as you walk.

FEET
With each step, plant your heel, roll onto the ball of your foot, and push off with your toes. Avoid rolling your foot inward or outward. To protect your feet and joints, wear good walking shoes. A proper fit means they feel great right out of the box. Make sure there's a finger width between the end of your longest toe and the inside of the front of the shoe.

CHRISTOPHER EDWIN NUZZACO/SHUTTERSTOCK

Live It Up!

Three small changes that can improve health and happiness

1 WALK IT OFF

Everybody gives in to temptation once in a while—the homemade biscuits, the mashed potatoes, the strawberry shortcake you just can't turn away. But that can make blood sugar rise too high later. While it's not a magic eraser, going for short after-meal strolls can work wonders for the body, studies have shown. And walking after eating dinner might be especially good for controlling blood sugar.

TIP: *If foot problems make walking difficult, invest in an inexpensive "pedaler"—a set of bike pedals on a frame that you use while sitting in a chair.*

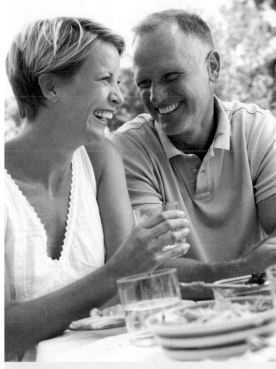

2 TALK IT OUT

Do a brief daily check-in with an online diabetes support group, or just post a comment or observation on a diabetes message board. It really can help you stay on track, blow off steam, and get much-needed encouragement from the real experts—people just like you who live with blood-sugar control challenges every day. Plus, you get the chance to reach out to someone else and share your own tips and experiences. The American Diabetes Association, the Joslin Diabetes Center, and the website PatientsLikeMe all host online boards or groups.

TIP: *Load your smartphone with apps that help you track your blood sugar and remind you to take medications on time.*

3 LAUGH IT UP

Deciding between a silly comedy and an action flick for movie night? Go for funny. Laughter helps your body process blood sugar more efficiently and relaxes your arteries. Indulging regularly even protects against heart attacks—good news for people with diabetes whose tickers are at higher risk for trouble.

ADDITIONAL RESOURCES

American Diabetes Association
1-800-Diabetes (1-800-342-2383)
Diabetes.org

American Association of Diabetes Educators
Diabeteseducator.org

Academy of Nutrition and Dietetics
Eatright.org

The Diabetic Newsletter
Diabeticnewsletter.com

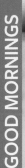

**ENGLISH MUFFIN EGG
SANDWICH, PAGE 29**

Good Mornings

It's time to rise and shine! Start the day off right with
a healthy breakfast featuring good-for-you ingredients.
From weekday quick fixes to lazy Sunday brunches,
enjoy sandwiches, stratas, smoothies and other
can't-beat breakfast favorites.

LEMON-RASPBERRY
RICOTTA PANCAKES

STRAWBERRY-CARROT SMOOTHIES

My children aren't big veggie fans, but they love smoothies. This smoothie packs in lots of good-for-you fruits and veggies, but to my kids, it's just a super delicious breakfast.

—ELISABETH LARSEN PLEASANT GROVE, UT

START TO FINISH: 5 MIN.
MAKES: 5 SERVINGS

- 2 cups (16 ounces) reduced-fat plain Greek yogurt
- 1 cup carrot juice
- 1 cup orange juice
- 1 cup frozen pineapple chunks
- 1 cup frozen unsweetened sliced strawberries

Place all ingredients in a blender; cover and process until smooth.
Per 1 cup: 141 cal., 2g fat (1g sat. fat), 5mg chol., 79mg sod., 20g carb. (15g sugars, 1g fiber), 10g pro.
Diabetic Exchanges: 1 fruit, ½ reduced-fat milk.

★ ★ ★ ★ ★ **READER REVIEW**

"These were great! Now I just wish I had bought more yogurt, so I could make them again tonight!"
SSTETZEL TASTEOFHOME.COM

FAST FIX

LEMON-RASPBERRY RICOTTA PANCAKES

I was raised in a home with a Sunday pancake tradition which I keep alive, making pancakes for my own family.

—ANITA ARCHIBALD AURORA, ON

START TO FINISH: 30 MIN.
MAKES: 24 PANCAKES

- 1½ cups cake or all-purpose flour
- ¼ cup sugar
- 2 teaspoons baking powder
- ¼ teaspoon salt
- ¼ teaspoon ground cinnamon
- 1 cup unsweetened almond milk
- 1 cup part-skim ricotta cheese
- 3 large eggs, separated
- 2 teaspoons grated lemon peel
- 3 tablespoons lemon juice
- 1 teaspoon almond extract
- 1 cup fresh or frozen raspberries
  Optional toppings: Whipped cream, maple syrup and additional raspberries

1. In a large bowl, whisk flour, sugar, baking powder, salt and cinnamon. In another bowl, whisk the almond milk, ricotta, egg yolks, lemon peel, lemon juice and extract until blended. Add to the dry ingredients, stirring just until moistened. In a clean small bowl, beat egg whites until stiff but not dry. Fold into batter. Gently stir in raspberries.
2. Lightly grease a griddle; heat over medium heat. Pour batter by ¼ cupfuls onto griddle. Cook until bubbles on top begin to pop and bottoms are golden brown. Turn; cook until second side is golden brown. If desired, serve the pancakes with whipped cream, syrup and additional raspberries.
Per 3 pancakes without toppings: 203 cal., 5g fat (2g sat. fat), 79mg chol., 254mg sod., 31g carb. (7g sugars, 2g fiber), 8g pro.
Diabetic Exchanges: 2 starch, 1 medium-fat meat.

FULL GARDEN FRITTATA

I was cooking for a health-conscious friend and wanted to serve a frittata. To brighten it up, I added classic bruschetta toppings. This has become a staple in my recipe book.

—**MELISSA ROSENTHAL** VISTA, CA

PREP: 25 MIN. • **BAKE:** 10 MIN.
MAKES: 2 SERVINGS

- 4   large eggs
- ⅓   cup 2% milk
- ¼   teaspoon salt, divided
- ⅛   teaspoon coarsely ground pepper
- 2   teaspoons olive oil
- ½   medium zucchini, chopped
- ½   cup chopped baby portobello mushrooms
- ¼   cup chopped onion
- 1   garlic clove, minced
- 2   tablespoons minced fresh basil
- 1   teaspoon minced fresh oregano
- 1   teaspoon minced fresh parsley
  Optional toppings: halved grape tomatoes, small fresh mozzarella cheese balls and thinly sliced fresh basil

1. Preheat oven to 375°. In a bowl, whisk eggs, milk, ⅛ teaspoon salt and pepper. In an 8-in. ovenproof skillet, heat oil over medium-high heat. Add zucchini, mushrooms and onion; cook and stir until tender. Add garlic, herbs and the remaining salt; cook 1 minute longer. Pour in egg mixture.

2. Bake, uncovered, 10-15 minutes or until eggs are set. Cut into four wedges. If desired, serve with toppings.

Per 2 wedges without toppings: 227 cal., 15g fat (4g sat. fat), 375mg chol., 463mg sod., 7g carb. (5g sugars, 1g fiber), 15g pro.

Diabetic Exchanges: 2 medium-fat meat, 1 vegetable, 1 fat.

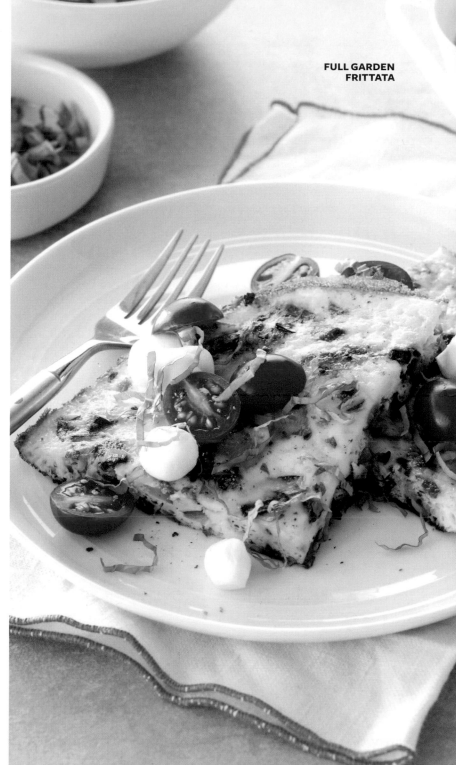

FULL GARDEN FRITTATA

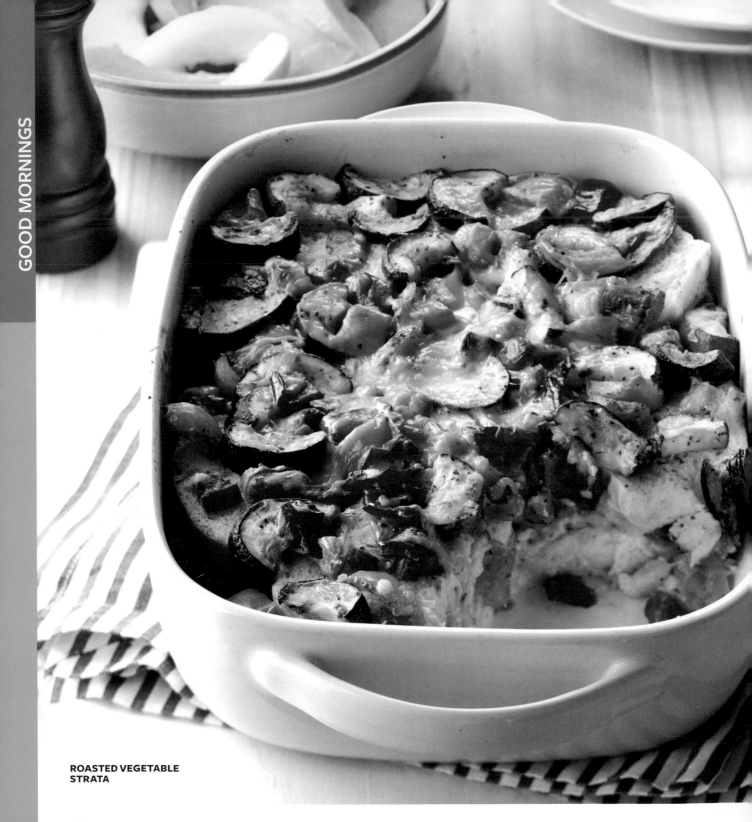

ROASTED VEGETABLE STRATA

ROASTED VEGETABLE STRATA

With the abundance of zucchini we have in fall, this makes the perfect breakfast dish that's sure to please!
—COLLEEN DOUCETTE TRURO, NS

PREP: 55 MIN. + CHILLING • **BAKE:** 40 MIN.
MAKES: 8 SERVINGS

- 3 large zucchini, halved lengthwise and cut into ¾-inch slices
- 1 each medium red, yellow and orange peppers, cut into 1-inch pieces
- 2 tablespoons olive oil
- 1 teaspoon dried oregano
- ½ teaspoon salt
- ½ teaspoon pepper
- ½ teaspoon dried basil
- 1 medium tomato, chopped
- 1 loaf (1 pound) unsliced crusty Italian bread
- ½ cup shredded sharp cheddar cheese
- ½ cup shredded Asiago cheese
- 6 large eggs
- 2 cups fat-free milk

1. Preheat oven to 400°. Toss zucchini and peppers with oil and seasonings; transfer to a 15x10x1-in. pan. Roast until tender, 25-30 minutes, stirring once. Stir in tomato; cool slightly.
2. Trim ends from bread; cut into 1-in. slices. In a greased 13x9-in. baking dish, layer half of each of the following: bread, roasted vegetables and cheeses. Repeat layers. Whisk together eggs and milk; pour evenly over top. Refrigerate, covered, 6 hours or overnight.
3. Preheat oven to 375°. Remove casserole from refrigerator while oven heats. Bake, uncovered, until golden brown, 40-50 minutes. Let stand 5-10 minutes before cutting.

To freeze: Cover and freeze unbaked casserole. To use, partially thaw in the refrigerator overnight. Remove from refrigerator 30 minutes before baking. Preheat oven to 375°. Bake casserole as directed, increasing time as necessary to heat through and for a thermometer inserted in center to read 165°.
Per piece: 349 cal., 14g fat (5g sat. fat), 154mg chol., 642mg sod., 40g carb. (9g sugars, 4g fiber), 17g pro.
Diabetic Exchanges: 2 starch, 1 medium-fat meat, 1 vegetable, 1 fat.

FAST FIX
HONEY-YOGURT BERRY SALAD

I wanted my family to eat more fruit but not more sugary ingredients. This berry salad lets you play with different low-fat yogurts and fruits.
—BETSY KING DULUTH, MN

START TO FINISH: 10 MIN.
MAKES: 8 SERVINGS

- 1½ cups sliced fresh strawberries
- 1½ cups fresh raspberries
- 1½ cups fresh blueberries
- 1½ cups fresh blackberries
- 1 cup (8 ounces) reduced-fat plain yogurt
- 1 tablespoon honey
- ¼ teaspoon grated orange peel
- 1 tablespoon orange juice

Place berries in a glass bowl; toss to combine. In a small bowl, mix remaining ingredients. Spoon over berries.
Per ¾ cup fruit with 2 tablespoons yogurt mixture: 76 cal., 1g fat (0 sat. fat), 2mg chol., 23mg sod., 16g carb. (11g sugars, 4g fiber), 3g pro.
Diabetic Exchanges: 1 fruit.

FAST FIX
POTATO-CHEDDAR FRITTATA

I like to serve this protein-packed frittata with toasted rustic bread. You can also use leftovers instead of the refrigerated potatoes with onions.
—DONNA RYAN TOPSFIELD, MA

START TO FINISH: 30 MIN.
MAKES: 4 SERVINGS

- 8 large egg whites
- 4 large eggs
- ½ cup shredded cheddar cheese
- ½ cup fat-free milk
- 2 green onions, chopped
- 2 teaspoons minced fresh parsley
- ¼ teaspoon salt
- ¼ teaspoon pepper
- 1 tablespoon canola oil
- 1½ cups refrigerated diced potatoes with onion

1. Preheat broiler. In a large bowl, whisk the first eight ingredients. In a 10-in. ovenproof skillet, heat oil over medium-high heat. Add the potatoes with onion; cook and stir for 3-4 minutes or until tender. Reduce heat; pour in the egg mixture. Cook, covered, 5-7 minutes or until nearly set.
2. Broil 3-4 in. from heat 2-3 minutes or until eggs are completely set. Let stand 5 minutes. Cut into wedges.
Per wedge: 241 cal., 13g fat (5g sat. fat), 201mg chol., 555mg sod., 11g carb. (2g sugars, 1g fiber), 19g pro.
Diabetic Exchanges: 2 medium-fat meat, 1 starch, 1 fat.

FAST FIX

GREEK VEGGIE OMELET

This is a family favorite in my house. It's very quick and satisfying, not to mention yummy!

—SHARON MANNIX WINDSOR, NY

START TO FINISH: 20 MIN.
MAKES: 2 SERVINGS

- 4 large eggs
- 2 tablespoons fat-free milk
- ⅛ teaspoon salt
- 3 teaspoons olive oil, divided
- 2 cups sliced baby portobello mushrooms
- ¼ cup finely chopped onion
- 1 cup fresh baby spinach
- 3 tablespoons crumbled feta cheese
- 2 tablespoons sliced ripe olives
  Freshly ground pepper

1. Whisk together eggs, milk and salt. In a large nonstick skillet, heat 2 teaspoons oil over medium-high heat; saute mushrooms and onion until golden brown, 5-6 minutes. Stir in spinach until wilted; remove from pan.
2. In same pan, heat remaining oil over medium-low heat. Pour in egg mixture. As eggs set, push cooked portions toward the center, letting uncooked eggs flow underneath. When eggs are thickened and no liquid egg remains, spoon vegetables on one side; sprinkle with cheese and olives. Fold to close; cut in half to serve. Sprinkle with freshly ground pepper.
Per serving: 271 cal., 19g fat (5g sat. fat), 378mg chol., 475mg sod., 7g carb. (3g sugars, 2g fiber), 18g pro.
Diabetic Exchanges: 2 medium-fat meat, 2 fat, 1 vegetable.

RASPBERRY PEACH PUFF PANCAKE

Here's a simple, satisfying treat that's perfect for company for brunch. And it's elegant enough to serve it for dessert at other meals.

—*TASTE OF HOME* TEST KITCHEN

PREP: 15 MIN. • **BAKE:** 20 MIN.
MAKES: 4 SERVINGS

- 2 medium peaches, peeled and sliced
- ½ teaspoon sugar
- ½ cup fresh raspberries
- 1 tablespoon butter
- 3 large eggs, lightly beaten
- ½ cup fat-free milk
- ⅛ teaspoon salt
- ½ cup all-purpose flour
- ¼ cup vanilla yogurt

1. Preheat oven to 400°. In a small bowl, toss peaches with sugar; gently stir in raspberries.
2. Place butter in a 9-in. pie plate; heat in oven 2-3 minutes or until butter is melted. Meanwhile, in a small bowl, whisk eggs, milk and salt until blended; gradually whisk in in flour. Remove pie plate from the oven; tilt carefully, coating bottom and sides with butter. Immediately pour in egg mixture.
3. Bake 18-22 minutes or until puffed and browned. Remove pancake from the oven. Serve immediately with fruit mixture and yogurt.
Per 1 piece with ½ cup fruit and 1 tablespoon yogurt: 199 cal., 7g fat (3g sat. fat), 149mg chol., 173mg sod., 25g carb. (11g sugars, 3g fiber), 9g pro.
Diabetic Exchanges: 1 medium-fat meat, 1 fruit, ½ starch, ½ fat.

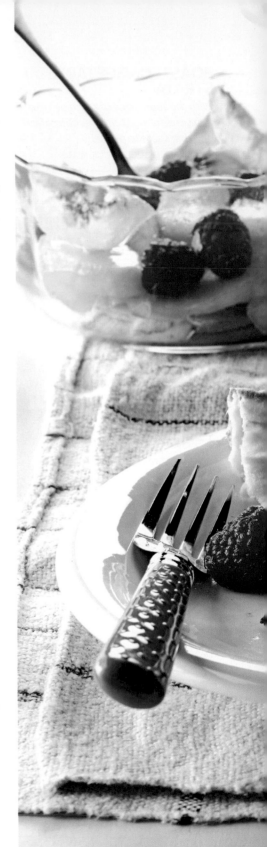

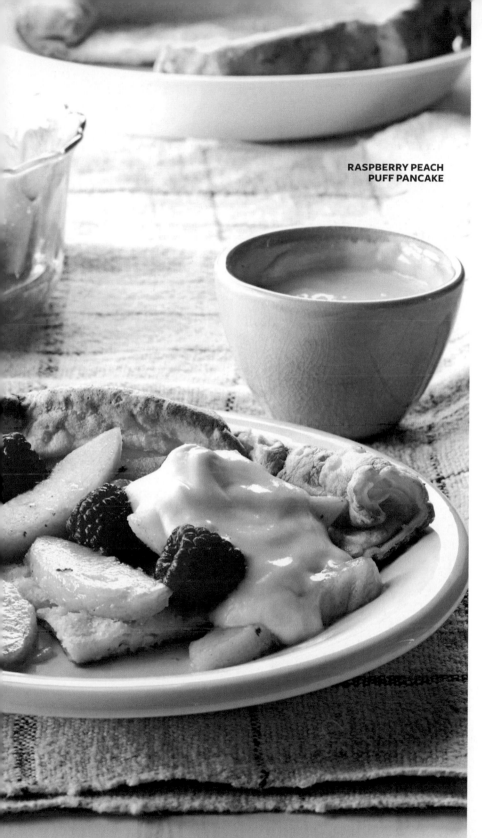

RASPBERRY PEACH PUFF PANCAKE

FAST FIX ▶

APPLE SPICED TEA

Take a moment to enjoy a cup of tea in the morning. After you try this sweetly spiced drink, you'll make it a regularly.
—SUSAN WESTERFIELD ALBUQUERQUE, NM

START TO FINISH: 10 MIN.
MAKES: 1 SERVING

- ½ cup apple cider or juice
- ¼ teaspoon minced fresh gingerroot
- 2 whole allspice
- 2 whole cloves
- 1 black tea bag
- ½ cup boiling water
- 1 tablespoon brown sugar

In a small bowl, combine the first five Ingredients. Add boiling water. Cover and steep for 5 minutes. Strain, discarding tea bag and spices. Stir in sugar. Serve immediately.

Per serving: 112 cal., 0 fat (0 sat. fat), 0 chol., 12mg sod., 28g carb. (27g sugars, 0 fiber), 0 pro.
Diabetic Exchanges: 1 starch, 1 fruit.

★ ★ ★ ★ ★ **READER REVIEW**

"This was delicious. We go through a lot of tea in winter, so we'll use this keeper of a recipe again and again."

BECKY66 TASTEOFHOME.COM

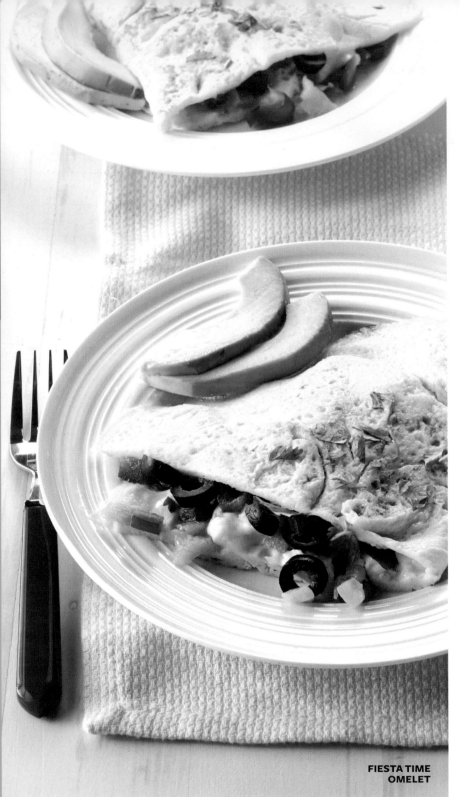

FIESTA TIME OMELET

FIESTA TIME OMELET

I created this dish when I needed to use up some black olives and jalapenos. With an abundance of vegetables, two of these large omelets can feed four people if served with side dishes.

—JENNINE VICTORY BEE BRANCH, AR

START TO FINISH: 15 MIN.
MAKES: 2 SERVINGS

- 4   large eggs
- ¼   cup fat-free milk
- ¼   teaspoon salt
- ¼   cup queso fresco
- ¼   cup canned diced jalapeno peppers or chopped green chilies
- 2   tablespoons finely chopped sweet red pepper
- 2   tablespoons sliced ripe olives
- 2   teaspoons chopped fresh cilantro
- ¼   medium ripe avocado, peeled and sliced

1. In a small bowl, whisk eggs, milk and salt until blended.

2. Place a 10-in. nonstick skillet coated with cooking spray over medium-high heat. Pour in egg mixture. The mixture should set immediately at edges. As eggs set, push cooked portions toward the center, letting uncooked eggs flow underneath. When eggs are thickened and no liquid egg remains, spoon the cheese, peppers, olives and cilantro on one side. Fold omelet in half. Cut in half; slide onto two plates. Top with avocado.

Per serving: 242 cal., 16g fat (5g sat. fat), 383mg chol., 601mg sod., 7g carb. (3g sugars, 2g fiber), 18g pro.
Diabetic Exchanges: 2 medium-fat meat, 1 fat, ½ starch.

FAST FIX

EGG & HASH BROWN BREAKFAST CUPS

When I want to deliver homey breakfast comfort, I turn sausage, eggs and hash browns into easy muffin-style cups. They're winners for dinner, too.
—**SUSAN STETZEL** GAINESVILLE, NY

START TO FINISH: 30 MIN.
MAKES: 2 SERVINGS

- 3 uncooked turkey breakfast sausage links (1 ounce each), casings removed
- 3 tablespoons chopped green pepper
- 2 tablespoons chopped onion
- ½ cup frozen cubed hash brown potatoes
- ⅓ cup fat-free milk
- ¼ cup egg substitute
- 3 tablespoons reduced-fat biscuit/baking mix
- ⅛ teaspoon pepper
- 2 tablespoons shredded reduced-fat cheddar cheese

1. Preheat oven to 400°. In a nonstick skillet coated with cooking spray, cook and stir sausage with green pepper and onion over medium heat until no longer pink, breaking sausage into small pieces. Stir in potatoes. Divide among four muffin cups coated with cooking spray.
2. Whisk together milk, egg substitute, baking mix and pepper; pour into cups. Sprinkle with cheese. Bake until a knife inserted in center comes out clean, 13-15 minutes.
Per 2 egg cups: 158 cal., 5g fat (2g sat. fat), 28mg chol., 435mg sod., 15g carb. (4g sugars, 1g fiber), 13g pro.
Diabetic Exchanges: 1 starch, 1 medium-fat meat.

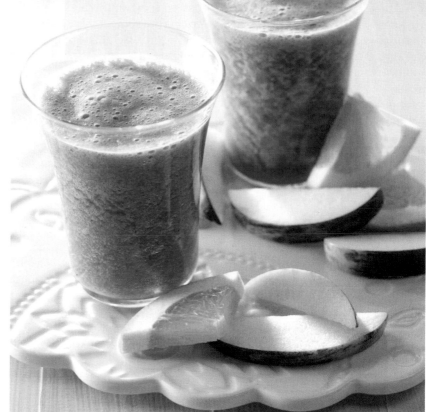

GINGER-KALE SMOOTHIES

FAST FIX

GINGER-KALE SMOOTHIES

Since I started drinking these spicy smoothies for breakfast every day, I honestly feel better! Substitute any fruit and juice you like to make this recipe your own healthy blend.
—**LINDA GREEN** KILAUEA, HI

START TO FINISH: 15 MIN.
MAKES: 2 SERVINGS

- 1¼ cups orange juice
- 1 teaspoon lemon juice
- 2 cups torn fresh kale
- 1 medium apple, peeled and coarsely chopped
- 1 tablespoon minced fresh gingerroot
- 4 ice cubes
- ⅛ teaspoon ground cinnamon
- ⅛ teaspoon ground turmeric or ¼-inch piece fresh turmeric, peeled and finely chopped
  Dash cayenne pepper

Place all ingredients in a blender; cover and process until blended. Serve the smoothie immediately.
Per 1 cup: 121 cal., 0 fat (0 sat. fat), 0 chol., 22mg sod., 29g carb. (21g sugars, 2g fiber), 1g pro.
Diabetic Exchanges: 1½ fruit, 1 vegetable.

SAUSAGE-EGG BURRITOS

My husband and I try to eat healthy, but finding new meals for breakfast is a challenge. By adding tomatoes, spinach and garlic to eggs with additional egg whites, we created a dish that is both satisfying and light.

—**WENDY G. BALL** BATTLE CREEK, MI

START TO FINISH: 20 MIN.
MAKES: 6 SERVINGS

- ½ pound bulk lean turkey breakfast sausage
- 3 large eggs
- 4 large egg whites
- 1 tablespoon olive oil
- 2 cups chopped fresh spinach
- 2 plum tomatoes, seeded and chopped
- 1 garlic clove, minced
- ¼ teaspoon pepper
- 6 whole wheat tortillas (8 inches), warmed
  Salsa, optional

1. In a large nonstick skillet coated with cooking spray, cook sausage over medium heat 4-6 minutes or until no longer pink, breaking into crumbles. Remove from pan.

2. In a small bowl, whisk eggs and egg whites until blended. In same pan, add eggs; cook and stir over medium heat until eggs are thickened and no liquid egg remains. Remove from pan; wipe skillet clean if necessary.

3. In a skillet, heat oil over medium-high heat. Add spinach, tomatoes and garlic; cook and stir for 2-3 minutes or until the spinach is wilted. Stir in sausage and eggs; heat through. Sprinkle mixture with pepper.

4. To serve, spoon ⅔ cup filling across center of each tortilla. Fold bottom and sides of tortilla over filling and roll up. If desired, serve with salsa.

Per 1 burrito without salsa: 258 cal., 10g fat (2g sat. fat), 134mg chol., 596mg sod., 24g carb. (1g sugars, 4g fiber), 20g pro.
Diabetic Exchanges: 2 medium-fat meat, 1½ starch, ½ fat.

FRESH FRUIT COMBO

Whenever I take this eye-catching fruit salad to a party, people ask for the recipe. Blueberries and cherries give it a distinctive flavor.

—**JULIE STERCHI** CAMPBELLSVLLE, KY

START TO FINISH: 20 MIN.
MAKES: 14 SERVINGS

- 2 cups cubed fresh pineapple
- 2 medium oranges, peeled and chopped
- 3 kiwifruit, peeled and sliced
- 1 cup sliced fresh strawberries
- 1 cup halved seedless red grapes
- 2 medium firm bananas, sliced
- 1 large red apple, cubed
- 1 cup fresh or frozen blueberries
- 1 cup fresh or canned pitted dark sweet cherries

In a large bowl, combine the first five ingredients; refrigerate until serving. When ready to serve, fold in bananas, apple, blueberries and cherries.

Per ¾ cup: 78 cal., 0 fat (0 sat. fat), 0 chol., 3mg sod., 20g carb. (13g sugars, 3g fiber), 1g pro.
Diabetic Exchanges: 1 fruit.

WHOLE WHEAT PECAN WAFFLES

We bought a new waffle iron, and along with it came a recipe. We finally decided to try it, and after a few changes we came up with these delicious waffles.

—**SARAH MORRIS** JOPLIN, MO

START TO FINISH: 30 MIN.
MAKES: 8 SERVINGS

- 2 cups whole wheat pastry flour
- 2 tablespoons sugar
- 3 teaspoons baking powder
- ½ teaspoon salt
- 2 large eggs, separated
- 1¾ cups fat-free milk
- ¼ cup canola oil
- ½ cup chopped pecans

1. Preheat the waffle maker. Whisk together the first four ingredients. In another bowl, whisk together egg yolks, milk and oil; add to the flour mixture, stirring just until moistened.

2. In a clean bowl, beat egg whites on medium speed until stiff but not dry. Fold into batter. Bake waffles according to the manufacturer's directions until golden brown, sprinkling batter with pecans after pouring.

To freeze: Cool waffles on wire racks. Freeze between layers of waxed paper in a resealable plastic freezer bag. Reheat waffles in a toaster or toaster oven on medium setting.

Per 2 (4-in.) waffles: 241 cal., 14g fat (1g sat. fat), 48mg chol., 338mg sod., 24g carb. (6g sugars, 3g fiber), 7g pro.
Diabetic Exchanges: 2½ fat, 1½ starch.

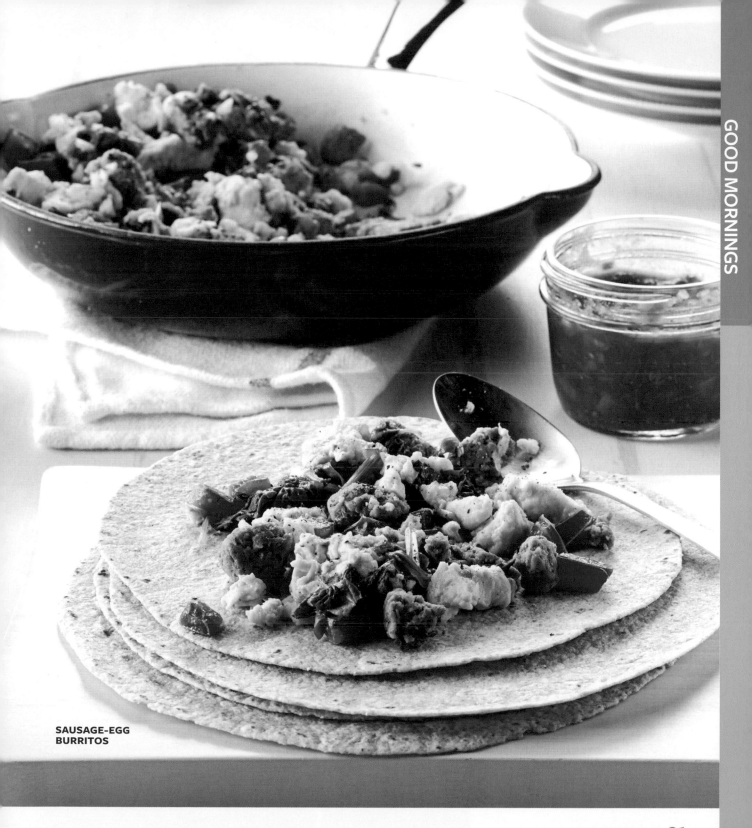

SAUSAGE-EGG BURRITOS

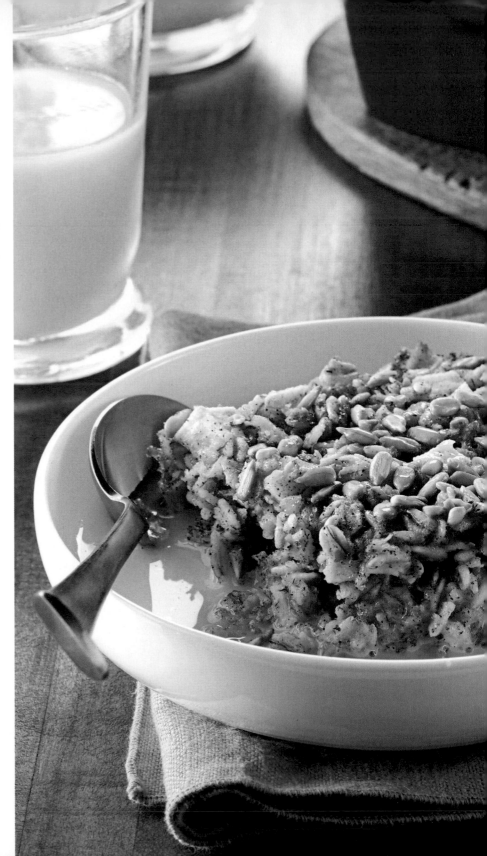

MAPLE APPLE BAKED OATMEAL

I've tried a number of different types of fruit for this recipe, but apple seems to be my family's favorite. I mix the dry and wet ingredients in separate bowls the night before and combine them the next morning when it's time to bake.

—**MEGAN BROOKS** SAINT LAZARE, QC

PREP: 20 MIN. • **BAKE:** 25 MIN.
MAKES: 8 SERVINGS

- 3 cups old-fashioned oats
- 2 teaspoons baking powder
- 1¼ teaspoons ground cinnamon
- ½ teaspoon salt
- ¼ teaspoon ground nutmeg
- 2 large eggs
- 2 cups fat-free milk
- ½ cup maple syrup
- ¼ cup canola oil
- 1 teaspoon vanilla extract
- 1 large apple, chopped
- ¼ cup sunflower kernels or pepitas

1. Preheat oven to 350°. In a large bowl, mix the first five ingredients. In a small bowl, whisk eggs, milk, syrup, oil and vanilla until blended; stir into dry ingredients. Let stand 5 minutes. Stir in apple.
2. Transfer to an 11x7-in. baking dish coated with cooking spray. Sprinkle with sunflower kernels. Bake, uncovered, 25-30 minutes or until set and edges are lightly browned.

Per piece: 305 cal., 13g fat (2g sat. fat), 48mg chol., 325mg sod., 41g carb. (20g sugars, 4g fiber), 8g pro.
Diabetic Exchanges: 3 starch, 1½ fat.

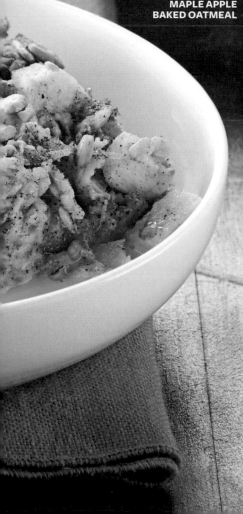

MAPLE APPLE BAKED OATMEAL

FAST FIX ▶

GRAPES WITH LEMON-HONEY YOGURT

We like to sweeten up Greek yogurt with honey, cinnamon and vanilla. It's a tasty counterpoint to plump grapes and crunchy nuts.

—JULIE STERCHI CAMPBELLSVLLE, KY

START TO FINISH: 10 MIN.
MAKES: 8 SERVINGS

- 1 cup fat-free plain Greek yogurt
- 2 tablespoons honey
- 1 teaspoon vanilla extract
- ½ teaspoon grated lemon peel
- ⅛ teaspoon ground cinnamon
- 3 cups seedless red grapes
- 3 cups green grapes
- 3 tablespoons sliced almonds, toasted

In a small bowl, combine the first five ingredients. Divide grapes among eight serving bowls. Top with yogurt mixture; sprinkle with almonds.

Note: To toast nuts, bake in a shallow pan in a 350° oven for 5-10 minutes or cook in a skillet over low heat until lightly browned, stirring occasionally.

Per ¾ cup grapes with 2 tablespoons yogurt mixture and about 1 teaspoon almonds: 138 cal., 2g fat (0 sat. fat), 0 chol., 20mg sod., 28g carb. (26g sugars, 2g fiber), 6g pro.
Diabetic Exchanges: 1½ fruit, ½ starch.

✳
TEST KITCHEN TIP
Greek yogurt boasts more protein and less sugars and carbs than traditional yogurt. Plus, its creamy, rich texture can't be beat.

ASPARAGUS-MUSHROOM FRITTATA

My Sicilian Aunt Paulina's cooking inspired this fluffy frittata.

—CINDY ESPOSITO BLOOMFIELD, NJ

PREP: 25 MIN. • **BAKE:** 20 MIN.
MAKES: 8 SERVINGS

- 8 large eggs
- ½ cup whole-milk ricotta cheese
- 2 tablespoons lemon juice
- ½ teaspoon salt
- ¼ teaspoon pepper
- 1 tablespoon olive oil
- 1 package (8 ounces) frozen asparagus spears, thawed
- 1 large onion, halved and thinly sliced
- ½ cup finely chopped sweet red or green pepper
- ¼ cup sliced baby portobello mushrooms

1. Preheat oven to 350°. In a bowl, whisk eggs, ricotta cheese, lemon juice, salt and pepper. In a 10-in. ovenproof skillet, heat oil over medium heat. Add the asparagus, onion, red pepper and mushrooms; cook and stir 6-8 minutes or until onion and pepper are tender.
2. Remove from heat; remove asparagus from skillet. Reserve eight spears; cut remaining asparagus into 2-in. pieces. Return cut asparagus to skillet; stir in egg mixture. Arrange the reserved asparagus spears over eggs to resemble spokes of a wheel.
3. Bake, uncovered, 20-25 minutes or until eggs are completely set. Let stand 5 minutes. Cut into 8 wedges.

Per wedge: 135 cal., 8g fat (3g sat. fat), 192mg chol., 239mg sod., 7g carb. (2g sugars, 1g fiber), 9g pro.
Diabetic Exchanges: 1 medium-fat meat, 1 vegetable, ½ fat.

BASIL VEGETABLE STRATA

I've been cooking this strata for years, and my family just can't get enough! The fresh basil gives this healthy brunch dish a real flavor boost.

—JEAN ECOS HARTLAND, WI

PREP: 40 MIN. + CHILLING
BAKE: 1 HOUR + STANDING
MAKES: 8 SERVINGS

- 3 teaspoons canola oil, divided
- ¾ pound sliced fresh mushrooms
- 1 cup finely chopped sweet onion
- 1 large sweet red pepper, cut into thin strips
- 1 large sweet yellow pepper, cut into thin strips
- 1 medium leek (white portion only), chopped
- ½ teaspoon salt
- ½ teaspoon pepper
- 10 slices whole wheat bread, cut into 1-inch cubes
- 1½ cups shredded part-skim mozzarella cheese
- ¼ cup grated Parmesan cheese
- 8 large eggs
- 4 large egg whites
- 2½ cups fat-free milk
- ¼ cup chopped fresh basil

1. In a large skillet, heat 1 teaspoon oil over medium-high heat. Add the mushrooms; cook and stir 8-10 minutes or until tender. Remove from pan.

✳

DID YOU KNOW?
Stale, day-old bread works perfectly in breakfast dishes like stratas and egg bakes. That's because its dry texture better soaks up egg-based custards, resulting in a casserole that holds together when eaten.

2. In same pan, heat 1 teaspoon oil over medium heat. Add onion; cook and stir 6-8 minutes or until golden brown. Add onion to mushrooms.
3. Add remaining oil to pan. Add peppers, leek, salt and pepper; cook and stir about 6-8 minutes or until leek pieces are tender. Stir in the sauteed mushrooms and onion.
4. In a 13x9-in. baking dish coated with cooking spray, layer half of each of the following: bread cubes, vegetable mixture, mozzarella cheese and Parmesan cheese. Repeat layers. In a large bowl, whisk eggs, egg whites and milk until blended; pour over layers. Sprinkle with basil. Refrigerate, covered, overnight.
5. Preheat oven to 350°. Remove the strata from refrigerator while oven heats.
6. Bake, covered, 50 minutes. Bake, uncovered, 10-15 minutes longer or until lightly browned and a knife inserted near the center comes out clean. Let strata stand 10 minutes before serving.

Per piece: 322 cal., 13g fat (5g sat. fat), 201 mg chol., 620mg sod., 28g carb. (9g sugars, 4g fiber), 24g pro.
Diabetic Exchanges: 2 medium-fat meat, 1½ starch, 1 vegetable, ½ fat.

FAST FIX

SOUTHWEST BREAKFAST POCKETS

I came up with this after the birth of my second son. The boys are 17 months apart, so I needed meals that were fast, delicious and kept us fueled all morning. This easy breakfast recipe can be a great lunch or even dinner, too.

—KOLEEN O'MALLEY-ELLINGSON
SIOUX FALLS, SD

START TO FINISH: 20 MIN.
MAKES: 2 SERVINGS

- 2 large eggs
- 2 large egg whites
- 1 teaspoon olive oil
- 1 small onion, chopped
- 1 garlic clove, minced
- ½ cup canned pinto beans, rinsed and drained
- 4 whole wheat pita pocket halves, warmed
- ¼ cup salsa
  Sliced avocado, optional

1. Whisk together eggs and egg whites. In a large nonstick skillet, heat oil over medium heat; saute onion until tender, 3-4 minutes. Add garlic; cook and stir 1 minute. Add eggs and beans; cook and stir until eggs are thickened and no liquid egg remains.
2. Spoon into pitas. Serve with salsa and, if desired, avocado.

Per 2 filled pita halves: 339 cal., 9g fat (2g sat. fat), 186mg chol., 580mg sod., 47g carb. (4g sugars, 7g fiber), 19g pro.
Diabetic Exchanges: 3 starch, 2 medium-fat meat.

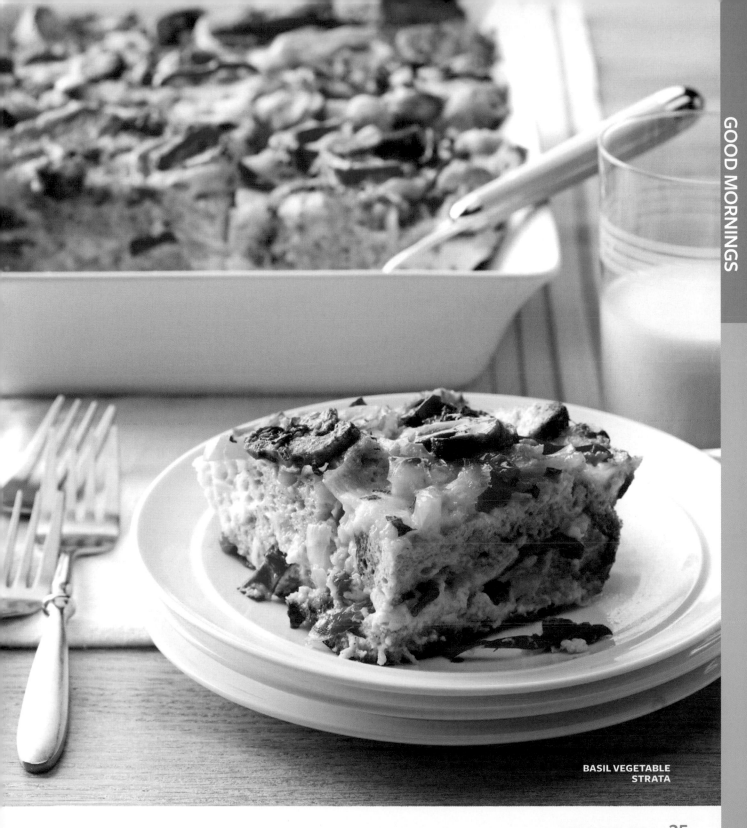

BASIL VEGETABLE STRATA

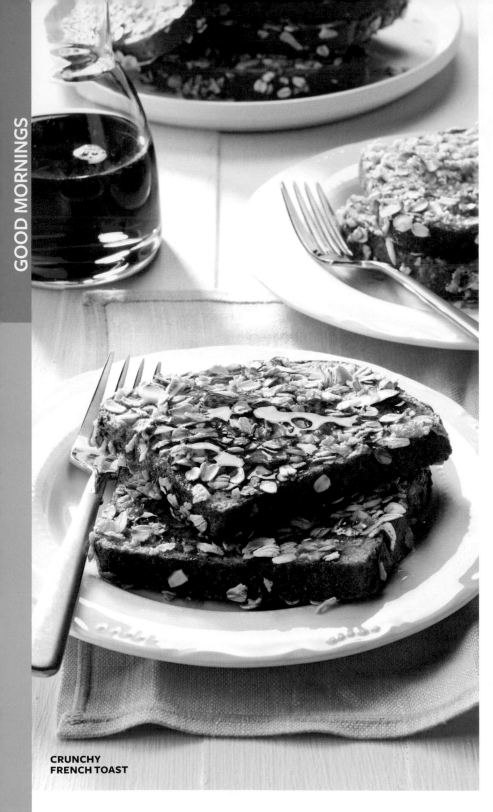

FAST FIX

CRUNCHY FRENCH TOAST

I like to eat healthy, so I always find time for breakfast. This light version of classic French toast is perfect for quick meals or Sunday brunches. My kids love it... and so do I!

—BARBARA ARNOLD SPOKANE, WA

START TO FINISH: 20 MIN.
MAKES: 4 SERVINGS

- 6 large eggs
- ⅓ cup fat-free milk
- 2 teaspoons vanilla extract
- ⅛ teaspoon salt
- 1 cup frosted cornflakes, crushed
- ½ cup old-fashioned oats
- ¼ cup sliced almonds
- 8 slices whole wheat bread
  Maple syrup, optional

1. In a shallow bowl, whisk eggs, milk, vanilla and salt until blended. In another shallow bowl, toss cornflakes with oats and almonds.

2. Heat a griddle coated with cooking spray over medium heat. Dip both sides of bread in egg mixture, then in cereal mixture, patting to help coating adhere. Place on griddle; toast 3-4 minutes on each side or until golden brown. If desired, serve with syrup.

Per 2 slices without syrup: 335 cal., 11g fat (2g sat. fat), 196mg chol., 436mg sod., 43g carb. (8g sugars, 5g fiber), 17g pro.

Diabetic Exchanges: 3 starch, 1 medium-fat meat, ½ fat.

CRUNCHY FRENCH TOAST

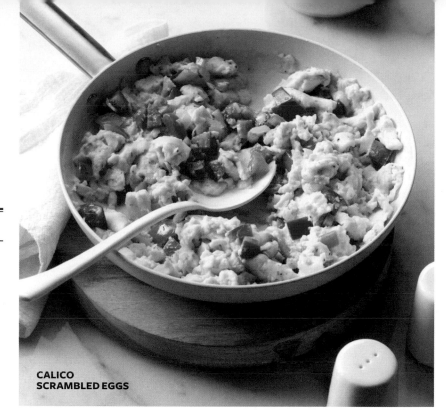

CALICO
SCRAMBLED EGGS

MIXED FRUIT WITH LEMON-BASIL DRESSING

A slightly savory lemony dressing really complements the sweet fruit in this recipe. I sometimes use the dressing on salad greens as well.

—**DIXIE TERRY** GOREVILLE, IL

START TO FINISH: 15 MIN.
MAKES: 8 SERVINGS

- 2 tablespoons lemon juice
- ½ teaspoon sugar
- ¼ teaspoon salt
- ¼ teaspoon ground mustard
- ⅛ teaspoon onion powder
  Dash pepper
- 6 tablespoons olive oil
- 4½ teaspoons minced fresh basil
- 1 cup cubed fresh pineapple
- 1 cup sliced fresh strawberries
- 1 cup sliced peeled kiwifruit
- 1 cup cubed seedless watermelon
- 1 cup fresh blueberries
- 1 cup fresh raspberries

1. In a blender, combine the lemon juice, sugar, salt, mustard, onion powder and pepper; cover and process for 5 seconds. While processing, gradually add oil in a steady stream. Stir in basil.

2. In a large bowl, combine the fruit. Drizzle with dressing and toss to coat. Refrigerate until serving.
Per ¾ cup: 145 cal., 11g fat (1g sat. fat), 0 chol., 76mg sod., 14g carb. (9g sugars, 3g fiber), 1g pro.
Diabetic Exchanges: 2 fat, 1 fruit.

CALICO SCRAMBLED EGGS

When you're short on time and really scrambling to get a meal on the table, this recipe is eggs-actly what you need. There's a short ingredient list, and cooking is kept to a minimum. Plus, with green pepper and tomato, it's colorful.

—*TASTE OF HOME* TEST KITCHEN

START TO FINISH: 15 MIN.
MAKES: 4 SERVINGS

- 8 large eggs
- ¼ cup 2% milk
- ⅛ to ¼ teaspoon dill weed
- ⅛ to ¼ teaspoon salt
- ⅛ to ¼ teaspoon pepper
- 1 tablespoon butter
- ½ cup chopped green pepper
- ¼ cup chopped onion
- ½ cup chopped fresh tomato

1. In a bowl, whisk the first five ingredients until blended. In a 12-in. nonstick skillet, heat butter over medium-high heat. Add green pepper and onion; cook and stir until tender. Remove from pan.

2. In same pan, pour in egg mixture; cook and stir over medium heat until eggs begin to thicken. Add tomato and pepper mixture; cook until heated through and no liquid egg remains, stirring gently.
Per 1 cup: 188 cal., 13g fat (5g sat. fat), 381mg chol., 248mg sod., 4g carb. (3g sugars, 1g fiber), 14g pro.
Diabetic Exchanges: 2 medium-fat meat, ½ fat.

COLORFUL BROCCOLI CHEDDAR CASSEROLE

When we have houseguests, we make broccoli and cheese strata the night before so we can relax and visit while it bubbles in the oven.

—**GALE LALMOND** DEERING, NH

PREP: 25 MIN. + CHILLING • **BAKE:** 50 MIN.
MAKES: 8 SERVINGS

- 1 tablespoon olive oil
- 6 green onions, sliced
- 2 cups fresh broccoli florets, chopped
- 1 medium sweet red pepper, finely chopped
- 2 garlic cloves, minced
- ⅛ teaspoon pepper
- 5 whole wheat English muffins, split, toasted and quartered
- 1½ cups shredded reduced-fat cheddar cheese, divided
- 8 large eggs
- 2½ cups fat-free milk
- 2 tablespoons Dijon mustard
- ½ teaspoon hot pepper sauce, optional

1. In a large skillet, heat the oil over medium-high heat. Add green onions; cook and stir until tender. Add broccoli, red pepper and garlic; cook and stir 4-5 minutes or until tender. Transfer to a large bowl; season with pepper.
2. Place English muffins in a greased 13x9-in. baking dish, cut sides up. Top muffins with vegetable mixture and sprinkle with 1 cup cheese.
3. In a large bowl, whisk together the eggs, milk, mustard and, if desired, hot sauce. Pour over the top. Refrigerate, covered, overnight.
4. Remove casserole from refrigerator 30 minutes before baking. Preheat oven to 350°. Bake, covered, 30 minutes.

Sprinkle with remaining cheese. Bake, uncovered, 20-30 minutes longer or until egg mixture is set. Let stand for 5 minutes before cutting.
Per piece: 273 cal., 12g fat (5g sat. fat), 228mg chol., 529mg sod., 25g carb. (9g sugars, 4g fiber), 19g pro.
Diabetic Exchanges: 2 medium-fat meat, 1½ starch, ½ fat.

⑤ INGREDIENTS **FAST FIX**
BLACKBERRY SMOOTHIES

Smoothies are a creamy treat that will get you going in the morning, too. I like to combine berries, yogurt, orange juice and honey.

—**VALERIE BELLEY** ST. LOUIS, MO

START TO FINISH: 10 MIN.
MAKES: 4 SERVINGS

- 1 cup orange juice
- 1 cup (8 ounces) plain yogurt
- 2 to 3 tablespoons honey
- 1½ cups fresh or frozen blackberries
- ½ cup frozen unsweetened mixed berries
  Additional blackberries and yogurt, optional

In a blender, combine the first five ingredients; cover and process for about 15 seconds or until smooth. Pour into chilled glasses; serve immediately. If desired top with additional blackberries and yogurt.
Per 1 cup without additional toppings: 130 cal., 2g fat (1g sat. fat), 8mg chol., 29mg sod., 26g carb. (21g sugars, 3g fiber), 3g pro.
Diabetic Exchanges: 1 starch, 1 fruit.

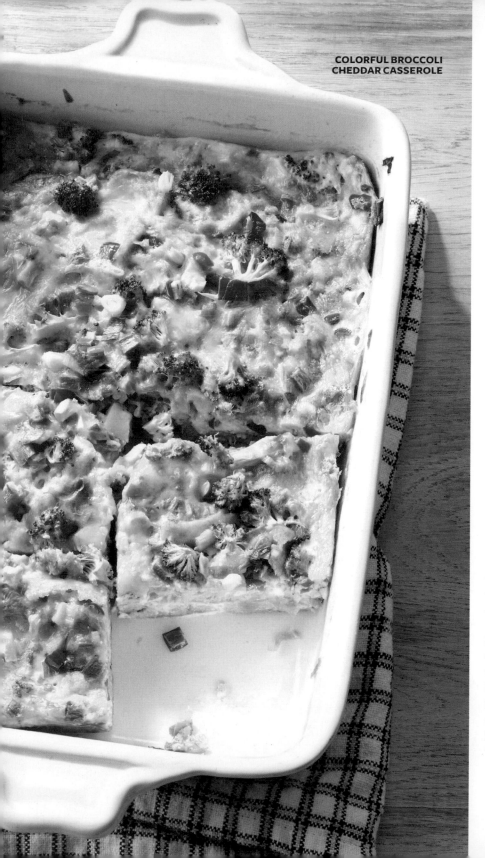

COLORFUL BROCCOLI CHEDDAR CASSEROLE

FAST FIX
ENGLISH MUFFIN EGG SANDWICH

You can't beat the delicious combination of mushrooms, onions, peppers and cream cheese! Leave out the red pepper flakes for a little less heat.
—**AMY LLOYD** MADISON, WI

START TO FINISH: 25 MIN.
MAKES: 8 SERVINGS

- ½ pound sliced fresh mushrooms
- 1 small sweet red pepper, chopped
- 1 small sweet onion, chopped
- ½ teaspoon garlic salt
- ¼ teaspoon pepper
- ¼ teaspoon crushed red pepper flakes, optional
- 7 large eggs, lightly beaten
- 8 whole wheat English muffins, split and toasted
- 4 ounces reduced-fat cream cheese

1. Place a large nonstick skillet coated with cooking spray over medium-high heat. Add mushrooms, red pepper, onion and seasonings; cook and stir 5-7 minutes or until mushrooms are tender. Remove from pan.
2. Wipe skillet clean and coat with cooking spray; place over medium heat. Add eggs; cook and stir just until eggs are thickened and no liquid egg remains. Add vegetables; heat through, stirring mixture gently.
3. Spread muffin bottoms with cream cheese; top with egg mixture. Replace the tops.
Per sandwich: 244 cal., 9g fat (4g sat. fat), 173mg chol., 425mg sod., 30g carb. (7g sugars, 5g fiber), 14g pro.
Diabetic Exchanges: 2 starch, 1 medium-fat meat, ½ fat.

**CURRIED CHICKEN
MEATBALL WRAPS, PAGE 36**

Starters & Snacks

· ·

When it's time to celebrate, these munchies
are made with fun in mind! From late-night light bites
to company-worthy appetizers that are sure to impress,
you'll find big taste in these little dips, wraps and plates.

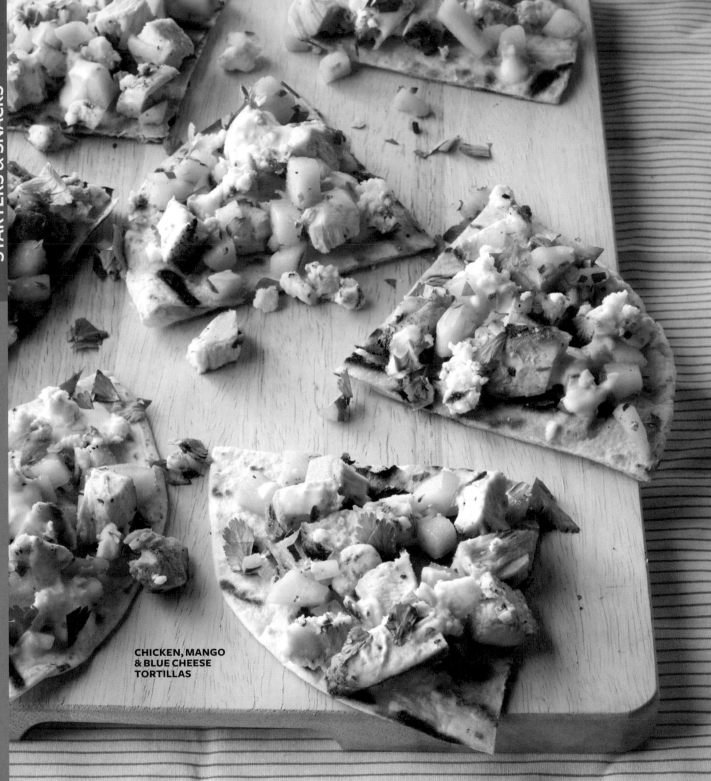

CHICKEN, MANGO
& BLUE CHEESE
TORTILLAS

FAST FIX ▶
CHICKEN, MANGO & BLUE CHEESE TORTILLAS

Tortillas packed with chicken, mango and blue cheese make a fantastic appetizer to welcome summer.
—**JOSEE LANZI** NEW PORT RICHEY, FL

START TO FINISH: 30 MIN.
MAKES: 16 APPEITZERS

- 1 boneless skinless chicken breast (8 ounces)
- 1 teaspoon blackened seasoning
- ¾ cup (6 ounces) plain yogurt
- 1½ teaspoons grated lime peel
- 2 tablespoons lime juice
- ¼ teaspoon salt
- ⅛ teaspoon pepper
- 1 cup finely chopped peeled mango
- ⅓ cup finely chopped red onion
- 4 flour tortillas (8 inches)
- ½ cup crumbled blue cheese
- 2 tablespoons minced fresh cilantro

1. Lightly oil grill rack with cooking oil. Sprinkle the chicken with blackened seasoning; grill, covered, over medium heat 6-8 minutes on each side or until a thermometer reads 165°.
2. In a bowl, mix yogurt, lime peel, lime juice, salt and pepper. Cool chicken slightly; finely chop and transfer to a small bowl. Stir in mango and onion.
3. Grill tortillas, uncovered, over medium heat 2-3 minutes, until puffed. Turn; top with chicken mixture and blue cheese. Grill, covered, 2-3 minutes, until bottoms are lightly browned. Drizzle with yogurt mixture; sprinkle with cilantro. Cut each into four wedges.
Per wedge: 85 cal., 3g fat (1g sat. fat), 12mg chol., 165mg sod., 10g carb. (2g sugars, 1g fiber), 5g pro.
Diabetic Exchanges: 1 lean meat, ½ starch.

⑤ INGREDIENTS   FAST FIX ▶
BALSAMIC-GOAT CHEESE GRILLED PLUMS

Make a real statement at your summer dinner party with this simple and elegant treat. Ripe plums are grilled, then dressed up with a balsamic reduction and sprinkled with tangy goat cheese.
—**ARIANA ABELOW** HOLLISTON, MA

START TO FINISH: 25 MIN.
MAKES: 8 SERVINGS

- 1 cup balsamic vinegar
- 2 teaspoons grated lemon peel
- 4 medium firm plums, halved and pitted
- ½ cup crumbled goat cheese

1. For glaze, in a small saucepan, combine vinegar and lemon peel; bring to a boil. Cook 10-12 minutes or until mixture is thickened and reduced to about ⅓ cup (do not overcook).
2. Grill plums, covered, over medium heat 2-3 minutes on each side or until tender. Drizzle with glaze; top with goat cheese.
Per plum half with 1 tablespoon cheese and 2 teaspoons glaze: 58 cal., 2g fat (1g sat. fat), 9mg chol., 41mg sod., 9g carb. (8g sugars, 1g fiber), 2g pro.
Diabetic Exchanges: ½ starch, ½ fat.

ROASTED RED PEPPER TAPENADE

I turn to this bright recipe often since it takes just 15 minutes to whip up. Sometimes I'll swap out the almonds for walnuts or pecans.
—**DONNA MAGLIARO** DENVILLE, NJ

PREP: 15 MIN. + CHILLING
MAKES: 2 CUPS

- 3 garlic cloves, peeled
- 2 cups roasted sweet red peppers, drained
- ½ cup blanched almonds
- ⅓ cup tomato paste
- 2 tablespoons olive oil
- ¼ teaspoon salt
- ¼ teaspoon pepper
  Minced fresh basil
  Toasted French bread baguette slices or water crackers

1. In a small saucepan, bring 2 cups water to a boil. Add garlic; cook, uncovered, 6-8 minutes or just until tender. Drain and pat dry. Place red peppers, almonds, tomato paste, oil, garlic, salt and pepper in a small food processor; process until blended. Transfer to a small bowl. Refrigerate at least 4 hours to allow flavors to blend.
2. Sprinkle with basil. Serve with baguette slices.
Per 2 tablespoons dip: 58 cal., 4g fat (0 sat. fat), 0 chol., 152mg sod., 3g carb. (2g sugars, 1g fiber), 1g pro.
Diabetic Exchanges: 1 fat.

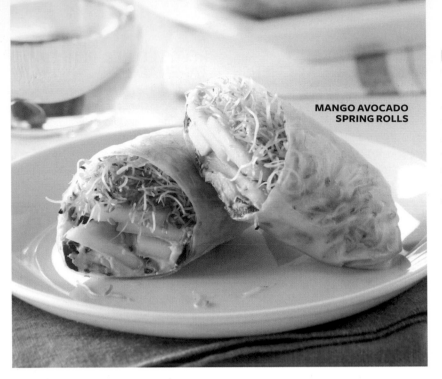

MANGO AVOCADO SPRING ROLLS

GARLICKY HERBED SHRIMP

Love shrimp? Love garlic? Love herbs? Cook 'em all up in butter and what could be better?

—DAVE LEVIN VAN NUYS, CA

START TO FINISH: 25 MIN.
MAKES: ABOUT 3 DOZEN

- 2 pounds uncooked jumbo shrimp, peeled and deveined
- 5 garlic cloves, minced
- 2 green onions, chopped
- ½ teaspoon garlic powder
- ½ teaspoon ground mustard
- ¼ teaspoon seasoned salt
- ¼ teaspoon crushed red pepper flakes
- ⅛ teaspoon pepper
- ½ cup butter, divided
- ¼ cup lemon juice
- 2 tablespoons minced fresh parsley
- 1 tablespoon minced fresh tarragon

1. In a large bowl, combine the first eight ingredients; toss to combine. In a large skillet, heat ¼ cup butter over medium-high heat. Add half of the shrimp mixture; cook and stir for 4-5 minutes or until shrimp turns pink. Transfer to a clean bowl.
2. Repeat with remaining butter and shrimp mixture. Return cooked shrimp to pan. Stir in lemon juice; heat through. Stir in herbs.
Per shrimp: 46 cal., 3g fat (2g sat. fat), 37mg chol., 61mg sod., 1g carb. (0 sugars, 0 fiber), 4g pro.
Diabetic Exchanges: ½ fat.

MANGO AVOCADO SPRING ROLLS

As a lover of both mangoes and avocados, I adore these wraps. Rice paper wraps can be hard to find, so I sometimes use tortillas instead.

—GENA STOUT RAVENDEN, AR

PREP: 40 MIN. • **MAKES:** 8 SPRING ROLLS

- 4 ounces reduced-fat cream cheese
- 2 tablespoons lime juice
- 1 teaspoon Sriracha Asian hot chili sauce or ½ teaspoon hot pepper sauce
- 1 medium sweet red pepper, finely chopped
- ⅔ cup cubed avocado
- 3 green onions, thinly sliced
- ⅓ cup chopped fresh cilantro
- 8 round rice paper wrappers (8 inches)
- 1 medium mango, peeled and thinly sliced
- 2 cups alfalfa sprouts

1. Mix cream cheese, lime juice and chili sauce; gently stir in pepper, avocado, green onions and cilantro.
2. Fill a large shallow dish partway with water. Dip a rice paper wrapper into water just until pliable, about 45 seconds (do not soften completely); allow excess water to drip off.
3. Place wrapper on a flat surface. Place cream cheese mixture, mango and sprouts across bottom third of wrapper. Fold in both ends of wrapper; fold bottom side over filling, then roll up tightly. Place on a serving plate, seam side down. Repeat with remaining ingredients. Serve immediately.
Per spring roll: 117 cal., 5g fat (2g sat. fat), 10mg chol., 86mg sod., 16g carb. (6g sugars, 2g fiber), 3g pro.
Diabetic Exchanges: 1 starch, 1 fat.

⑤ INGREDIENTS **FAST FIX**

MINI FETA PIZZAS

We usually have an abundance of pesto from the basil in our garden, which we use in our feta-covered mini pizzas. My family loves this dish, and we often add a little extra feta.

—NICOLE FILIZETTI STEVENS POINT, WI

START TO FINISH: 20 MIN.
MAKES: 4 SERVINGS

- 2 whole wheat English muffins, split and toasted
- 2 tablespoons reduced-fat cream cheese
- 4 teaspoons prepared pesto
- ½ cup thinly sliced red onion
- ¼ cup crumbled feta cheese

1. Preheat oven to 425°. Place muffins on a baking sheet.
2. Mix cream cheese and pesto; spread over muffins. Top with onion and feta cheese. Bake until lightly browned, 6-8 minutes.

Per pizza: 136 cal., 6g fat (3g sat. fat), 11mg chol., 294mg sod., 16g carb. (4g sugars, 3g fiber), 6g pro.
Diabetic Exchanges: 1 starch, 1 fat.

✽

TEST KITCHEN TIP
Punch up homemade pesto by adding flavorful ingredients such as fresh parsley, spinach or arugula. Or forgo the green and give sun-dried tomato or roasted red pepper pesto a try.

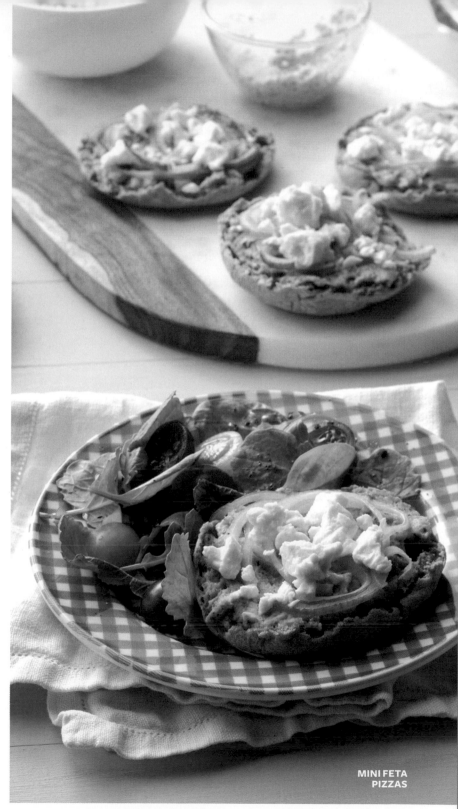

MINI FETA PIZZAS

CURRIED CHICKEN MEATBALL WRAPS

My kids love these easy meatball wraps topped with crunchy vegetables and a creamy dollop of yogurt.

—JENNIFER BECKMAN FALLS CHURCH, VA

PREP: 25 MIN. • **BAKE:** 20 MIN.
MAKES: 2 DOZEN

- 1 large egg, lightly beaten
- 1 small onion, finely chopped
- ½ cup Rice Krispies
- ¼ cup golden raisins
- ¼ cup minced fresh cilantro
- 2 teaspoons curry powder
- ½ teaspoon salt
- 1 pound lean ground chicken

SAUCE
- 1 cup (8 ounces) plain yogurt
- ¼ cup minced fresh cilantro

WRAPS
- 24 small Bibb or Boston lettuce leaves
- 1 medium carrot, shredded
- ½ cup golden raisins
- ½ cup chopped salted peanuts
  Additional minced fresh cilantro

1. Preheat oven to 350°. In a large bowl, combine first seven ingredients. Add chicken; mix lightly but thoroughly. With wet hands, shape mixture into 24 balls (about 1¼-in.).

2. Place meatballs on a greased rack in a 15x10x1-in. baking pan. Bake 17-20 minutes or until cooked through.

3. In a small bowl, mix the sauce ingredients. To serve, place 1 teaspoon sauce and one meatball in each lettuce leaf; top with remaining ingredients.

Per wrap: 72 cal., 3g fat (1g sat. fat), 22mg chol., 89mg sod., 6g carb. (4g sugars, 1g fiber), 6g pro.
Diabetic Exchanges: 1 lean meat, ½ starch.

FRESH FRUIT SALSA WITH CINNAMON CHIPS

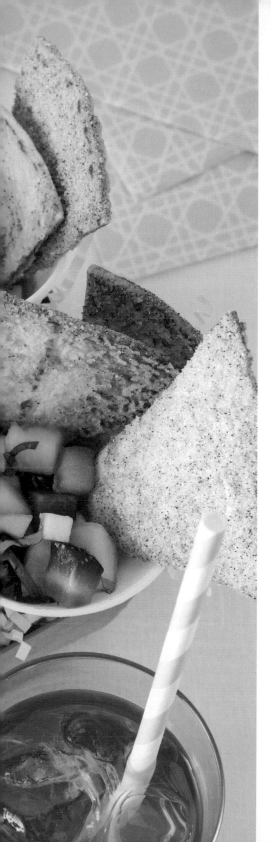

FRESH FRUIT SALSA WITH CINNAMON CHIPS

Lime and basil brighten the flavors in this colorful salsa. It's best when scooped up on a homemade cinnamon chip.

—**NAVALEE HYLTON** LAUDERHILL, FL

PREP: 30 MIN. • **BAKE:** 10 MIN.
MAKES: 4½ CUPS SALSA (64 CHIPS)

SALSA

- 1 medium pear, peeled and finely chopped
- 1 medium apple, peeled and finely chopped
- 1 medium kiwifruit, peeled and finely chopped
- 1 small peach, peeled and finely chopped
- ½ cup fresh blueberries
- ½ cup finely chopped fresh pineapple
- ½ cup finely chopped fresh strawberries
- 2 tablespoons honey
- 1 tablespoon lime juice
- ¾ teaspoon grated lime peel
- 3 small fresh basil leaves, thinly sliced
- 3 fresh mint leaves, thinly sliced

CINNAMON CHIPS

- 8 flour tortillas (8 inches)
  Cooking spray
- ½ cup sugar
- 1 teaspoon ground cinnamon

1. In a large bowl, combine the salsa ingredients; mix lightly. Refrigerate until ready to serve.

2. Lightly spritz both sides of tortillas with cooking spray; cut each into eight wedges. In a large bowl, combine sugar and cinnamon. Add tortillas and toss to coat.

3. Arrange wedges in a single layer on ungreased baking sheets. Bake at 350° for 10-12 minutes or until golden brown. Serve with salsa.

Per ¼ cup salsa with 4 chips: 124 cal., 2g fat (0 sat. fat), 0 chol., 118mg sod., 25g carb. (9g sugars, 2g fiber), 2g pro. **Diabetic Exchanges:** 1½ starch.

⑤ INGREDIENTS FAST FIX ▸

MOCHA PUMPKIN SEEDS

Roasted pumpkin seeds are a classic fall snack. Kick them up a notch with instant coffee and cocoa powder for a mix that's mocha genius.

—**REBEKAH BEYER** SABETHA, KS

START TO FINISH: 25 MIN.
MAKES: 3 CUPS

- 6 tablespoons sugar
- 2 tablespoons baking cocoa
- 1 tablespoon instant coffee granules
- 1 large egg white
- 2 cups salted shelled pumpkin seeds (pepitas)

1. Preheat oven to 325°. Place sugar, cocoa and coffee granules in a small food processor; cover and pulse until finely ground.

2. In a bowl, whisk egg white until frothy. Stir in pumpkin seeds. Sprinkle with sugar mixture; toss to coat evenly. Spread in a single layer in a parchment paper-lined 15x10x1-in. baking pan.

3. Bake 20-25 minutes or until dry and no longer sticky, stirring seeds every 10 minutes. Cool completely in pan. Store in an airtight container.

Per ¼ cup: 142 cal., 10g fat (2g sat. fat), 0 chol., 55mg sod., 10g carb. (7g sugars, 1g fiber), 6g pro. **Diabetic Exchanges:** 2 fat, ½ starch.

CHEESY SNACK MIX

Our love for Mexican food inspired me to add taco seasoning to my party mix. The flavor is so mild that it's even kid-friendly.

—ELIZABETH WYNNE AZTEC, NM

PREP: 10 MIN. • **COOK:** 5 MIN. + COOLING
MAKES: 2½ QUARTS

- 3 cups Corn Chex
- 3 cups Rice Chex
- 3 cups cheddar miniature pretzels
- ¼ cup butter, melted
- 1 envelope cheesy taco seasoning
- 2 cups white cheddar popcorn

1. In a large microwave-safe bowl, combine cereal and pretzels. In a small bowl, mix melted butter and taco seasoning; drizzle over cereal mixture and toss to coat.
2. Microwave, uncovered, on high 3-3½ minutes or until heated through, stirring once every minute. Stir in popcorn. Transfer to a baking sheet to cool completely. Store snack mix in an airtight container.

Note: This recipe was tested in a 1,100-watt microwave.
Per ¾ cup: 151 cal., 5g fat (3g sat. fat), 11mg chol., 362mg sod., 23g carb. (2g sugars, 1g fiber), 3g pro.
Diabetic Exchanges: 1½ starch, 1 fat.

MEATBALLS IN CHERRY SAUCE

A ruby-red cherry glaze gives my meatballs festive color. Everyone will love the zesty, sweet-tart flavors, too.

—RITA CHABOT-SCHULTZ BALLWIN, MO

PREP: 30 MIN. • **BAKE:** 15 MIN.
MAKES: ABOUT 3½ DOZEN

- 1 cup seasoned bread crumbs
- 1 small onion, chopped
- 1 large egg, lightly beaten
- 3 garlic cloves, minced
- 1 teaspoon salt
- ½ teaspoon pepper
- 1 pound lean ground beef (90% lean)
- 1 pound ground pork

SAUCE

- 1 can (21 ounces) cherry pie filling
- ⅓ cup sherry or chicken broth
- ⅓ cup cider vinegar
- ¼ cup steak sauce
- 2 tablespoons brown sugar
- 2 tablespoons reduced-sodium soy sauce
- 1 teaspoon honey

1. Preheat oven to 400°. In a large bowl, combine the first six ingredients. Add the beef and pork; mix lightly but thoroughly. Shape into 1-in. balls. Place on a greased rack in a shallow baking pan. Bake for 11-13 minutes or until cooked through. Drain on paper towels.
2. In a saucepan, combine the sauce ingredients. Bring to a boil over medium heat, stirring constantly. Reduce heat; simmer, uncovered, 2-3 minutes or until thickened. Add meatballs; heat through.
Per meatball: 76 cal., 3g fat (1g sat. fat), 19mg chol., 169mg sod., 7g carb. (5g sugars, 0 fiber), 5g pro.
Diabetic Exchanges: 1 lean meat, ½ starch.

FAST FIX

BLUEBERRY SALSA

This is a fruity and refreshing twist on salsa. Guests commonly line up to try it at parties, and they always leave happy and satisfied.

—KIMBERLY SORENSEN CARUTHERS, CA

START TO FINISH: 15 MIN.
MAKES: 1½ CUPS

- 1½ cups fresh blueberries
- ¼ cup chopped sweet red pepper
- 2 green onions, finely chopped
- 2 tablespoons minced seeded jalapeno pepper
- 2 tablespoons lemon juice
- 1 to 2 tablespoons minced fresh cilantro
- 1½ teaspoons sugar
- ¼ teaspoon salt
  Dash of pepper

Place blueberries in a food processor; pulse five times or until coarsely chopped. Transfer to a small bowl; stir in remaining ingredients. Refrigerate until serving.

Note: Wear disposable gloves when cutting hot peppers; the oils can burn skin. Avoid touching your face.
Per ¼ cup: 30 cal., 0 fat (0 sat. fat), 0 chol., 100mg sod., 8g carb. (5g sugars, 1g fiber), 0 pro.
Diabetic Exchanges: ½ fruit.

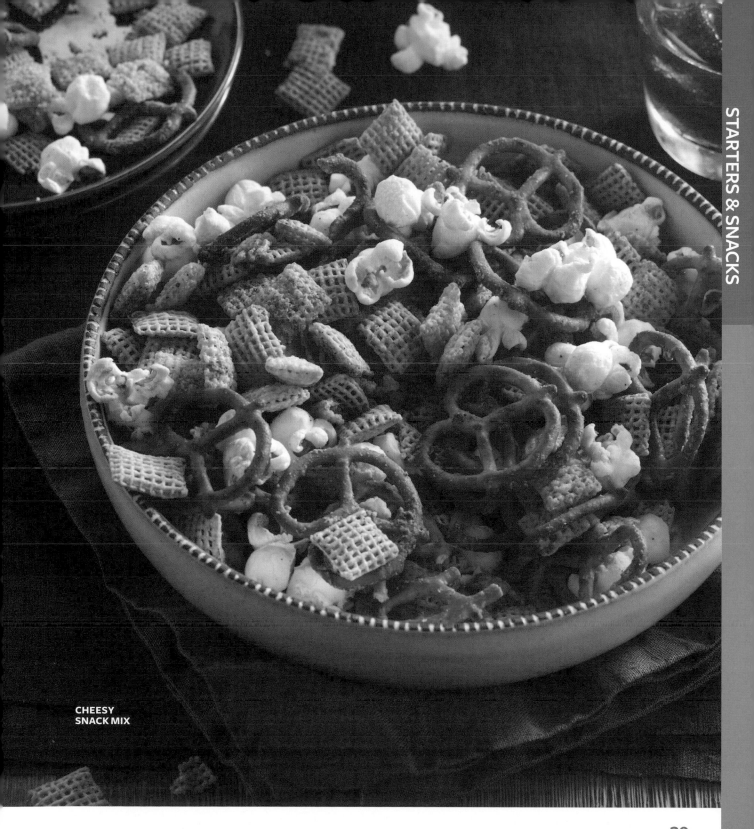

CHEESY
SNACK MIX

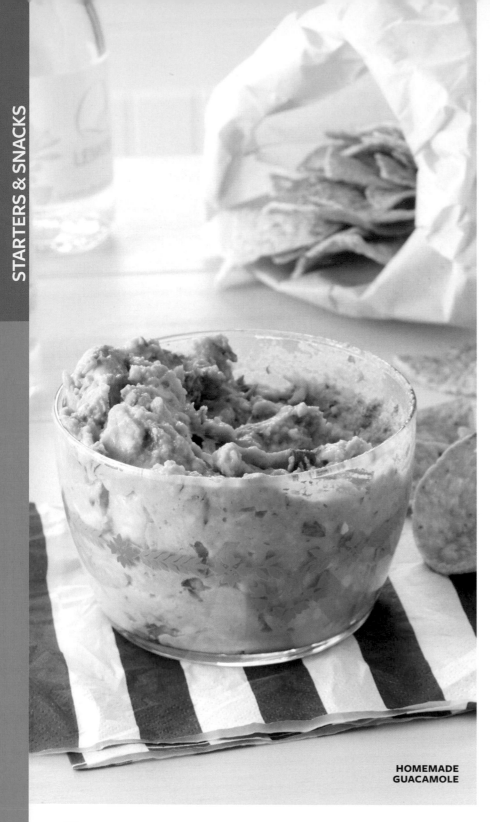

HOMEMADE GUACAMOLE

HOMEMADE GUACAMOLE

Nothing is better than fresh guacamole when you're eating something spicy. It's easy to whip together in a matter of minutes, and it quickly tames anything that's too spicy.

—JOAN HALLFORD
NORTH RICHLAND HILLS, TX

START TO FINISH: 10 MIN.
MAKES: 2 CUPS

- 3 medium ripe avocados, peeled and cubed
- 1 garlic clove, minced
- ¼ to ½ teaspoon salt
- 2 medium tomatoes, seeded and chopped, optional
- 1 small onion, finely chopped
- ¼ cup mayonnaise, optional
- 1 to 2 tablespoons lime juice
- 1 tablespoon minced fresh cilantro

Mash avocados with garlic and salt. Stir in remaining ingredients.
Per ¼ cup without chips: 111 calories, 10g fat (1g saturated fat), 0mg cholesterol, 43mg sodium, 6g carbohydrate (1g sugars, 5g fiber), 1g protein.
Diabetic Exchanges: ½ starch, 2 fat.

★ ★ ★ ★ ★ **READER REVIEW**

"My friends love this. I bring it to our monthly game nights because they always request it."
ERINPATTY TASTEOFHOME.COM

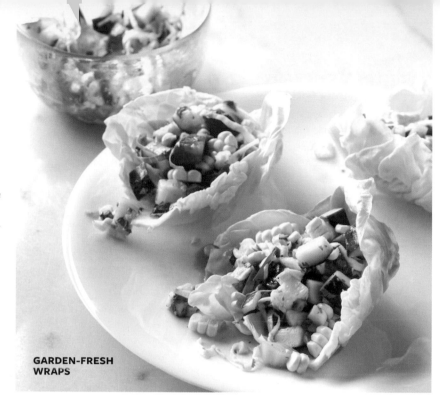

GARDEN-FRESH WRAPS

FAST FIX ▶
ARTICHOKE HUMMUS

Whenever I go to a party, the hostess asks me to bring my artichoke hummus. A versatile dip, it perfectly complements most other appetizers.
—HOLLY COLE PARRISH, FL

PREP/TOTAL TIME: 15 MIN.
MAKES: 2 CUPS

- 1 can (15 ounces) chickpeas, rinsed and drained
- 1 jar (7½ ounces) marinated quartered artichoke hearts, drained
- ¼ cup tahini
- 1 tablespoon capers, drained
- 2 tablespoons lemon juice
- 4 garlic cloves, minced
- 2 teaspoons grated lemon peel
- 1 teaspoon ground cumin
- ½ teaspoon garlic powder
- ⅛ teaspoon salt
  - Dash crushed red pepper flakes, optional
  - Dash pepper
- 2 fresh rosemary sprigs, chopped
  - Assorted fresh vegetables or baked pita chips

Place the first 12 ingredients in a food processor; cover and process until smooth. Transfer to a small bowl; stir in rosemary. Serve with vegetables.
Per 2 tablespoons without vegetables or chips: 75 cal., 5g fat (1g sat. fat), 0 chol., 116mg sod., 6g carb. (1g sugars, 2g fiber), 2g pro.
Diabetic Exchanges: ½ starch, ½ fat.

GARDEN-FRESH WRAPS

We moved into a house with a garden and used the herbs we found to make "freshtastic" wraps for our first dinner.
—CHRIS BUGHER ASHEVILLE, NC

PREP: 20 MIN. + STANDING
MAKES: 8 SERVINGS

- 1 medium ear sweet corn
- 1 medium cucumber, chopped
- 1 cup shredded cabbage
- 1 medium tomato, chopped
- 1 small red onion, chopped
- 1 jalapeno pepper, seeded and minced
- 1 tablespoon minced fresh basil
- 1 tablespoon minced fresh cilantro
- 1 tablespoon minced fresh mint
- ⅓ cup Thai chili sauce
- 3 tablespoons rice vinegar
- 2 teaspoons reduced-sodium soy sauce
- 2 teaspoons creamy peanut butter
- 8 Bibb or Boston lettuce leaves

1. Cut corn from cob and place in a large bowl. Add cucumber, cabbage, tomato, onion, jalapeno and herbs.
2. Whisk together chili sauce, vinegar, soy sauce and peanut butter. Pour over vegetable mixture; toss to coat. Let stand 20 minutes.
3. Using a slotted spoon, place ½ cup salad in each lettuce leaf. Fold lettuce over filling.
Note: Wear disposable gloves when cutting hot peppers; the oils can burn skin. Avoid touching your face.
Per wrap: 64 cal., 1g fat (0 sat. fat), 0 chol., 319mg sod., 13g carb. (10g sugars, 2g fiber), 2g pro.
Diabetic Exchanges: 1 vegetable, ½ starch.

BAKED POT STICKERS WITH DIPPING SAUCE

Twisting these wontons like little candy wrappers makes them a snap to assemble. The dipping sauce is packed with lip-smacking sweet heat.

—TAYLOR MARSH ALGONA, IA

PREP: 30 MIN. • **BAKE:** 15 MIN./BATCH
MAKES: 4 DOZEN

- 2 **cups finely chopped cooked chicken breast**
- 1 **can (8 ounces) water chestnuts, drained and chopped**
- 4 **green onions, thinly sliced**
- ¼ **cup shredded carrots**
- ¼ **cup reduced-fat mayonnaise**
- 1 **large egg white**
- 1 **tablespoon reduced-sodium soy sauce**
- 1 **garlic clove, minced**
- 1 **teaspoon grated fresh gingerroot**
- 48 **wonton wrappers**
  Cooking spray

SAUCE
- ½ **cup jalapeno pepper jelly**
- ¼ **cup rice vinegar**
- 2 **tablespoons reduced-sodium soy sauce**

1. Preheat the oven to 425°. In a large bowl, combine the first nine ingredients. Place 2 teaspoons of filling in the center of a wonton wrapper. Cover the rest of wrappers with a damp paper towel until ready to use.
2. Moisten filled wrapper edges with water. Fold edge over filling and roll to form a log; twist ends to seal. Repeat with remaining wrappers and filling.
3. Place pot stickers on a baking sheet coated with cooking spray; spritz each with cooking spray. Bake 12-15 minutes or until edges are golden brown.

4. Meanwhile, place jelly in a small microwave-safe bowl; microwave, covered, on high until melted. Stir in vinegar and soy sauce. Serve sauce with pot stickers.
Per pot sticker with ¾ teaspoon sauce: 52 cal., 1g fat (0 sat. fat), 6mg chol., 101mg sod., 8g carb. (2g sugars, 0 fiber), 3g pro.
Diabetic Exchanges: ½ starch.

⑤INGREDIENTS FAST FIX

RAISIN & HUMMUS PITA WEDGES

The best part about this easy hummus appetizer is you can make your own hummus, or if you don't have time, you can purchase some at the store. It's a year-round food that everyone enjoys.

—HELENE STEWART-RAINVILLE SACKETS HARBOR, NY

START TO FINISH: 15 MIN.
MAKES: 8 SERVINGS

- ¼ **cup golden raisins**
- 1 **tablespoon chopped dates**
- ½ **cup boiling water**
- 2 **whole wheat pita breads (6 inches)**
- ⅔ **cup hummus**
  Snipped fresh dill or dill weed, optional

1. Place raisins and dates in a small bowl. Cover with boiling water; let stand for 5 minutes. Drain well.
2. Cut each pita into four wedges. Spread with hummus; top with raisins, dates and, if desired, dill.
Per wedge: 91 cal., 2g fat (0 sat. fat), 0 chol., 156mg sod., 16g carb. (4g sugars, 3g fiber), 3g pro.
Diabetic Exchanges: 1 starch.

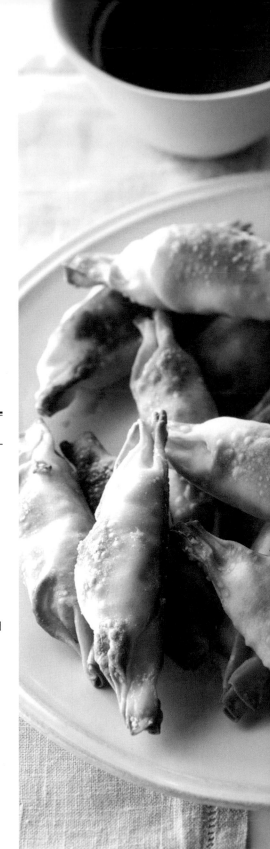

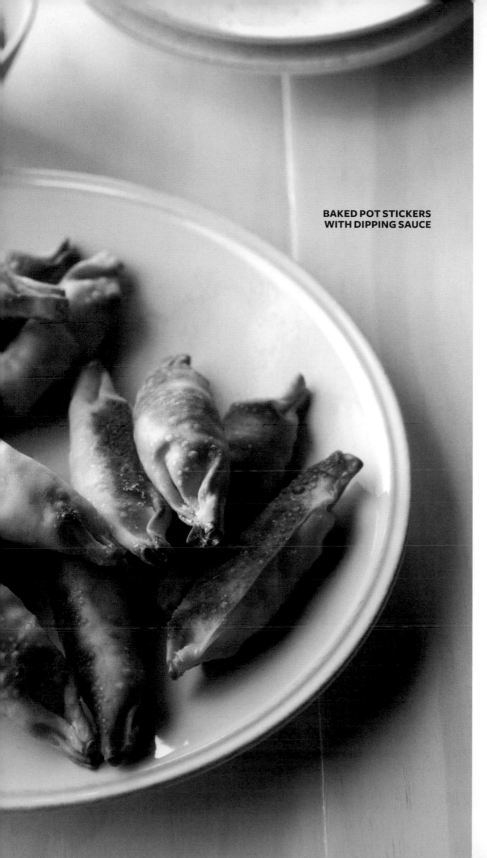

**BAKED POT STICKERS
WITH DIPPING SAUCE**

⑤INGREDIENTS **FAST FIX**

GORGONZOLA POLENTA BITES

For a New Year's Day party, I needed a brand-new appetizer. I covered polenta with Gorgonzola and a tangy sauce. That's how you spread holiday cheer.

—MARGEE BERRY WHITE SALMON, WA

START TO FINISH: 25 MIN.
MAKES: 16 APPETIZERS

⅓ cup balsamic vinegar
1 tablespoon orange marmalade
½ cup panko (Japanese) bread crumbs
1 tube (18 ounces) polenta, cut into 16 slices
2 tablespoons olive oil
½ cup crumbled Gorgonzola cheese
3 tablespoons dried currants, optional

1. In a small saucepan, combine vinegar and marmalade. Bring to a boil; cook 5-7 minutes or until liquid is reduced to 2 tablespoons.
2. Meanwhile, place bread crumbs in a shallow bowl. Press both sides of the polenta slices in bread crumbs. In a large skillet, heat oil over medium-high heat. Add polenta in batches; cook for 2-4 minutes on each side or until slices are golden brown.
3. Arrange polenta on a serving platter; spoon cheese over top. If desired, sprinkle with currants; drizzle with vinegar mixture. Serve bites warm or at room temperature.
Per appetizer: 67 cal., 3g fat (1g sat. fat), 3mg chol., 161mg sod., 9g carb. (3g sugars, 0 fiber), 1g pro.
Diabetic Exchanges: ½ starch, ½ fat.

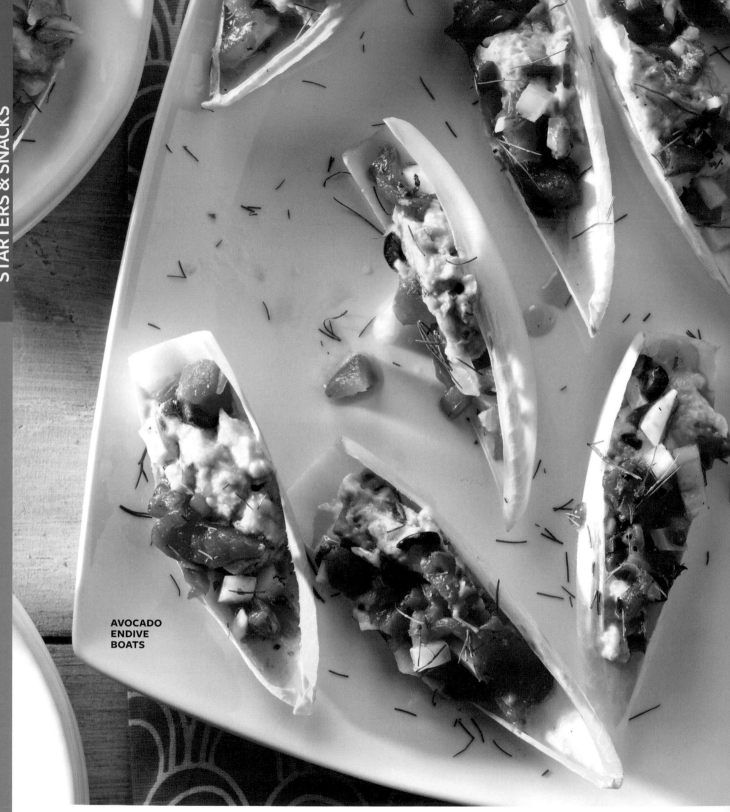

AVOCADO
ENDIVE
BOATS

AVOCADO ENDIVE BOATS

I jazz up guacamole by serving it on endive leaves with homemade salsa.

—**GILDA LESTER** MILLSBORO, DE

PREP: 45 MIN. • **MAKES:** 2½ DOZEN

- 1 jar (12 ounces) roasted sweet red peppers, drained and finely chopped
- 1 cup finely chopped fennel bulb
- ¼ cup sliced ripe olives, finely chopped
- 2 tablespoons olive oil
- 1 tablespoon minced fresh cilantro
- ½ teaspoon salt, divided
- ½ teaspoon pepper, divided
- 2 medium ripe avocados, peeled and pitted
- 3 tablespoons lime juice
- 2 tablespoons diced jalapeno pepper
- 1 green onion, finely chopped
- 1 garlic clove, minced
- ½ teaspoon ground cumin
- ¼ teaspoon hot pepper sauce
- 2 plum tomatoes, choppped
- 30 endive leaves
  Chopped fennel fronds

1. In a small bowl, combine first five ingredients; stir in ¼ teaspoon each salt and pepper.
2. In another bowl, mash avocados with a fork. Stir in next six ingredients and the remaining salt and pepper. Stir in tomatoes.
3. Spoon about 1 tablespoon avocado mixture onto each endive leaf; top each with about 1 tablespoon pepper mixture. Sprinkle with fennel fronds.
Per appetizer: 43 cal., 3g fat (0 sat. fat), 0 chol., 109mg sod., 4g carb. (1g sugars, 3g fiber), 1g pro.
Diabetic Exchanges: 1 vegetable, ½ fat.

---

⑤ INGREDIENTS

TOMATO-JALAPENO GRANITA

Everyone will be wowed after one taste of this icy refresher. Even my grandchildren enjoy the tomato, mint and lime flavors.

—**PAULA MARCHESI** LENHARTSVILLE, PA

PREP: 15 MIN. + FREEZING
MAKES: 6 SERVINGS

- 2 cups tomato juice
- ⅓ cup sugar
- 4 mint sprigs
- 1 jalapeno pepper, sliced
- 2 tablespoons lime juice
  Fresh mint leaves, optional

1. In a small saucepan, bring the tomato juice, sugar, mint sprigs and jalapeno to a boil. Cook and stir until sugar is dissolved. Remove from the heat; cover and let stand 15 minutes.
2. Strain and discard solids. Stir in lime juice. Transfer to a 1-qt. dish; cool to room temperature. Freeze for 1 hour; stir with a fork.
3. Freeze 2-3 hours longer or until completely frozen, stirring every 30 minutes. Scrape granita with a fork just before serving; spoon into dessert dishes. If desired garnish with additional mint leaves.
Note: Wear disposable gloves when cutting hot peppers; the oils can burn skin. Avoid touching your face.
Per ⅓ cup: 59 cal., 0 fat (0 sat. fat), 0 chol., 205mg sod., 15g carb. (13g sugars, 0 fiber), 1g pro.
Diabetic Exchanges: 1 starch.

ROASTED GRAPE CROSTINI

A trip to Spain introduced me to its culinary treasures, like Manchego cheese and sherry. This appetizer always impresses the friends who have never tasted roasted grapes. They're amazing!

—**JANICE ELDER** CHARLOTTE, NC

PREP: 35 MIN. • **BROIL:** 5 MIN.
MAKES: 2 DOZEN

- 3 cups seedless red or green grapes, halved lengthwise
- 2 tablespoons sherry vinegar or rice vinegar
- 2 tablespoons olive oil
- ½ teaspoon salt
- ¼ teaspoon freshly ground pepper
- 1 teaspoon grated orange peel
- 24 slices French bread baguette (cut diagonally ½ inch thick)
- ½ cup shaved manchego cheese or Romano cheese
  Thinly sliced fresh basil leaves

1. Preheat oven to 400°. Toss the first five ingredients; spread in a greased 15x10x1-in. pan. Roast until grapes are lightly browned and softened, 30-35 minutes. Stir in orange peel.
2. Preheat broiler. Arrange bread slices on an ungreased baking sheet. Broil 3-4 in. from heat until lightly browned, 1-2 minutes per side. Top with warm grape mixture; sprinkle with cheese and basil.
Per appetizer: 52 cal., 2g fat (1g sat. fat), 2mg chol., 110mg sod., 8g carb. (3g sugars, 0 fiber), 1g pro.
Diabetic Exchanges: ½ starch, ½ fat.

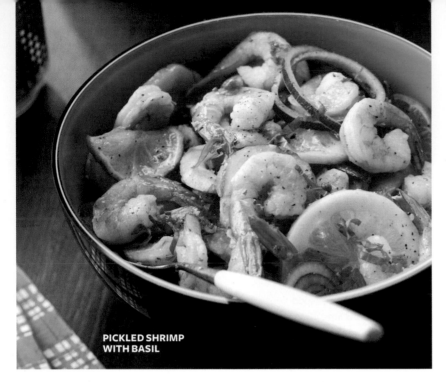

PICKLED SHRIMP
WITH BASIL

PICKLED SHRIMP WITH BASIL

Red wine vinegar plus the freshness of citrus and basil perk up shrimp, and there's hardly any prep. Serve over greens for a super salad.

—JAMES SCHEND PLEASANT PRAIRIE, WI

PREP: 15 MIN. + MARINATING
MAKES: 20 SERVINGS

- ½ cup red wine vinegar
- ½ cup olive oil
- 2 teaspoons seafood seasoning
- 2 teaspoons stone-ground mustard
- 1 garlic clove, minced
- 2 pounds peeled and deveined cooked shrimp (31-40 per pound)
- 1 medium lemon, thinly sliced
- 1 medium lime, thinly sliced
- ½ medium red onion, thinly sliced
- ¼ cup thinly sliced fresh basil
- 2 tablespoons capers, drained
- ¼ cup minced fresh basil
- ½ teaspoon kosher salt
- ¼ teaspoon coarsely ground pepper

1. In a large bowl, whisk the first five ingredients. Add shrimp, lemon, lime, onion, sliced basil and capers; toss gently to coat. Refrigerate, covered, up to 8 hours, stirring occasionally.

2. Just before serving, stir minced basil, salt and pepper into the shrimp mixture. Serve with a slotted spoon.

Per ½ cup: 64 cal., 2g fat (0 sat. fat), 69mg chol., 111mg sod., 1g carb. (0 sugars, 0 fiber), 9g pro.
Diabetic Exchanges: 1 lean meat, ½ fat.

FAST FIX ▶
WICKED DEVILED EGGS

My stepdaughter gave me the recipe for this delicious variation on deviled eggs. They make a tasty start to any party or get-together. I think they're even better when made the day before.

—JANICE L. PARKER HUMBOLDT, IA

START TO FINISH: 30 MIN.
MAKES: 2 DOZEN

- 12 hard-cooked eggs, peeled
- ½ cup Miracle Whip
- 2 tablespoons cider vinegar
- 2 tablespoons prepared mustard
- 1 tablespoon minced fresh parsley or 1 teaspoon dried parsley flakes
- 1 tablespoon butter, melted
- 1 tablespoon sweet pickle relish
- 2 teaspoons Worcestershire sauce
- 1 teaspoon sweet pickle juice
- ½ teaspoon salt
- ½ teaspoon cayenne pepper
- ½ teaspoon pepper
  Paprika

1. Cut eggs in half lengthwise. Remove yolks; set whites aside. In a small bowl, mash yolks. Add the Miracle Whip, vinegar, mustard, parsley, butter, relish, Worcestershire sauce, pickle juice, salt, cayenne and pepper; mix well. Stuff or pipe into egg whites.

2. Refrigerate until serving. Sprinkle with paprika.

Per deviled egg half: 61 cal., 5g fat (1g sat. fat), 109mg chol., 151mg sod., 1g carb. (1g sugars, 0 fiber), 3g pro.
Diabetic Exchanges: 1 fat.

✱
DID YOU KNOW?
Want to learn how to make a perfect hard-boiled egg? The *Taste of Home* Test Kitchen shows you how at: *Tasteofhome.com/recipes/hard-cooked-eggs.*

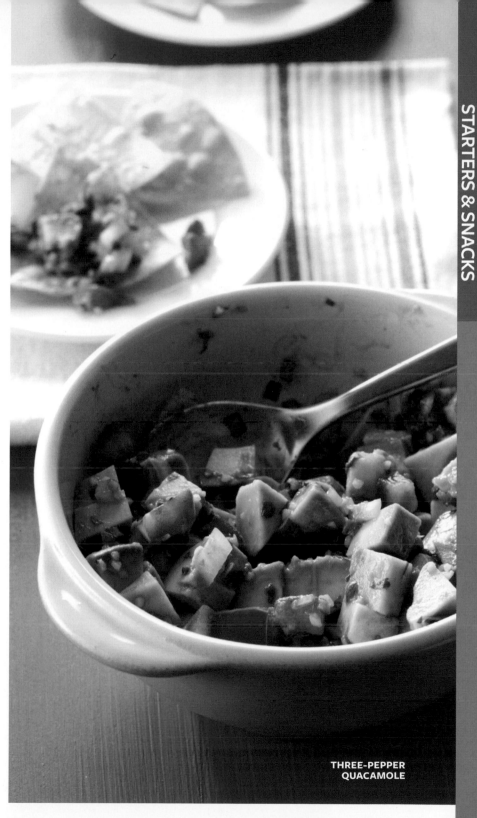

FAST FIX ▶
THREE-PEPPER GUACAMOLE

If you're serious about guacamole, use a molcajete. The lava stone makes a big difference in the pepper paste, and it's fun for guests.

—LAURA LEVY LYONS, CO

START TO FINISH: 25 MIN.
MAKES: 4 CUPS

- 3 tablespoons plus ¼ cup minced fresh cilantro, divided
- 4 tablespoons finely chopped onion, divided
- 3 tablespoons minced seeded jalapeno pepper
- 1 tablespoon minced seeded serrano pepper
- 2 to 3 teaspoons chopped chipotle pepper in adobo sauce
- 3 garlic cloves, minced
- ½ teaspoon salt
- 4 medium ripe avocados, peeled and cubed
- ⅓ cup finely chopped tomatoes
  Tortilla chips

In a large bowl, combine 3 tablespoons cilantro, 2 tablespoons onion, peppers, garlic and salt; mash together with a fork. Stir in avocados; fold in tomatoes and remaining cilantro and onion. Serve immediately with chips.

Note: Wear disposable gloves when cutting hot peppers; the oils can burn skin. Avoid touching your face.

Per ¼ cup without chips: 76 cal., 7g fat (1g sat. fat), 0 chol., 82mg sod., 4g carb. (0 sugars, 3g fiber), 1g pro.
Diabetic Exchanges: 1½ fat.

**THREE-PEPPER
QUACAMOLE**

**COLD-DAY
CHICKEN NOODLE
SOUP, PAGE 63**

Heartwarming Soups

Let's ladle out some comfort!
Treat your family to bowlfuls of happiness
with any of the sensational soups found here.
From chili and chowder to bisque and gazpacho,
there's something to satisfy everyone in this
colorful collection of hearty and healthy greats!

SALMON DILL SOUP

This is the best soup I have ever made, according to my husband who loves salmon so much that he could eat it every day. Salmon is a treat for both of us, so when I get it, I try to make a very special dish like this one.
—HIDEMI WALSH PLAINFIELD, IN

START TO FINISH: 30 MIN.
MAKES: 2 SERVINGS

- 1 large potato, peeled and cut into 1½-inch pieces
- 1 large carrot, cut into ½-inch-thick slices
- 1½ cups water
- 1 cup reduced-sodium chicken broth
- 5 medium fresh mushrooms, halved
- 1 tablespoon all-purpose flour
- ¼ cup reduced-fat evaporated milk
- ¼ cup shredded part-skim mozzarella cheese
- ½ pound salmon fillet, cut into 1½-inch pieces
- ¼ teaspoon pepper
- ⅛ teaspoon salt
- 1 tablespoon chopped fresh dill

1. Place first four ingredients in a saucepan; bring to a boil. Reduce heat to medium; cook, uncovered, until vegetables are tender, 10-15 minutes.
2. Add mushrooms. In a small bowl, mix flour and milk until smooth; stir into soup. Return to a boil; cook and stir until mushrooms are tender. Reduce the heat to medium; stir in the cheese until melted.
3. Reduce heat to medium-low. Add salmon; cook, uncovered, until fish just begins to flake easily with a fork, 3-4 minutes. Stir in pepper and salt. Sprinkle with dill.

Per 2½ cups: 398 cal., 14g fat (4g sat. fat), 71mg chol., 647mg sod., 37g carb. (7g sugars, 3g fiber), 30g pro.
Diabetic Exchanges: 3 lean meat, 2½ starch.

TURKEY & VEGETABLE BARLEY SOUP

Using ingredients I had on hand, I stirred up this turkey- and veggie-packed soup. If you have them, corn, beans or celery make great additions!
—LISA WIGER ST. MICHAEL, MN

START TO FINISH: 30 MIN.
MAKES: 6 SERVINGS

- 1 tablespoon canola oil
- 5 medium carrots, chopped
- 1 medium onion, chopped
- ⅔ cup quick-cooking barley
- 6 cups reduced-sodium chicken broth
- 2 cups cubed cooked turkey breast
- 2 cups fresh baby spinach
- ½ teaspoon pepper

1. In a large saucepan, heat oil over medium-high heat. Add carrots and onion; cook and stir 4-5 minutes or until carrots are crisp-tender.
2. Stir in barley and broth; bring to a boil. Reduce heat; simmer, covered, 10-15 minutes or until carrots and barley are tender. Stir in the turkey, spinach and pepper; heat through.

Per 1⅓ cups: 208 cal., 4g fat (1g sat. fat), 37mg chol., 662mg sod., 23g carb. (4g sugars, 6g fiber), 21g pro.
Diabetic Exchanges: 2 lean meat, 1 starch, 1 vegetable, ½ fat.

CREAMY CHICKEN RICE SOUP

I came up with this flavorful soup while making some adjustments to a favorite stovetop chicken casserole. We like this dish for lunch with a crisp roll and fresh fruit.
—JANICE MITCHELL AURORA, CO

START TO FINISH: 30 MIN.
MAKES: 4 SERVINGS

- 1 tablespoon canola oil
- 1 medium carrot, chopped
- 1 celery rib, chopped
- ½ cup chopped onion
- ½ teaspoon minced garlic
- ⅓ cup uncooked long grain rice
- ¾ teaspoon dried basil
- ¼ teaspoon pepper
- 2 cans (14½ ounces each) reduced-sodium chicken broth
- 3 tablespoons all-purpose flour
- 1 can (5 ounces) evaporated milk
- 2 cups cubed cooked chicken

1. In a large saucepan, heat oil over medium-high heat; saute carrot, celery and onion until tender. Add garlic; cook and stir 1 minute. Stir in rice, seasonings and broth; bring to a boil. Reduce heat; simmer, covered, until rice is tender, about 15 minutes.
2. Mix flour and milk until smooth; stir into soup. Bring to a boil; cook and stir until thickened, about 2 minutes. Stir in chicken; heat through.

Per 1¼ cups: 322 cal., 11g fat (3g sat. fat), 73mg chol., 630mg sod., 26g carb. (6g sugars, 1g fiber), 28g pro.
Diabetic Exchanges: 3 lean meat, 2 starch, 1 fat.

SALMON
DILL SOUP

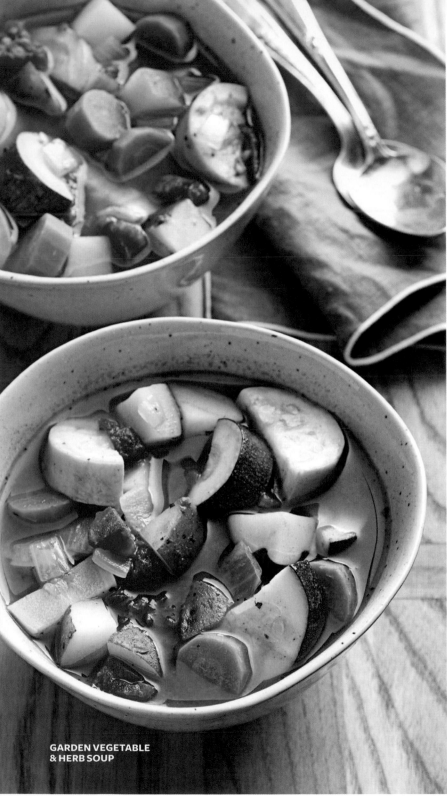

GARDEN VEGETABLE & HERB SOUP

GARDEN VEGETABLE & HERB SOUP

I make this hearty soup whenever my family needs a good dose of veggies.

—**JODY SAULNIER** NORTH WOODSTOCK, NH

PREP: 20 MIN. • **COOK:** 30 MIN.
MAKES: 8 SERVINGS

- 2 tablespoons olive oil
- 2 medium onions, chopped
- 1 pound red potatoes (about 3 medium), cubed
- 2 large carrots, sliced
- 2 cups water
- 1 can (14½ ounces) diced tomatoes in sauce
- 1½ cups vegetable broth
- 1½ teaspoons garlic powder
- 1 teaspoon dried basil
- ½ teaspoon salt
- ½ teaspoon paprika
- ¼ teaspoon dill weed
- ¼ teaspoon pepper
- 1 medium yellow summer squash, halved and sliced
- 1 medium zucchini, halved and sliced

1. In a large saucepan, heat oil over medium heat. Add onions; cook and stir for 4-6 minutes or until tender. Add potatoes and carrots. Stir in the water, tomatoes, broth and seasonings. Bring to a boil. Reduce heat; simmer, uncovered, 12-15 minutes or until potatoes and carrots are tender.

2. Add sliced yellow squash and zucchini; cook 8-10 minutes longer or until tender.

Per 1 cup: 115 cal., 4g fat (1g sat. fat), 0 chol., 525mg sod., 19g carb. (6g sugars, 3g fiber), 2g pro.
Diabetic Exchanges: 1 vegetable, 1 fat, ½ starch.

COCONUT CURRY VEGETABLE SOUP

I've been a vegetarian since high school, so modifying recipes to fit my meatless requirements is a challenge I enjoy. This soup tastes rich and creamy, and it's packed with nutrients!

—CARISSA SUMNER WASHINGTON, DC

PREP: 15 MIN. • **COOK:** 25 MIN.
MAKES: 6 SERVINGS

- 1 tablespoon canola oil
- 2 celery ribs, chopped
- 2 medium carrots, chopped
- 6 garlic cloves, minced
- 1 tablespoon minced fresh gingerroot
- 2 teaspoons curry powder
- ½ teaspoon ground turmeric
- 1 can (14½ ounces) vegetable broth
- 1 can (13.66 ounces) light coconut milk
- 1 medium potato (about 8 ounces), peeled and chopped
- ½ teaspoon salt
- 1 package (8.8 ounces) ready-to-serve brown rice
  Lime wedges, optional

1. In a large saucepan, heat oil over medium heat. Add celery and carrots; cook and stir 6-8 minutes or until tender. Add garlic, ginger, curry powder and turmeric; cook 1 minute longer.
2. Add broth, coconut milk, potato and salt; bring to a boil. Reduce heat; cook, uncovered, 10-15 minutes or until potato is tender. Meanwhile, heat rice according to package directions.
3. Stir rice into soup. If desired, serve with lime wedges.
Per ¾ cup: 186 cal., 8g fat (4g sat. fat), 0 chol., 502mg sod., 22g carb. (3g sugars, 2g fiber), 3g pro.
Diabetic Exchanges: 1½ starch, 1½ fat.

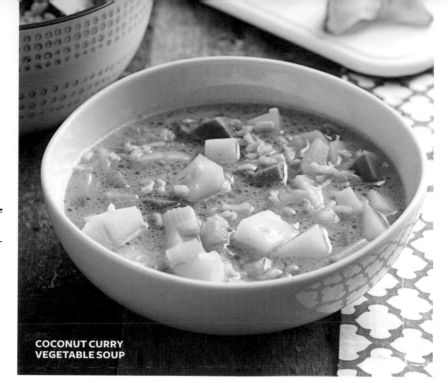

COCONUT CURRY VEGETABLE SOUP

BLACK BEAN-TOMATO CHILI

My daughter Kayla saw a black bean chili dish while watching a cooking show and called me about it, because it looked so good. We messed with our own recipe until we got this easy winner.

—LISA BELCASTRO VINEYARD HAVEN, MA

PREP: 10 MIN. • **COOK:** 35 MIN.
MAKES: 6 SERVINGS

- 2 tablespoons olive oil
- 1 large onion, chopped
- 1 medium green pepper, chopped
- 3 garlic cloves, minced
- 1 teaspoon ground cinnamon
- 1 teaspoon ground cumin
- 1 teaspoon chili powder
- ¼ teaspoon pepper
- 3 cans (14½ ounces each) diced tomatoes, undrained
- 2 cans (15 ounces each) black beans, rinsed and drained
- 1 cup orange juice or juice from 3 medium oranges

1. In a Dutch oven, heat the oil over medium-high heat. Add onion and green pepper; cook and stir for 8-10 minutes or until tender. Add garlic and seasonings; cook 1 minute longer.
2. Stir in remaining ingredients; bring to a boil. Reduce heat; simmer, covered, 20-25 minutes to allow flavors to blend, stirring occasionally.
Per 1½ cups: 232 cal., 5g fat (1g sat. fat), 0 chol., 608mg sod., 39g carb. (13g sugars, 10g fiber), 9g pro.
Diabetic Exchanges: 2 vegetable, 1½ starch, 1 lean meat, 1 fat.

✳

TEST KITCHEN TIP
It's important to drain and rinse canned beans because the thick, cloudy liquid inside often contains excess sodium and starch. Doing this can improve the taste, texture and nutritional content of a dish.

SHRIMP PAD THAI SOUP

Pad thai is one of my favorite foods, but it is often loaded with extra calories. This version is a healthier option!
—JULIE MERRIMAN SEATTLE, WA

PREP: 15 MIN. • **COOK:** 30 MIN.
MAKES: 8 SERVINGS

- 1 tablespoon sesame oil
- 2 shallots, thinly sliced
- 1 Thai chili pepper or serrano pepper, seeded and finely chopped
- 1 can (28 ounces) no-salt-added crushed tomatoes
- ¼ cup creamy peanut butter
- 2 tablespoons reduced-sodium soy sauce or fish sauce
- 6 cups reduced-sodium chicken broth
- 1 pound uncooked shrimp (31-40 per pound), peeled and deveined
- 6 ounces uncooked thick rice noodles
- 1 cup bean sprouts
- 4 green onions, sliced
  Chopped peanuts and additional chopped Thai chili pepper, optional
  Lime wedges

1. In a 6-qt. stockpot, heat oil over medium heat. Add shallots and chili pepper; cook and stir 4-6 minutes or until tender. Stir in crushed tomatoes, peanut butter and soy sauce until blended; add broth. Bring to a boil; cook, uncovered, 15 minutes to allow flavors to blend.

2. Add shrimp and noodles; cook 4-6 minutes longer or until shrimp turn pink and noodles are tender. Top each serving with bean sprouts, green onions and, if desired, chopped peanuts and additional chopped chili pepper. Serve with lime wedges.

Per 1⅓ cups without optional ingredients: 252 cal., 7g fat (1g sat. fat), 69mg chol., 755mg sod., 31g carb. (5g sugars, 4g fiber), 17g pro.
Diabetic Exchanges: 2 lean meat, 1½ starch, 1 vegetable, 1 fat.

CREAMY BUTTERNUT SOUP

Topped with chives and a drizzle of sour cream, my thick and velvety soup looks as special as it tastes.
—AMANDA SMITH CINCINNATI, OH

PREP: 15 MIN. • **COOK:** 20 MIN.
MAKES: 10 SERVINGS

- 1 medium butternut squash, peeled, seeded and cubed (about 6 cups)
- 3 medium potatoes (about 1 pound), peeled and cubed
- 1 large onion, diced
- 2 chicken bouillon cubes
- 2 garlic cloves, minced
- 5 cups water
  Sour cream and minced fresh chives, optional

1. In a 6-qt. stockpot, combine first six ingredients; bring to a boil. Reduce heat; simmer, covered, until vegetables are tender, 15-20 minutes.

2. Puree soup using an immersion blender. Or, cool slightly and puree soup in batches in a blender; return to pan and heat through. If desired, serve with sour cream and chives.

Per 1 cup without sour cream: 112 cal., 0 fat (0 sat. fat), 0 chol., 231mg sod., 27g carb. (5g sugars, 4g fiber), 3g pro.
Diabetic Exchanges: 2 starch.

FAST FIX
SATISFYING TOMATO SOUP

I made up my own recipe to satisfy a craving for tomato soup. My sister Joan loves this soup chunky-style, so she doesn't need to use a blender. Maybe you will prefer it that way, too!
—MARIAN BROWN MISSISSAUGA, ON

START TO FINISH: 30 MIN.
MAKES: 4 SERVINGS

- 2 teaspoons canola oil
- ¼ cup finely chopped onion
- ¼ cup finely chopped celery
- 2 cans (14½ ounces each) diced tomatoes, undrained
- 1½ cups water
- 2 teaspoons brown sugar
- ½ teaspoon salt
- ½ teaspoon dried basil
- ¼ teaspoon dried oregano
- ¼ teaspoon coarsely ground pepper

1. In a large saucepan, heat oil over medium-high heat. Add the onion and celery; cook and stir 2-4 minutes or until tender. Add the remaining ingredients. Bring to a boil. Reduce heat; simmer, uncovered, 10 minutes to allow flavors to blend.

2. Puree soup using an immersion blender. Or, cool the soup slightly and puree in batches in a blender; return to pan and heat through.

To freeze: Freeze the cooled soup in freezer containers. To use, partially thaw in refrigerator overnight. Heat through in a saucepan, stirring occasionally and adding a little water if necessary.

Per 1¼ cups: 76 cal., 2g fat (0 sat. fat), 0 chol., 627mg sod., 13g carb. (9g sugars, 4g fiber), 2g pro.
Diabetic Exchanges: 2 vegetable, ½ fat.

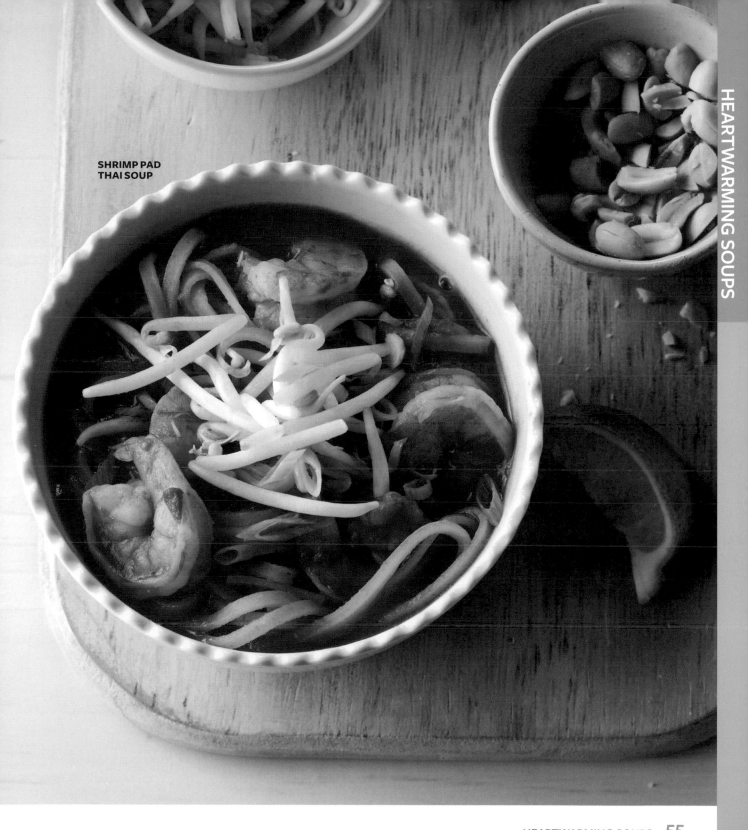

SHRIMP PAD THAI SOUP

FAST FIX ▶

EASY WHITE CHICKEN CHILI

We like to use chicken and white beans for a twist on traditional red chili. It's soothing comfort food at its best.

—**RACHEL LEWIS** DANVILLE, VA

START TO FINISH: 30 MIN.
MAKES: 6 SERVINGS

- 1 pound lean ground chicken
- 1 medium onion, chopped
- 2 cans (15 ounces each) cannellini beans, rinsed and drained
- 1 can (4 ounces) chopped green chilies
- 1 teaspoon ground cumin
- ½ teaspoon dried oregano
- ¼ teaspoon pepper
- 1 can (14½ ounces) reduced-sodium chicken broth
  Optional toppings: reduced-fat sour cream, shredded cheddar cheese and chopped fresh cilantro

1. In a large saucepan, cook chicken and onion over medium-high heat 6-8 minutes or until chicken is no longer pink, breaking up chicken into crumbles.

2. Place one can of beans in a small bowl; mash slightly. Stir mashed beans, the remaining can of beans, chilies, seasonings and broth into chicken mixture; bring to a boil. Reduce heat; simmer, covered, 12-15 minutes or until flavors are blended. Serve with toppings as desired.

Per 1 cup without toppings: 228 cal., 5g fat (1g sat. fat), 54mg chol., 504mg sod., 23g carb. (1g sugars, 6g fiber), 22g pro.

Diabetic Exchanges: 3 lean meat, 1½ starch.

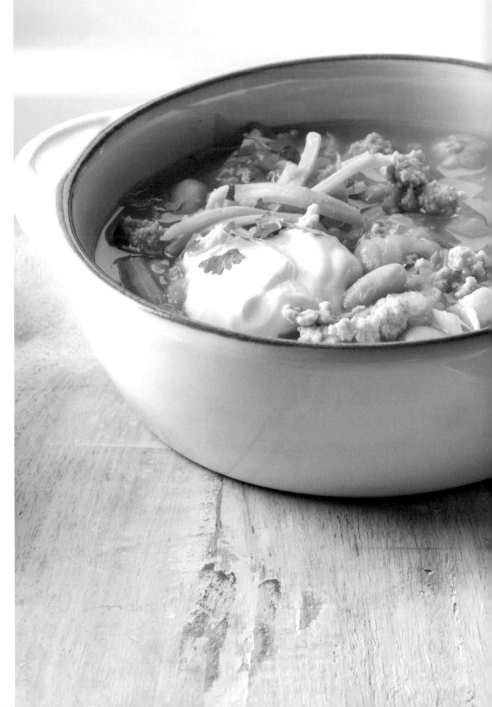

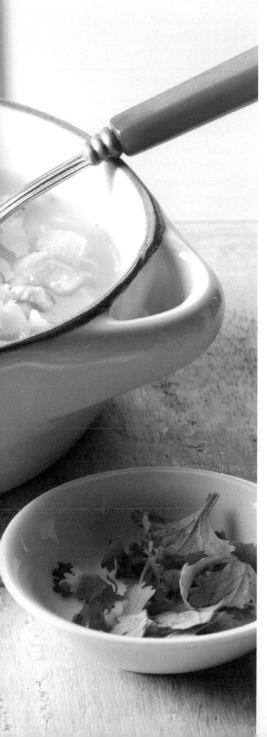

EASY WHITE CHICKEN CHILI

COMFORTING BEEF BARLEY SOUP

When the weather outside is cool, we want a bowl of soup that's chock full of beef, barley and veggies. It's the most delicious way to warm up.
—**SUE JURACK** MEQUON, WI

PREP: 10 MIN. • **COOK:** 35 MIN.
MAKES: 8 SERVINGS

- 1 tablespoon butter
- 1 medium carrot, chopped
- 1 celery rib, chopped
- ½ cup chopped onion
- 4 cups beef broth
- 4 cups water
- 2 cups chopped cooked roast beef
- 1 can (14½ ounces) diced tomatoes, undrained
- 1 cup quick-cooking barley
- ½ teaspoon dried basil
- ½ teaspoon dried oregano
- ½ teaspoon pepper
- ¼ teaspoon salt
- ½ cup frozen peas

1. In a 6-qt. stockpot, heat butter over medium-high heat; saute carrot, celery and onion until tender, 4-5 minutes.
2. Add broth, water, beef, tomatoes, barley and seasonings; bring to a boil. Reduce heat; simmer soup, covered, for 20 minutes, stirring occasionally. Add peas; heat through, about 5 minutes.
Per 1½ cups: 198 cal., 4g fat (2g sat. fat), 36mg chol., 652mg sod., 23g carb. (3g sugars, 6g fiber), 18g pro.
Diabetic Exchanges: 2 lean meat, 1½ starch, ½ fat.

SUMMER SQUASH SOUP

Delicate and lemony, this squash soup sets the stage for memorable ladies luncheons. It's the best of late summer in a bowl.
—**HEIDI WILCOX** LAPEER, MI

PREP: 35 MIN. • **COOK:** 15 MIN.
MAKES: 8 SERVINGS

- 2 large sweet onions, chopped
- 1 medium leek (white portion only), chopped
- 2 tablespoons olive oil
- 6 garlic cloves, minced
- 6 medium yellow summer squash, seeded and cubed (about 6 cups)
- 4 cups reduced-sodium chicken broth
- 4 fresh thyme sprigs
- ¼ teaspoon salt
- 2 tablespoons lemon juice
- ⅛ teaspoon hot pepper sauce
- 1 tablespoon shredded Parmesan cheese
- 2 teaspoons grated lemon peel

1. In a large saucepan, saute onions and leek in oil until tender. Add garlic; cook 1 minute longer. Add squash; saute 5 minutes. Stir in the broth, thyme and salt. Bring to a boil. Reduce heat; cover and simmer for 15-20 minutes or until squash is tender.
2. Discard thyme sprigs. Cool slightly. In a blender, process soup in batches until smooth. Return all to the pan. Stir in lemon juice and hot pepper sauce; heat through. Sprinkle each serving with cheese and lemon peel.
Per 1 cup: 90 cal., 4g fat (1g sat. fat), 0 chol., 377mg sod., 12g carb. (6g sugars, 3g fiber), 4g pro.
Diabetic Exchanges: 1 starch, ½ fat.

ITALIAN VEGGIE
BEEF SOUP

CHICKEN BUTTERNUT CHILI

We just love a hearty chili with bold flavors! You can even prepare it in a slow cooker. Just add ingredients to the cooker and simmer for about 4 hours.
—**COURTNEY STULTZ** WEIR, KS

PREP: 20 MIN. • **COOK:** 35 MIN.
MAKES: 4 SERVINGS

- 1 tablespoon canola oil
- 2 medium carrots, chopped
- 2 celery ribs, chopped
- 1 medium onion, chopped
- 2 cups cubed peeled butternut squash
- 1 medium tomato, chopped
- 2 tablespoons tomato paste
- 1 envelope reduced-sodium chili seasoning mix
- 2 cups chicken stock
- 1 cup cubed cooked chicken breast Chopped fresh cilantro

1. In a large saucepan, heat oil over medium heat; saute carrots, celery and onion until tender, 6-8 minutes.
2. Stir in the squash, tomato, tomato paste, seasoning mix and stock; bring to a boil. Reduce heat; simmer, covered, until squash is tender, 20-25 minutes. Stir in chicken; heat through. Sprinkle with cilantro.

To freeze: Freeze cooled chili in freezer containers. To use, partially thaw in refrigerator overnight. Heat through in a saucepan, stirring occasionally.
Per 1¼ cups: 201 cal., 5g fat (1g sat. fat), 27mg chol., 591mg sod., 25g carb. (8g sugars, 4g fiber), 15g pro.
Diabetic Exchanges: 2 lean meat, 1 starch, 1 vegetable, ½ fat.

FAST FIX
ITALIAN VEGGIE BEEF SOUP

My sweet father-in-law, Pop Pop, would bring this satisfying chunky soup to our house when we were under the weather.
—**SUE WEBB** REISTERSTOWN, MD

START TO FINISH: 30 MIN.
MAKES: 12 SERVINGS

- 1½ pounds lean ground beef (90% lean)
- 2 medium onions, chopped
- 4 cups chopped cabbage
- 1 package (16 ounces) frozen mixed vegetables
- 1 can (28 ounces) crushed tomatoes
- 1 bay leaf
- 3 teaspoons Italian seasoning
- 1 teaspoon salt
- ½ teaspoon pepper
- 2 cartons (32 ounces each) reduced-sodium beef broth

1. In a 6-qt. stockpot, cook ground beef and onions over medium-high heat for 6-8 minutes or until the beef is no longer pink, breaking up the beef into crumbles; drain.
2. Add cabbage, mixed vegetables, tomatoes, seasonings and broth; bring to a boil. Reduce heat; simmer soup, uncovered, for 10-15 minutes or until the cabbage is crisp-tender. Remove bay leaf.

To freeze: Freeze the cooled soup in freezer containers. To use, partially thaw in refrigerator overnight. Heat through in a saucepan, stirring occasionally and adding a little broth if necessary.
Per 1⅓ cups: 159 cal., 5g fat (2g sat. fat), 38mg chol., 646mg sod., 14g carb. (6g sugars, 4g fiber), 15g pro.
Diabetic Exchanges: 2 lean meat, 1 vegetable, ½ starch.

GOLDEN SUMMER PEACH GAZPACHO

Since peaches and tomatoes are in season together, I like to blend them into a cool, delicious soup.
—**JULIE HESSION** LAS VEGAS, NV

PREP: 20 MIN. + CHILLING
MAKES: 8 SERVINGS

- 3 cups sliced peeled fresh or frozen peaches, thawed
- 3 medium yellow tomatoes, chopped
- 1 medium sweet yellow pepper, chopped
- 1 medium cucumber, peeled and chopped
- ½ cup chopped sweet onion
- 1 garlic clove, minced
- ⅓ cup lime juice
- 2 tablespoons rice vinegar
- 1 tablespoon marinade for chicken
- 1 teaspoon salt
- ¼ teaspoon hot pepper sauce
- 1 to 3 teaspoons sugar, optional
  Chopped peaches, cucumber and tomatoes

1. Place the first six ingredients in a food processor; process until blended. Add lime juice, vinegar, marinade for chicken, salt and pepper sauce; process until smooth. If desired, stir in sugar.

2. Refrigerate, covered, for at least 4 hours. Top individual servings with additional chopped peaches, cucumber and tomatoes.

Note: This recipe was tested with Lea & Perrins Marinade for Chicken.

Per ⅔ cup: 56 cal., 0 fat (0 sat. fat), 0 chol., 342mg sod., 13g carb. (8g sugars, 2g fiber), 2g pro.

Diabetic Exchanges: 1 vegetable, ½ fruit.

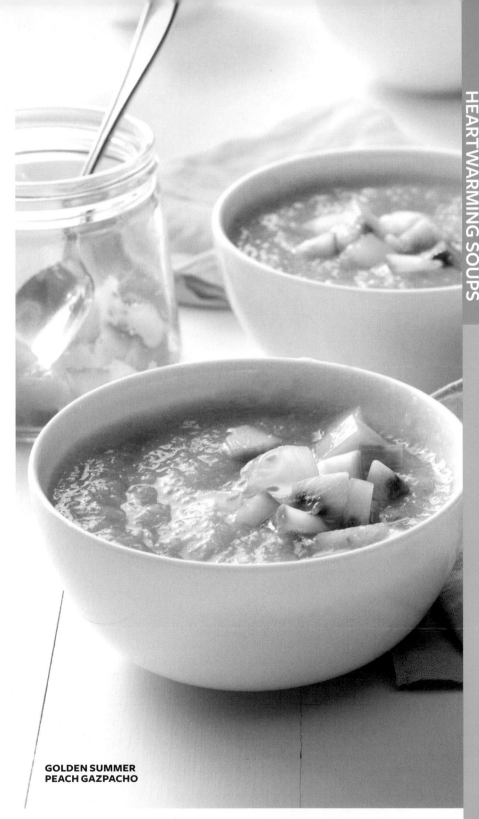

**GOLDEN SUMMER
PEACH GAZPACHO**

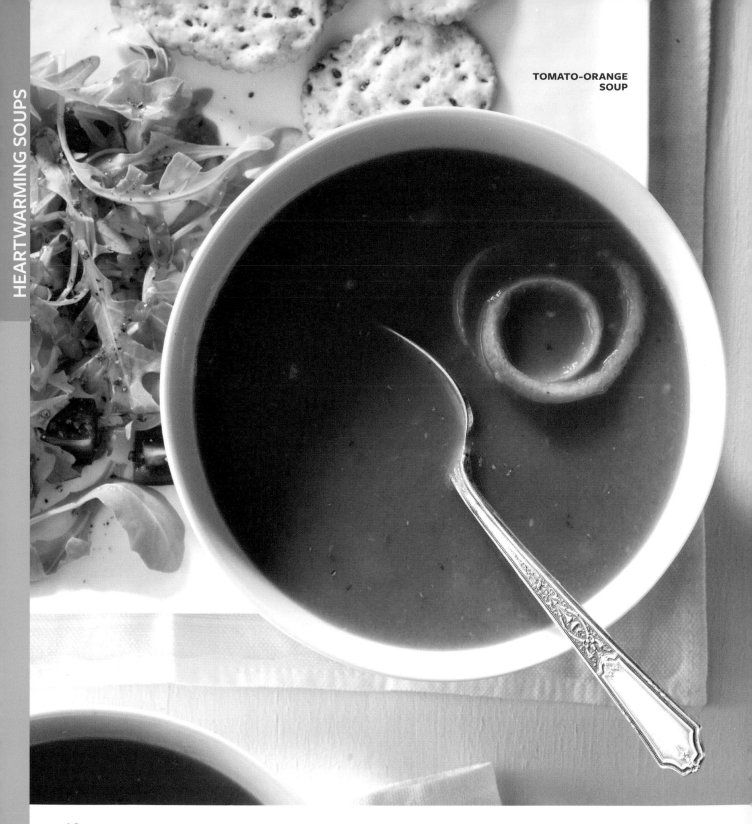

TOMATO-ORANGE
SOUP

TOMATO-ORANGE SOUP

Who knew orange and tomato were such a good pair? Whenever I serve this, I keep the recipe handy for requests.

—**BARBARA WOOD** ST. JOHN'S, NL

PREP: 30 MIN. • **COOK:** 1 HOUR
MAKES: 6 SERVINGS

- 3 pounds tomatoes, halved
- 2 tablespoons canola oil, divided
- 2 medium onions, chopped
- 2 garlic cloves, minced
- 3 cups reduced-sodium chicken broth
- 1 cup orange juice
- 2 tablespoons tomato paste
- 4 teaspoons grated orange peel
- 1 tablespoon butter
- 1 tablespoon minced fresh cilantro
- 1 tablespoon honey
- ¼ teaspoon salt

1. Preheat oven to 450°. Place the tomatoes in a 15x10x1-in. baking pan, cut side down; brush tomato tops with 1 tablespoon oil. Roast 20-25 minutes or until skins are blistered and charred. Remove and discard skins.

2. In a 6-qt. stockpot, heat remaining oil over medium-high heat. Add onions; cook and stir until tender. Add garlic; cook 1 minute longer. Stir in broth, orange juice, tomato paste and roasted tomatoes; bring to a boil. Reduce heat; simmer, uncovered, 45 minutes.

3. Stir in orange peel, butter, cilantro, honey and salt. Remove from heat; cool slightly. Process soup in batches in a blender until smooth. Return to pot; heat through.

Per 1 cup: 160 cal., 7g fat (2g sat. fat), 5mg chol., 419mg sod., 22g carb. (15g sugars, 4g fiber), 5g pro.
Diabetic Exchanges: 2 vegetable, 1½ fat, ½ starch.

FRESH CORN & POTATO CHOWDER

This soup was one of my favorites as a child in upstate New York, and I still love it to this day. For extra depth, place the spent cob in the soup, simmer, then simply remove it.

—**TRACY BIVINS** KNOB NOSTER, MO

PREP: 15 MIN. • **COOK:** 25 MIN.
MAKES: 6 SERVINGS

- 1 tablespoon butter
- 1 medium onion, chopped
- 1 pound red potatoes (about 3 medium), cubed
- 1½ cups fresh or frozen corn (about 7 ounces)
- 3 cups reduced-sodium chicken broth
- 1¼ cups half-and-half cream, divided
- 2 green onions, thinly sliced
- ½ teaspoon salt
- ¼ teaspoon freshly ground pepper
- 3 tablespoons all-purpose flour
- 1 tablespoon minced fresh parsley

1. In a large saucepan, heat butter over medium-high heat. Add the onion; cook and stir 2-4 minutes or until tender. Add the potatoes, corn, broth, 1 cup cream, green onions, salt and pepper; bring to a boil. Reduce heat; simmer, covered, about 12-15 minutes or until potatoes are tender.

2. In a small bowl, mix the flour and remaining cream until smooth; stir into soup. Return to a boil, stirring soup constantly; cook and stir 1-2 minutes or until slightly thickened. Stir in parsley.

Per 1 cup: 200 cal., 8g fat (5g sat. fat), 30mg chol., 534mg sod., 26g carb. (6g sugars, 3g fiber), 7g pro.
Diabetic Exchanges: 2 starch, 1½ fat.

MUSHROOM & BROCCOLI SOUP

Here's how I get my family to eat right without sacrificing flavor.

—**MARIA DAVIS** FLOWER MOUND, TX

PREP: 20 MIN. • **COOK:** 45 MIN.
MAKES: 8 SERVINGS

- 1 bunch broccoli (about 1½ pounds)
- 1 tablespoon canola oil
- ½ pound sliced fresh mushrooms
- 1 tablespoon reduced-sodium soy sauce
- 2 medium carrots, finely chopped
- 2 celery ribs, finely chopped
- ¼ cup finely chopped onion
- 1 garlic clove, minced
- 4 cups vegetable broth
- 2 cups water
- 2 tablespoons lemon juice

1. Cut broccoli florets into bite-size pieces. Peel and chop stalks.

2. In a large saucepan, heat oil over medium-high heat; saute mushrooms until tender, 4-6 minutes. Stir in soy sauce; remove from pan.

3. In same pan, combine broccoli stalks, carrots, celery, onion, garlic, broth and water; bring to a boil. Reduce heat; simmer, uncovered, until the vegetables are softened, 25-30 minutes.

4. Puree soup using an immersion blender. Or, cool slightly and puree soup in a blender; return to pan. Stir in florets and mushrooms; bring to a boil. Reduce heat to medium; cook until broccoli is tender, 8-10 minutes, stirring occasionally. Stir in lemon juice.

Per ¾ cup: 69 cal., 2g fat (0 sat. fat), 0 chol., 574mg sod., 11g carb. (4g sugars, 3g fiber), 4g pro.
Diabetic Exchanges: 2 vegetable, ½ fat.

GARDEN VEGETABLE BEEF SOUP

This soup is my go-to healthy lunch option. It's a great way to eat my vegetables, and it's so comforting during the cold winter months.
—**DAWN DONALD** HERRON, MI

PREP: 20 MIN. • **COOK:** 55 MIN.
MAKES: 8 SERVINGS

- 1½ pounds lean ground beef (90% lean)
- 1 medium onion, chopped
- 2 garlic cloves, minced
- 1 package (10 ounces) julienned carrots
- 2 celery ribs, chopped
- ¼ cup tomato paste
- 1 can (14½ ounces) diced tomatoes, undrained
- 1½ cups shredded cabbage
- 1 medium zucchini, coarsely chopped
- 1 medium red potato (about 5 ounces), finely chopped
- ½ cup fresh or frozen cut green beans
- 1 teaspoon dried basil
- ½ teaspoon dried oregano
- ¼ teaspoon salt
- ¼ teaspoon pepper
- 4 cans (14½ ounces each) reduced-sodium beef broth
  Grated Parmesan cheese, optional

1. In a 6-qt. stockpot, cook beef, onion and garlic over medium heat for 6-8 minutes or until beef is no longer pink, breaking up beef into crumbles; drain. Add carrots and celery; cook and stir 6-8 minutes or until tender. Stir in tomato paste; cook 1 minute longer.
2. Add tomatoes, cabbage, zucchini, potato, green beans, seasonings and broth; bring to a boil. Reduce heat; simmer, covered, 35-45 minutes or until vegetables are tender. If desired, top each serving with cheese.

Per 1¾ cups without cheese: 207 cal., 7g fat (3g sat. fat), 57mg chol., 621mg sod., 14g carb. (7g sugars, 3g fiber), 21g pro.
Diabetic Exchanges: 3 lean meat, 2 vegetable.

---

⑤ INGREDIENTS **FAST FIX**
SPICY PUMPKIN & CORN SOUP

A seriously quick dish, this can satisfy a hungry household in 20 minutes. My family loves it alongside hot corn bread.
—**HEATHER ROREX** WINNEMUCCA, NV

START TO FINISH: 20 MIN.
MAKES: 8 SERVINGS

- 1 can (15 ounces) solid-pack pumpkin
- 1 can (15 ounces) black beans, rinsed and drained
- 1½ cups frozen corn
- 1 can (10 ounces) diced tomatoes and green chilies
- 2 cans (14½ ounces each) reduced-sodium chicken broth
- ¼ teaspoon pepper

In a large saucepan, mix all ingredients. Bring to a boil. Reduce heat; simmer, uncovered, 10-15 minutes or until slightly thickened, stirring occasionally.
To freeze: Freeze the cooled soup in freezer containers. To use, partially thaw in refrigerator overnight. Heat through in a saucepan, stirring occasionally and adding a little broth if necessary.
Per ¾ cup: 100 cal., 0 fat (0 sat. fat), 0 chol., 542mg sod., 20g carb. (3g sugars, 5g fiber), 6g pro.
Diabetic Exchanges: 1 starch.

GARDEN VEGETABLE BEEF SOUP

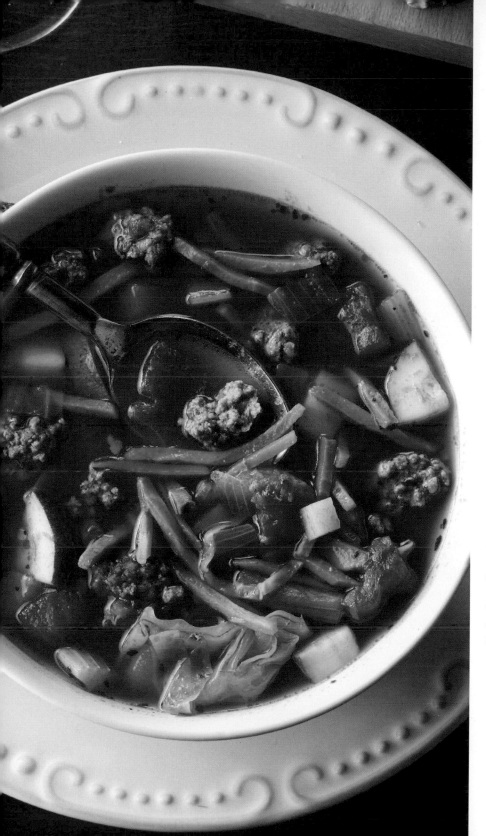

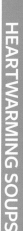

COLD-DAY CHICKEN NOODLE SOUP

When I was sick, my mom would stir up a heartwarming chicken noodle soup. It's so soothing for colds—and for those cold-weather days.

—ANTHONY GRAHAM OTTAWA, IL

PREP: 15 MIN. • **COOK:** 25 MIN.
MAKES: 8 SERVINGS

- 1 tablespoon canola oil
- 2 celery ribs, chopped
- 2 medium carrots, chopped
- 1 medium onion, chopped
- 8 cups reduced-sodium chicken broth
- ½ teaspoon dried basil
- ¼ teaspoon pepper
- 3 cups uncooked whole wheat egg noodles (about 4 ounces)
- 3 cups coarsely chopped rotisserie chicken
- 1 tablespoon minced fresh parsley

1. In a 6-qt. stockpot, heat oil over medium-high heat. Add celery, carrots and onion; cook and stir 5-7 minutes or until tender.

2. Add broth, basil and pepper; bring to a boil. Stir in the noodles; cook 12-14 minutes or until al dente. Stir in chicken and parsley; heat through.

Per 1½ cups: 195 cal., 6g fat (1g sat. fat), 47mg chol., 639mg sod., 16g carb. (2g sugars, 3g fiber), 21g pro.
Diabetic Exchanges: 2 lean meat, 1 starch, ½ fat.

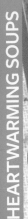

AUTUMN
BISQUE

AUTUMN BISQUE

I like cozy comfort soups that taste creamy, but without the cream. This one's full of goodies such as rutabagas, leeks, fresh herbs and almond milk.

—MERRY GRAHAM NEWHALL, CA

PREP: 25 MIN. • **COOK:** 50 MIN.
MAKES: 12 SERVINGS

- ¼ cup buttery spread
- 2 teaspoons minced fresh chives
- 2 teaspoons minced fresh parsley
- ½ teaspoon grated lemon peel

BISQUE

- 2 tablespoons olive oil
- 2 large rutabagas, peeled and cubed (about 9 cups)
- 1 large celery root, peeled and cubed (about 3 cups)
- 3 medium leeks (white portion only), chopped (about 2 cups)
- 1 large carrot, cubed (about ⅔ cup)
- 3 garlic cloves, minced
- 7 cups vegetable stock
- 2 teaspoons minced fresh thyme
- 1½ teaspoons minced fresh rosemary
- 1 teaspoon salt
- ½ teaspoon coarsely ground pepper
- 2 cups almond milk
- 2 tablespoons minced fresh chives

1. Mix first four ingredients. Using a melon baller or 1-teaspoon measuring spoon, shape mixture into 12 balls. Freeze on a waxed paper-lined baking sheet until firm. Transfer to a freezer container; freeze up to 2 months.
2. In a 6-qt. stock pot, heat oil over medium heat; saute rutabagas, celery root, leeks and carrot 8 minutes. Add garlic; cook and stir 2 minutes. Stir in stock, herbs, salt and pepper; bring to a boil. Reduce heat; simmer the soup, covered, until vegetables are tender, 30-35 minutes.
3. Puree soup using an immersion blender. Or, cool slightly and puree soup in batches in a blender; return to pan. Stir in milk; heat through. Top each serving with chives and herbed buttery spread ball.

Per 1 cup: 146 cal., 7g fat (2g sat. fat), 0 chol., 672mg sod., 20g carb. (9g sugars, 5g fiber), 3g pro.
Diabetic Exchanges: 1 starch, 1 fat.

ROASTED CAULIFLOWER & RED PEPPER SOUP

When cooler weather comes, soup is one of our favorite meals. I wanted to develop a healthier version of all the cream-based soups out there for my husband and me. After a bit of trial and error, this is the keeper.

—ELIZABETH BRAMKAMP GIG HARBOR, WA

PREP: 50 MIN. + STANDING
COOK: 25 MIN. • **MAKES:** 6 SERVINGS

- 2 medium sweet red peppers, halved and seeded
- 1 large head cauliflower, broken into florets (about 7 cups)
- 4 tablespoons olive oil, divided
- 1 cup chopped sweet onion
- 2 garlic cloves, minced
- 2½ teaspoons minced fresh rosemary or ¾ teaspoon dried rosemary, crushed
- ½ teaspoon paprika
- ¼ cup all-purpose flour
- 4 cups chicken stock
- 1 cup 2% milk
- ½ teaspoon salt
- ¼ teaspoon pepper
- ⅛ to ¼ teaspoon cayenne pepper
  Shredded Parmesan cheese, optional

1. Preheat broiler. Place peppers on a foil-lined baking sheet, skin side up. Broil 4 in. from heat until skins are blistered, about 5 minutes. Transfer to a bowl; let stand, covered, 20 minutes. Change oven setting to bake; preheat oven to 400°.
2. Toss cauliflower with 2 tablespoons oil; spread in a 15x10x1-in. pan. Roast until tender, 25-30 minutes, stirring occasionally. Remove skin and seeds from peppers; chop peppers.
3. In a 6-qt. stockpot, heat remaining oil over medium heat. Add onion; cook until golden and softened, 6-8 minutes, stirring occasionally. Add the garlic, rosemary and paprika; cook and stir 1 minute. Stir in flour until blended; cook and stir 1 minute. Gradually stir in stock. Bring to a boil, stirring constantly; cook and stir until thickened.
4. Stir in cauliflower and peppers. Puree soup using an immersion blender. Or, cool slightly and puree in batches in a blender; return to pot. Stir in milk and remaining seasonings; heat through. If desired, serve with cheese.

To freeze: Freeze the cooled soup in freezer containers. To use, partially thaw in refrigerator overnight. Heat through in a saucepan, stirring occasionally and adding a little stock or milk if necessary.
Per 1 cup: 193 cal., 10g fat (2g sat. fat), 3mg chol., 601mg sod., 19g carb. (8g sugars, 4g fiber), 8g pro.
Diabetic Exchanges: 2 vegetable, 2 fat, ½ starch.

✳

DID YOU KNOW?
Roasting is one of the healthiest methods for cooking vegetables. It often uses less fat than sauteing and helps retain more nutrients than boiling would.

FAST FIX ▶
BROCCOLI & POTATO SOUP

If I don't have frozen broccoli on hand, I can always toss in some frozen spinach or chopped carrots and celery instead.
—MARY PRICE YOUNGSTOWN, OH

START TO FINISH: 30 MIN.
MAKES: 3 SERVINGS

- 3 cups cubed peeled potatoes
- 1 medium onion, chopped
- 2 garlic cloves, minced
- 2 cups reduced-sodium chicken broth
- 1 cup water
   Dash pepper
- ⅛ teaspoon salt
- 3 cups frozen broccoli florets
- 3 tablespoons all-purpose flour
- ⅓ cup fat-free milk
- ½ cup shredded reduced-fat sharp cheddar cheese
   Minced fresh parsley

1. In a large saucepan, combine the first seven ingredients; bring to a boil. Reduce heat; simmer, covered, 10-15 minutes or until potatoes are tender. Stir in broccoli; return to a boil.

2. In a small bowl, whisk flour and milk until smooth; stir into soup. Cook and stir for 2 minutes or until thickened. Remove from heat; cool slightly.

3. Process in batches in a blender until smooth. Return to pan; heat through. Sprinkle servings with cheddar cheese and parsley.

Per 2 cups: 262 cal., 4g fat (3g sat. fat), 14mg chol., 636mg sod., 44g carb. (9g sugars, 5g fiber), 14g pro.

Diabetic Exchanges: 2 starch, 1 medium-fat meat, 1 vegetable.

HEARTY VEGETABLE LENTIL SOUP

My mother has diabetes so I often make this veggie-and-fiber-packed dish for her. Lentils, a handful of spices and a little bacon really hit the spot on cool autumn nights.
—NICOLE HOPPING PINOLE, CA

PREP: 15 MIN. • **COOK:** 45 MIN.
MAKES: 6 SERVINGS

- 6 bacon strips, chopped
- 1 pound red potatoes (about 3 medium), chopped
- 2 medium carrots, chopped
- 1 medium onion, chopped
- 6 garlic cloves, minced
- ¾ teaspoon ground cumin
- ½ teaspoon salt
- ½ teaspoon rubbed sage
- ½ teaspoon dried thyme
- ¼ teaspoon pepper
- 1½ cups dried lentils, rinsed
- 4 cups chicken stock

1. In a large saucepan, cook the bacon over medium heat until crisp, stirring occasionally. Remove with a slotted spoon; drain on paper towels. Discard drippings, reserving 1 tablespoon in pan. Add potatoes, carrots and onion; cook and stir 6-8 minutes or until the carrots and onion are tender. Add garlic and seasonings; cook 1 minute longer.

2. Add lentils and stock; bring to a boil. Reduce heat; simmer, covered, 30-35 minutes or until lentils and potatoes are tender. Top each serving with bacon.

Per 1 cup: 314 cal., 6g fat (2g sat. fat), 10mg chol., 708mg sod., 47g carb. (4g sugars, 17g fiber), 20g pro.

Diabetic Exchanges: 3 starch, 2 lean meat.

SAUSAGE & GREENS SOUP

I found a winner with this colorful dish!
—ANGIE PITTS CHARLESTON, SC

PREP: 20 MIN. • **COOK:** 20 MIN.
MAKES: 6 SERVINGS

- 1 tablespoon olive oil
- 2 Italian turkey sausage links (4 ounces each), casings removed
- 1 medium onion, chopped
- 1 celery rib, chopped
- 1 medium carrot, chopped
- 1 garlic clove, minced
- 6 ounces Swiss chard, stems removed, chopped (about 4 cups)
- 1 can (14½ ounces) no-salt-added diced tomatoes, undrained
- 1 bay leaf
- 1 teaspoon rubbed sage
- 1 teaspoon Italian seasoning
- ½ teaspoon pepper
- 1 carton (32 ounces) reduced-sodium chicken broth
- 1 can (15 ounces) no-salt-added cannellini beans, rinsed and drained
- 1 tablespoon lemon juice

1. In a 6-qt. stockpot, heat oil over medium-high heat. Add the next four ingredients; cook 6-8 minutes or until sausage is no longer pink and vegetables are tender. Add garlic; cook 1 minute.

2. Stir in Swiss chard, tomatoes, bay leaf and seasonings. Add broth; bring to a boil. Reduce heat; simmer, covered, 10-12 minutes or until Swiss chard is tender. Stir in beans and lemon juice; heat through. Remove bay leaf.

Per 1½ cups: 155 cal., 5g fat (1g sat. fat), 14mg chol., 658mg sod., 18g carb. (5g sugars, 5g fiber), 11g pro.

Diabetic Exchanges: 1 medium-fat meat, 1 vegetable, ½ starch, ½ fat.

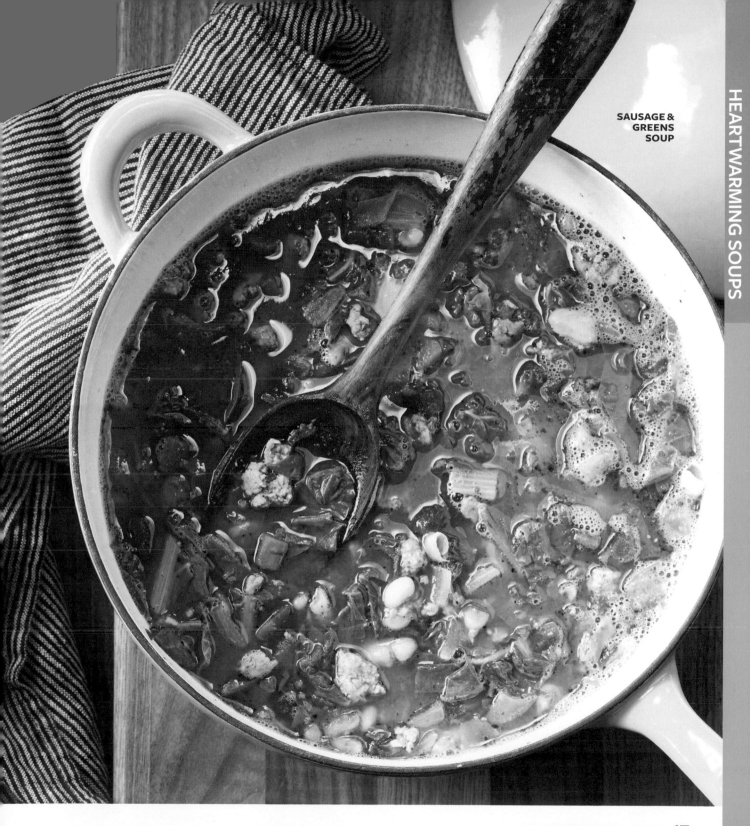

SAUSAGE & GREENS SOUP

**RED, WHITE & BLUE
POTATO SALAD, PAGE 81**

Sensational Side Salads

Packing a picnic? Invited to a potluck? Looking to add
a bit of color to mealtime lineups? Featuring tender
greens, fresh fruit and loads of other flavorful favorites,
these creative takes on traditional side salads are sure
to please everyone!

FAST FIX

RAINBOW VEGGIE SALAD

Every salad should be colorful and crunchy like this one with its bright tomatoes, carrots, peppers and sassy spring mix. Toss with your best dressing.
—**LIZ BELLVILLE** JACKSONVILLE, NC

START TO FINISH: 25 MIN.
MAKES: 8 SERVINGS

- ½ English cucumber, cut lengthwise in half and sliced
- 2 medium carrots, thinly sliced
- 1 cup each red and yellow cherry tomatoes, halved
- ¾ cup pitted ripe olives, halved
- 1 celery rib, thinly sliced
- ¼ cup each chopped sweet yellow, orange and red pepper
- ¼ cup thinly sliced red onion
- ⅛ teaspoon garlic salt
  Dash coarsely ground pepper
- 1 package (5 ounces) spring mix salad greens
- ⅔ cup reduced-fat buttermilk ranch salad dressing

1. Place cucumber, carrots, tomatoes, olives, celery, sweet peppers, onion, garlic salt and pepper in a large bowl; toss to combine.
2. Just before serving, add salad greens. Drizzle with dressing and toss gently to combine.
Per 1 cup: 64 cal., 3g fat (1g sat. fat), 0 chol., 232mg sod., 7g carb. (3g sugars, 2g fiber), 2g pro.
Diabetic Exchanges: 1 vegetable, ½ fat.

CARAWAY COLESLAW WITH CITRUS MAYONNAISE

I always get requests to bring a big batch of this unique coleslaw to potlucks—proof positive that it's a keeper! I like to make it a day ahead so the flavors blend.
—**LILY JULOW** LAWRENCEVILLE, GA

PREP: 20 MIN. + CHILLING
MAKES: 12 SERVINGS

- 1 medium head cabbage, finely shredded
- 1 tablespoon sugar
- 2 teaspoons salt
  DRESSING
- ⅔ cup reduced-fat mayonnaise
- ⅓ cup orange juice
- 3 tablespoons cider vinegar
- 2 tablespoons caraway seeds
- 2 teaspoons grated orange peel
- ¼ teaspoon salt
- ¼ teaspoon pepper

1. Place cabbage in a colander over a plate. Sprinkle with sugar and salt; toss to coat. Let stand 1 hour.
2. In a small bowl, whisk the dressing ingredients until blended. Rinse cabbage and drain well; place in a large bowl. Add dressing; toss to coat. Refrigerate, covered, overnight.
Per ⅔ cup: 75 cal., 5g fat (1g sat. fat), 5mg chol., 366mg sod., 8g carb. (5g sugars, 2g fiber), 1g pro.
Diabetic Exchanges: 1 vegetable, 1 fat.

FAST FIX

HEIRLOOM TOMATO & ZUCCHINI SALAD

Tomato wedges give this salad a juicy bite. It's a smart use of fresh herbs and veggies from your own garden or the farmers market.
—**MATTHEW HASS** FRANKLIN, WI

START TO FINISH: 25 MIN.
MAKES: 12 SERVINGS

- 7 large heirloom tomatoes (about 2½ pounds), cut into wedges
- 3 medium zucchini, halved lengthwise and thinly sliced
- 2 medium sweet yellow peppers, thinly sliced
- ⅓ cup cider vinegar
- 3 tablespoons olive oil
- 1 tablespoon sugar
- 1½ teaspoons salt
- 1 tablespoon each minced fresh basil, parsley and tarragon

1. In a large bowl, combine tomatoes, zucchini and peppers. In a small bowl, whisk vinegar, oil, sugar and salt until blended. Stir in herbs.
2. Just before serving, drizzle dressing over salad; toss gently to coat.
Per 1 cup: 68 cal., 4g fat (1g sat. fat), 0 chol., 306mg sod., 8g carb. (5g sugars, 2g fiber), 2g pro.
Diabetic Exchanges: 1 vegetable, ½ fat.

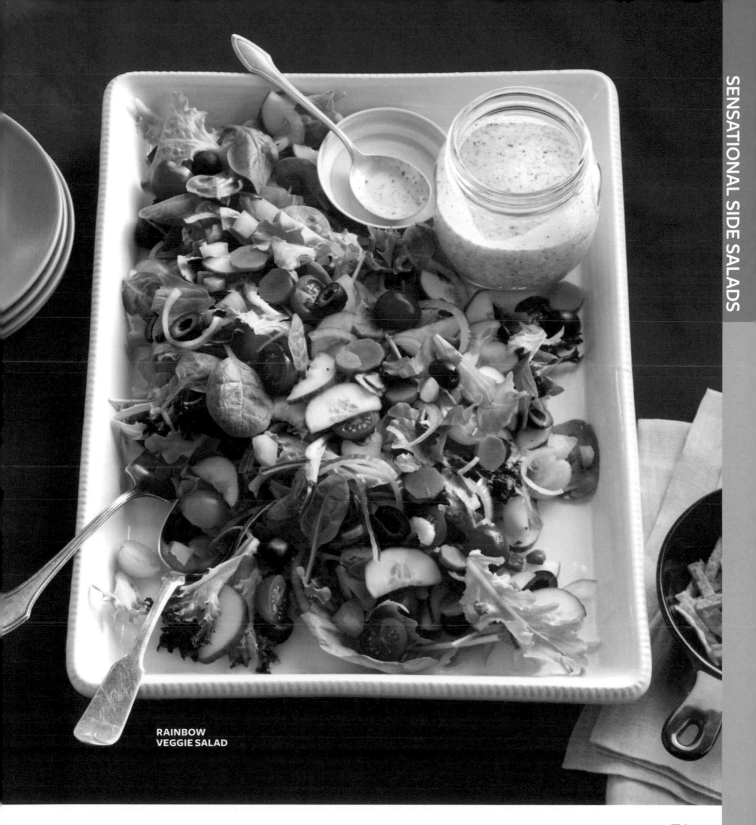

RAINBOW
VEGGIE SALAD

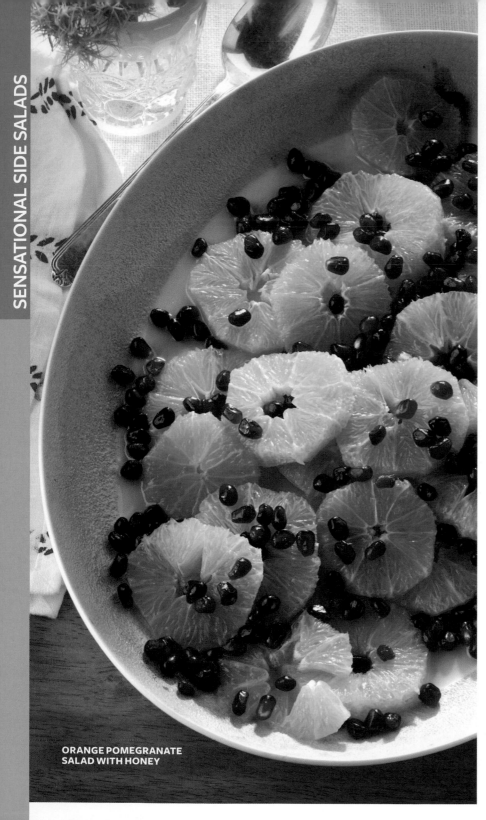

**ORANGE POMEGRANATE
SALAD WITH HONEY**

(5)INGREDIENTS   FAST FIX▶

ORANGE POMEGRANATE
SALAD WITH HONEY

*I discovered this fragrant salad in a
cooking class. If you can, try to find
orange flower water (also called orange
blossom water), which perks up the
orange segments. But orange juice adds
a nice zip, too!*

—CAROL RICHARDSON MARTY
LYNWOOD, WA

START TO FINISH: 15 MIN.
MAKES: 6 SERVINGS

- 5 medium oranges or
  10 clementines
- ½ cup pomegranate seeds
- 2 tablespoons honey
- 1 to 2 teaspoons orange flower
  water or orange juice

1. Cut a thin slice from the top and
bottom of each orange; stand orange
upright on a cutting board. With a knife,
cut off peel and outer membrane from
oranges. Cut crosswise into ½-in. slices.
2. Arrange orange slices on a serving
platter; sprinkle with pomegranate
seeds. In a small bowl, mix honey and
orange flower water; drizzle over fruit.
Per ⅔ cup: 62 cal., 0 fat (0 sat. fat),
0 chol., 2mg sod., 15g carb. (14g
sugars, 0 fiber), 1g pro.
Diabetic Exchanges: 1 fruit.

CHERRY TOMATO SALAD

This recipe evolved from a need to use up the bumper crop of cherry tomatoes that we regularly grow. It's become a summer favorite, especially at cookouts.

—SALLY SIBLEY ST. AUGUSTINE, FL

PREP: 15 MIN. + MARINATING
MAKES: 6 SERVINGS

- 1 quart cherry tomatoes, halved
- ¼ cup canola oil
- 3 tablespoons white vinegar
- ½ teaspoon salt
- ½ teaspoon sugar
- ¼ cup minced fresh parsley
- 1 to 2 teaspoons minced fresh basil
- 1 to 2 teaspoons minced fresh oregano

Place tomatoes in a shallow bowl. In a small bowl, whisk oil, vinegar, salt and sugar until blended; stir in herbs. Pour over tomatoes; gently toss to coat. Refrigerate, covered, overnight.
Per ¾ cup: 103 cal., 10g fat (1g sat. fat), 0 chol., 203mg sod., 4g carb. (3g sugars, 1g fiber), 1g pro.
Diabetic Exchanges: 2 fat, 1 vegetable.

★ ★ ★ ★ ★ **READER REVIEW**

"This was delicious ... good and tangy. I used dried herbs, sprinkled in grated Parmesan cheese and topped with seasoned croutons."

CHRISD1717 TASTEOFHOME.COM

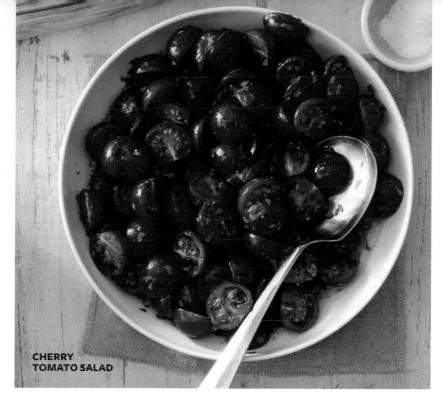

CHERRY TOMATO SALAD

FAST FIX
ALL-SPICED UP RASPBERRY & MUSHROOM SALAD

Here's a refreshing salad for summertime or anytime. Make a homemade vinaigrette with just raspberry vinegar, olive oil, jalapeno jelly and allspice.

—ROXANNE CHAN ALBANY, CA

START TO FINISH: 30 MIN.
MAKES: 4 SERVINGS

- 2 tablespoons raspberry vinegar
- 2 tablespoons olive oil, divided
- 1 tablespoon red jalapeno pepper jelly
- ¼ teaspoon ground allspice
- 1 pound small fresh mushrooms, halved
- 4 cups spring mix salad greens
- 1 cup fresh raspberries
- 2 tablespoons chopped red onion
- 2 tablespoons minced fresh mint
- 2 tablespoons sliced almonds, toasted
- ¼ cup crumbled goat cheese

1. In a small bowl, whisk vinegar, 1 tablespoon oil, pepper jelly and allspice until blended. In a large skillet, heat remaining oil over medium-high heat. Add mushrooms; cook and stir until tender; cool slightly.
2. In a large bowl, combine salad greens, raspberries, onion, mint and almonds. Just before serving, add mushrooms and vinaigrette; toss to combine. Top with cheese.
Note: To toast nuts, bake in a shallow pan in a 350° oven for 5-10 minutes or cook in a skillet over low heat until lightly browned, stirring occasionally.
Per serving: 168 cal., 11g fat (2g sat. fat), 9mg chol., 54mg sod., 15g carb. (6g sugars, 6g fiber), 6g pro.
Diabetic Exchanges: 2 fat, 1 starch.

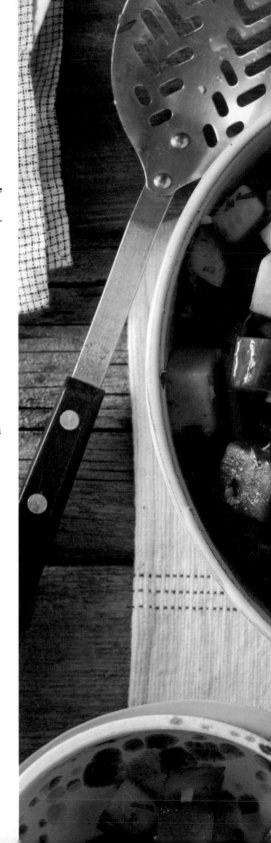

FAST FIX

FAUX POTATO SALAD

Make your potato salad super healthy by taking out the potatoes. It may sound crazy, but cauliflower is a tasty alternative to spuds.

—**MIKE SCHULZ** TAWAS CITY, MI

START TO FINISH: 30 MIN.
MAKES: 8 SERVINGS

- 1 medium head cauliflower, broken into florets
- 1 medium carrot, chopped
- 2 hard-cooked large eggs, chopped
- 4 green onions, chopped
- 1 celery rib, chopped
- ¼ cup pitted green olives, halved lengthwise
- ¼ cup thinly sliced radishes
- ¼ cup chopped dill pickle
- ¼ cup fat-free mayonnaise
- 1 tablespoon Dijon mustard
- ¼ teaspoon salt
- ⅛ teaspoon pepper

1. In a large saucepan, bring 1 in. of water to a boil. Add cauliflower florets; cook, covered, 5-8 minutes or until tender. Drain and rinse in cold water. Pat dry and place in a large bowl. Add carrot, eggs, green onions, celery, olives, radishes and pickle.

2. In a small bowl, mix the remaining ingredients. Add to cauliflower mixture; toss to coat. Refrigerate until serving.

Per ¾ cup: 61 cal., 2g fat (0 sat. fat), 54mg chol., 375mg sod., 7g carb. (3g sugars, 3g fiber), 3g pro.
Diabetic Exchanges: 1 vegetable, ½ starch.

FAST FIX

WATERMELON & SPINACH SALAD

Now's the perfect time to toss up my melon salad. You'd never expect it, but spinach is awesome here. Eat it and feel cool on even the hottest days.

—**MARJORIE AU** HONOLULU, HI

START TO FINISH: 30 MIN.
MAKES: 8 SERVINGS

- ¼ cup rice vinegar or white wine vinegar
- 1 tablespoon grated lime peel
- 2 tablespoons lime juice
- 2 tablespoons canola oil
- 4 teaspoons minced fresh gingerroot
- 2 garlic cloves, minced
- ½ teaspoon salt
- ¼ teaspoon sugar
- ¼ teaspoon pepper

SALAD

- 4 cups fresh baby spinach or arugula
- 3 cups cubed seedless watermelon
- 2 cups cubed cantaloupe
- 2 cups cubed English cucumber
- ½ cup chopped fresh cilantro
- 2 green onions, chopped

In a small bowl, whisk the first nine ingredients. In a large bowl, combine salad ingredients. Drizzle with dressing and toss to coat; serve immediately.

Per 1 cup: 84 cal., 4g fat (0 sat. fat), 0 chol., 288mg sod., 13g carb. (10g sugars, 1g fiber), 1g pro.
Diabetic Exchanges: 1 vegetable, 1 fat, ½ fruit.

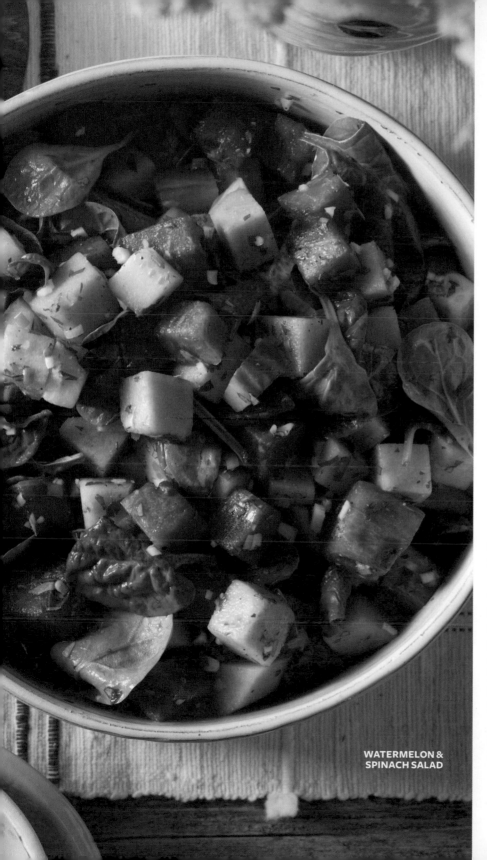

**WATERMELON &
SPINACH SALAD**

FAST FIX

MICHIGAN CHERRY SALAD

This salad reminds me what I love about my home state: apple picking with my children, buying greens at the farmers market and tasting cherries.

—JENNIFER GILBERT BRIGHTON, MI

START TO FINISH: 15 MIN.
MAKES: 8 SERVINGS

- 7 ounces fresh baby spinach (about 9 cups)
- 3 ounces spring mix salad greens (about 5 cups)
- 1 large apple, chopped
- ½ cup coarsely chopped pecans, toasted
- ½ cup dried cherries
- ¼ cup crumbled Gorgonzola cheese

DRESSING
- ¼ cup fresh raspberries
- ¼ cup red wine vinegar
- 3 tablespoons cider vinegar
- 3 tablespoons cherry preserves
- 1 tablespoon sugar
- 2 tablespoons olive oil

1. In a large bowl, combine the first six ingredients.

2. Place the raspberries, vinegars, preserves and sugar in a blender. While processing, gradually add oil in a steady stream. Drizzle over salad; toss to coat.

Note: To toast nuts, bake in a shallow pan in a 350° oven for 5-10 minutes or cook in a skillet over low heat until lightly browned, stirring occasionally.

Per 1½ cups: 172 cal., 10g fat (2g sat. fat), 3mg chol., 78mg sod., 21g carb. (16g sugars, 3g fiber), 3g pro.

Diabetic Exchanges: 2 vegetable, 2 fat, 1 starch.

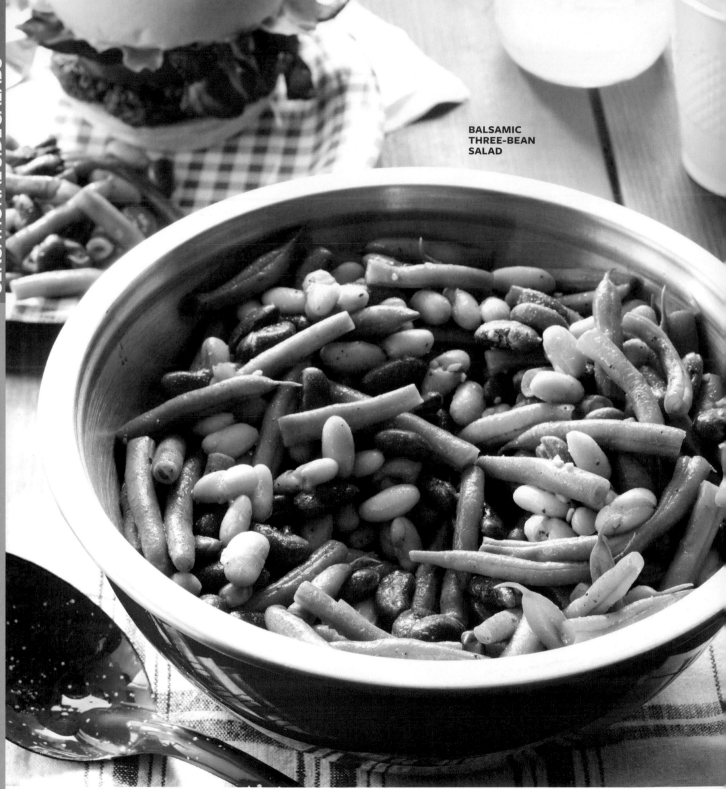

BALSAMIC THREE-BEAN SALAD

BALSAMIC THREE-BEAN SALAD

Here's my little girl's favorite salad. She eats it just about as fast as I can make it. Prepare it ahead so the flavors have time to get to know each other.
—STACEY FEATHER JAY, OK

PREP: 25 MIN. + CHILLING
MAKES: 12 SERVINGS

- 2 pounds fresh green beans, trimmed and cut into 2-inch pieces
- ½ cup balsamic vinaigrette
- ¼ cup sugar
- 1 garlic clove, minced
- ¾ teaspoon salt
- 2 cans (16 ounces each) kidney beans, rinsed and drained
- 2 cans (15 ounces each) cannellini beans, rinsed and drained
- 4 fresh basil leaves, torn

1. Fill a Dutch oven three-fourths full with water; bring to a boil. Add green beans; cook, uncovered, 3-6 minutes or until crisp-tender. Drain and immediately drop into ice water. Drain and pat dry.
2. In a large bowl, whisk vinaigrette, sugar, garlic and salt until sugar is dissolved. Add canned beans and green beans; toss to coat. Refrigerate, covered, at least 4 hours. Stir in basil just before serving.
Per ¾ cup: 190 cal., 3g fat (0 sat. fat), 0 chol., 462mg sod., 33g carb. (8g sugars, 9g fiber), 9g pro.
Diabetic Exchanges: 1½ starch, 1 very lean meat, 1 vegetable, ½ fat.

FAST FIX ▶

BABY KALE SALAD WITH AVOCADO-LIME DRESSING

We pull a bunch of ingredients from our garden when we make this salad of greens, zucchini and sweet onion. The yogurt dressing layers on big lime flavor.
—SUZANNA ESTHER STATE COLLEGE, PA

START TO FINISH: 20 MIN.
MAKES: 4 SERVINGS

- 6 cups baby kale salad blend
- 1 cup julienned zucchini
- ½ cup thinly sliced sweet onion
- ½ cup fat-free plain yogurt
- 2 tablespoons lime juice
- 1 garlic clove, minced
- ¼ teaspoon salt
- ⅛ teaspoon pepper
- ½ medium ripe avocado, peeled
- 3 green onions, chopped
- 2 tablespoons minced fresh parsley

In a large bowl, combine salad blend, zucchini and sweet onion. Place the remaining ingredients in a blender; cover and process until smooth. Divide salad mixture among four plates; drizzle with dressing.
Per 1½ cups salad with 3 tablespoons dressing: 74 cal., 3g fat (1g sat. fat), 1mg chol., 197mg sod., 10g carb. (4g sugars, 4g fiber), 4g pro.
Diabetic Exchanges: 2 vegetable, ½ fat.

✱

DID YOU KNOW?
If you've never been a fan of kale because the mature leaves seem too tough, try the baby variety. Available at most supermarkets, the leaves are more tender, mild and palatable. Use it in anything from salads to omelets to wraps.

FAST FIX ▶

SUMMER BUZZ FRUIT SALAD

For picnics, cookouts and showers, we make a sweet salad of watermelon, cherries, blueberries and microgreens. No matter where I take it, it always delivers the wow factor.
—KALISKA RUSSELL TALKEETNA, AK

START TO FINISH: 15 MIN
MAKES: 6 SERVINGS

- 2 cups watermelon balls
- 2 cups fresh sweet cherries, pitted and halved
- 1 cup fresh blueberries
- ½ cup cubed English cucumber
- ½ cup microgreens or torn mixed salad greens
- ½ cup crumbled feta cheese
- 3 fresh mint leaves, thinly sliced
- ¼ cup honey
- 1 tablespoon lemon juice
- 1 teaspoon grated lemon peel

Combine the first seven ingredients. In a small bowl, whisk together remaining ingredients. Drizzle over salad; toss.
Per ¾ cup: 131 cal., 2g fat (1g sat. fat), 5mg chol., 94mg sod., 28g carb. (24g sugars, 2g fiber), 3g pro.
Diabetic Exchanges: 1 starch, 1 fruit.

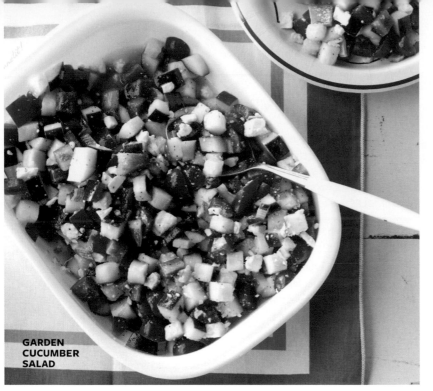

GARDEN CUCUMBER SALAD

GARDEN CUCUMBER SALAD

If you like cucumber salad as I do, this one's a cool pick. It's a mix of fresh veggies, feta and Greek seasoning. It's so refreshing when the sun's beating down.

—**KATIE STANCZAK** HOOVER, AL

PREP: 10 MIN. + CHILLING
MAKES: 12 SERVINGS

- 4 medium cucumbers, cut into ½-inch pieces (about 7 cups)
- 2 medium sweet red peppers, chopped
- 1 cup cherry tomatoes, halved
- 1 cup crumbled feta cheese
- ½ cup finely chopped red onion
- ½ cup olive oil
- ¼ cup lemon juice
- 1 tablespoon Greek seasoning
- ½ teaspoon salt

Place all of the ingredients in a large bowl; toss gently to combine. Refrigerate, covered, for at least 30 minutes before serving.
Per ¾ cup: 125 cal., 11g fat (2g sat. fat), 5mg chol., 431mg sod., 5g carb. (3g sugars, 2g fiber), 3g pro.
Diabetic Exchanges: 2 fat, 1 vegetable.

★ ★ ★ ★ ★ **READER REVIEW**

"I thought this was delicious exactly as is. A nice, light, simple salad that's healthy and easy to make."

REMENEC TASTEOFHOME.COM

GREEN BEAN & POTATO SALAD

For family reunions, my mom would always make everybody's favorite green bean and potato salad. Now I'm the one who brings it!

—**CONNIE DICAVOLI** SHAWNEE, KS

PREP: 15 MIN. • **COOK:** 20 MIN. + CHILLING
MAKES: 10 SERVINGS

- 2 pounds red potatoes (about 6 medium), cubed
- 1 pound fresh green beans, trimmed and halved
- 1 small red onion, halved and thinly sliced
- ¼ cup chopped fresh mint, optional

DRESSING

- ½ cup canola oil
- ¼ cup white vinegar
- 2 tablespoons lemon juice
- 1 teaspoon salt
- ½ teaspoon garlic powder
- ¼ teaspoon pepper

1. Place cubed potatoes in a 6-qt. stockpot; add water to cover. Bring to a boil. Reduce heat; cook, uncovered, 10-15 minutes or until tender, adding green beans during the last 4 minutes of cooking. Drain.
2. Transfer potatoes and green beans to a large bowl; add onion and, if desired, mint. In a small bowl, whisk dressing ingredients until blended. Pour over potato mixture; toss gently to coat. Refrigerate, covered, at least 2 hours before serving.
Per ¾ cup: 183 cal., 11g fat (1g sat. fat), 0 chol., 245mg sod., 19g carb. (2g sugars, 3g fiber), 3g pro.
Diabetic Exchanges: 2½ fat, 1 starch.

FAST FIX ▸

LEMON CRANBERRY QUINOA SALAD

Change up this salad by substituting diced fresh mango for the cranberries, cilantro for the parsley, and lime for the lemon juice and zest.

—**MARY SHENK** DEKALB, IL

START TO FINISH: 30 MIN.
MAKES: 8 SERVINGS

- ¼ cup olive oil
- 2 teaspoons grated lemon peel
- 2 tablespoons lemon juice
- 2 teaspoons minced fresh gingerroot
- ¾ teaspoon salt

SALAD

- 2 cups reduced-sodium chicken broth
- 1 cup quinoa, rinsed
- 1 cup chopped peeled jicama or tart apple
- 1 cup chopped seeded cucumber
- ¾ cup dried cranberries
- ½ cup minced fresh parsley
- 1 green onion, thinly sliced
- 1 cup cubed avocado

1. For dressing, in a small bowl, whisk the first five ingredients until blended.
2. In a small saucepan, bring broth to a boil. Add quinoa. Reduce heat; simmer, covered, 12-15 minutes or until liquid is absorbed. Remove from heat; fluff with a fork. Transfer to a large bowl.
3. Add jicama, cucumber, cranberries, parsley and green onion to quinoa. Drizzle with dressing and toss to coat. Serve warm or refrigerate and serve cold. Stir in avocado before serving.
Per ¾ cup: 218 cal., 11g fat (2g sat. fat), 0 chol., 370mg sod., 27g carb. (8g sugars, 5g fiber), 5g pro.
Diabetic Exchanges: 2 starch, 2 fat.

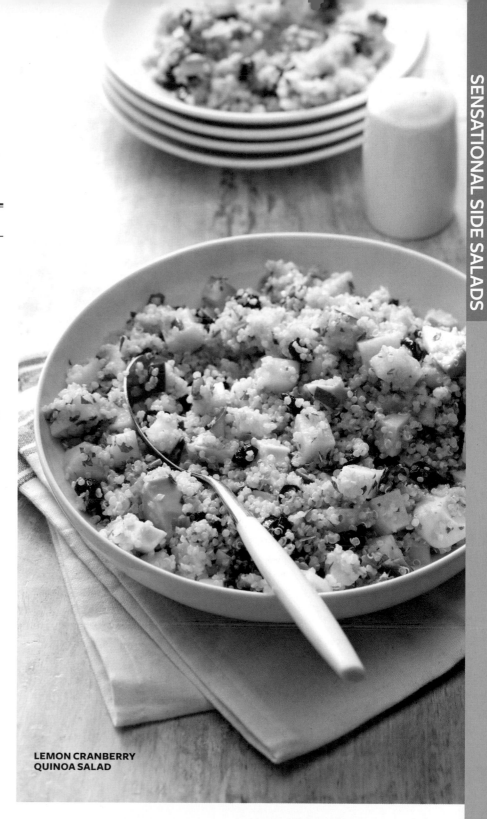

LEMON CRANBERRY QUINOA SALAD

FAST FIX ▶

ITALIAN SALAD WITH LEMON VINAIGRETTE

For an Italian twist on salad, I mix greens with red onion, mushrooms, olives, pepperoncini, lemon juice and a little seasoning. Add tomatoes and carrots for a splash of color if you like.

—**DEBORAH LOOP** CLINTON TOWNSHIP, MI

START TO FINISH: 20 MIN.
MAKES: 8 SERVINGS

- 1 package (5 ounces) spring mix salad greens
- 1 small red onion, thinly sliced
- 1 cup sliced fresh mushrooms
- 1 cup assorted olives, pitted and coarsely chopped
- 8 pepperoncini
  Optional toppings: chopped tomatoes, shredded carrots and grated Parmesan cheese

VINAIGRETTE

- ⅓ cup extra virgin olive oil
- 3 tablespoons lemon juice
- 1 teaspoon Italian seasoning
- ¼ teaspoon salt
- ¼ teaspoon pepper

1. In a large bowl, combine the first five ingredients; toss lightly. If desired, add the optional toppings.

2. In a small bowl, whisk vinaigrette ingredients until blended. Serve with the salad.

Per 1¼ cups: 109 cal., 11g fat (1g sat. fat), 0 chol., 343mg sod., 4g carb. (1g sugars, 1g fiber), 1g pro.

Diabetic Exchanges: 2 fat, 1 vegetable.

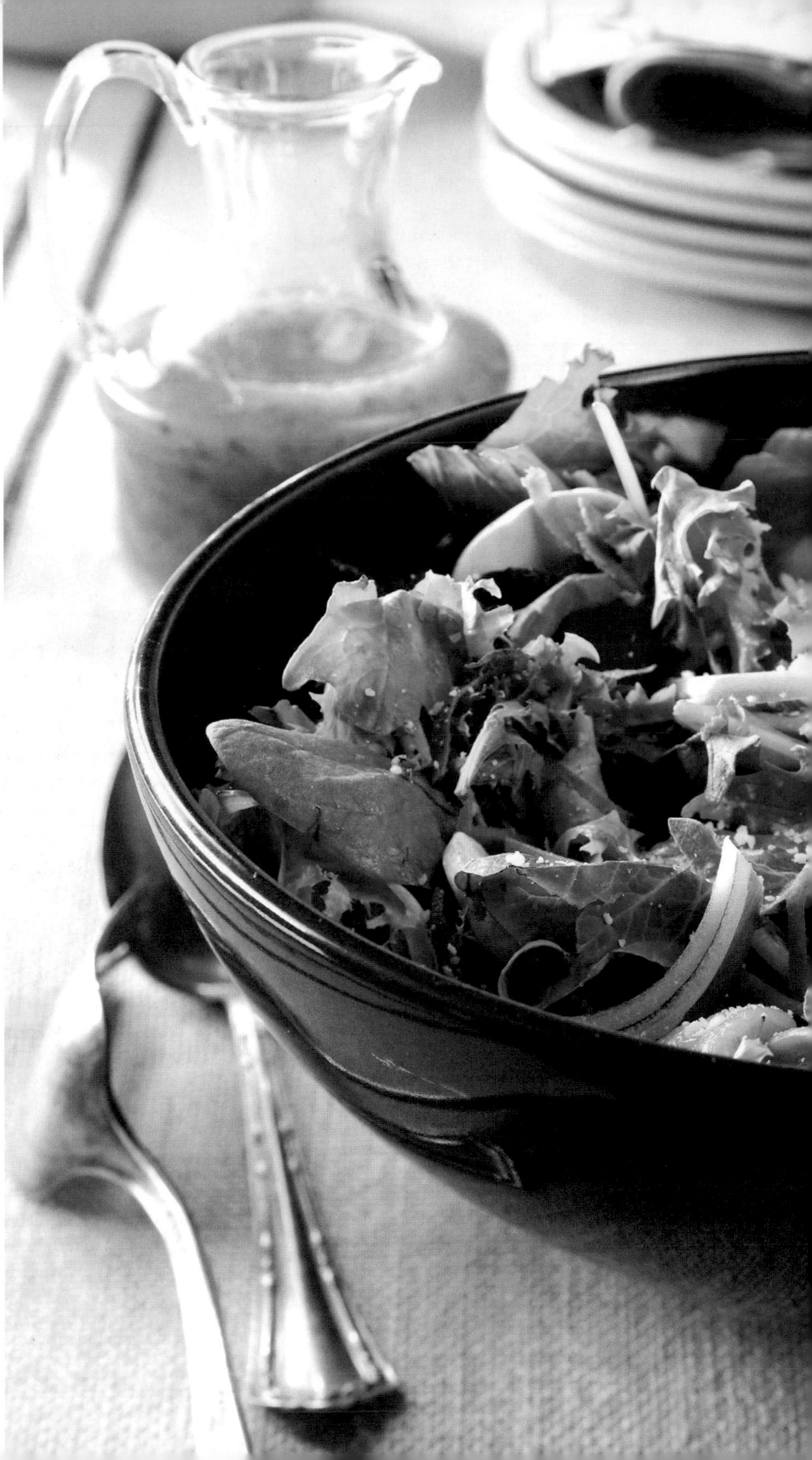

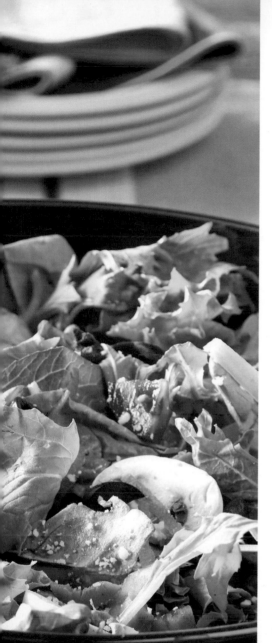

ITALIAN SALAD WITH LEMON VINAIGRETTE

RED, WHITE & BLUE POTATO SALAD

Tossing the cooked potatoes with stock and wine right after you drain them infuses them with flavor. The liquid absorbs like magic.
—GEORGE LEVINTHAL GOLETA, CA

PREP: 40 MIN. • **COOK:** 10 MIN.
MAKES: 12 SERVINGS

- 1¼ pounds small purple potatoes (about 11), quartered
- 1 pound small Yukon Gold potatoes (about 9), quartered
- 1 pound small red potatoes (about 9), quartered
- ½ cup chicken stock
- ¼ cup white wine or additional chicken stock
- 2 tablespoons sherry vinegar
- 2 tablespoons white wine vinegar
- 1½ teaspoons Dijon mustard
- 1½ teaspoons stone-ground mustard
- ¾ teaspoon salt
- ½ teaspoon coarsely ground pepper
- 6 tablespoons olive oil
- 3 celery ribs, chopped
- 1 small sweet red pepper, chopped
- 8 green onions, chopped
- ¾ pound bacon strips, cooked and crumbled
- 3 tablespoons each minced fresh basil, dill and parsley
- 2 tablespoons toasted sesame seeds

1. Place all potatoes in a Dutch oven; add water to cover. Bring to a boil. Reduce heat; cook, uncovered, 10-15 minutes or until tender. Drain; transfer to a large bowl. Drizzle potatoes with stock and wine; toss gently, allowing liquids to absorb.

2. In a small bowl, whisk vinegars, mustards, salt and pepper. Gradually whisk in oil until blended. Add the vinaigrette, vegetables, bacon and herbs to the potato mixture; toss to combine. Sprinkle with sesame seeds. Serve warm.

Per 1 cup: 221 cal., 12g fat (2g sat. fat), 10mg chol., 405mg sod., 22g carb. (2g sugars, 3g fiber), 7g pro.
Diabetic Exchanges: 2 fat, 1½ starch.

FAST FIX ▶
BROCCOLI & APPLE SALAD

Even my picky daughter loves this one! My yogurt dressing on crunchy veggie salad makes a cool and creamy side dish.
—LYNN CLUFF LITTLEFIELD, AZ

START TO FINISH: 15 MIN.
MAKES: 6 SERVINGS

- 3 cups small fresh broccoli florets
- 3 medium apples, chopped
- ½ cup chopped mixed dried fruit
- 1 tablespoon chopped red onion
- ½ cup reduced-fat plain yogurt
- 4 bacon strips, cooked and crumbled

In a large bowl, combine broccoli, apples, dried fruit and onion. Add yogurt; toss to coat. Sprinkle with bacon. Refrigerate until serving.
Per 1 cup: 124 cal., 3g fat (1g sat. fat), 7mg chol., 134mg sod., 22g carb. (17g sugars, 3g fiber), 4g pro.
Diabetic Exchanges: 1½ starch, ½ fat.

FAST FIX
CHILLED SHRIMP PASTA SALAD

This chilled salad is just the thing for a hot summer day. It also makes a nice side dish for sharing anytime.

—MARY PRICE YOUNGSTOWN, OH

START TO FINISH: 30 MIN.
MAKES: 12 SERVINGS

- 3 cups uncooked small pasta shells
- ½ cup sour cream
- ½ cup mayonnaise
- ¼ cup horseradish sauce
- 2 tablespoons grated onion
- 1½ teaspoons seasoned salt
- ¾ teaspoon pepper
- 1 pound peeled and deveined cooked small shrimp
- 1 large cucumber, seeded and chopped
- 3 celery ribs, thinly sliced
  Red lettuce leaves, optional

1. Cook pasta according to package directions. Drain; rinse with cold water.
2. In a large bowl, mix sour cream, mayonnaise, horseradish sauce, onion, seasoned salt and pepper. Stir in the shrimp, cucumber, celery and pasta. Refrigerate until serving. If desired, serve on lettuce.

Per ¾ cup without lettuce: 239 cal., 12g fat (2g sat. fat), 72mg chol., 344mg sod., 20g carb. (3g sugars, 1g fiber), 11g pro.
Diabetic Exchanges: 2 fat, 1 starch, 1 lean meat.

FAST FIX
CHUNKY VEGGIE SLAW

So much for same ol' slaw—this classic coleslaw gets a fresh approach when you add broccoli, cucumbers, snap peas and crunchy walnuts.

—NICHOLAS KING DULUTH, MN

START TO FINISH: 25 MIN.
MAKES: 14 SERVINGS

- 1 small head cabbage, chopped
- 6 cups fresh broccoli florets
- 1 medium cucumber, chopped
- 2 celery ribs, sliced
- 12 fresh sugar snap peas, halved
- 1 small green pepper, chopped
- ¾ cup buttermilk
- ½ cup reduced-fat mayonnaise
- 3 tablespoons cider vinegar
- 2 tablespoons sugar
- ½ teaspoon salt
- 1 cup chopped walnuts, toasted
- 2 green onions, thinly sliced

In a large bowl, combine the first six ingredients. In a small bowl, whisk buttermilk, mayonnaise, vinegar, sugar and salt. Pour over salad; toss to coat. Top with walnuts and green onions. Refrigerate leftovers.
Note: To toast nuts, bake in a shallow pan in a 350° oven for 5-10 minutes or cook in a skillet over low heat until lightly browned, stirring occasionally.

Per 1 cup: 125 cal., 9g fat (1g sat. fat), 4mg chol., 189mg sod., 10g carb. (6g sugars, 3g fiber), 4g pro.
Diabetic Exchanges: 2 vegetable, 1½ fat.

FAST FIX
SPINACH, APPLE & PECAN SALAD

Company was on the way, and I forgot to buy salad fixings. Scavenging the fridge for ingredients, I pulled this together and invented a salad superstar.

—KELLY WALSH AVISTON, IL

START TO FINISH: 15 MIN.
MAKES: 16 SERVINGS

- 2 packages (6 ounces each) fresh baby spinach
- 1 medium apple, chopped
- 1 cup (4 ounces) crumbled feta cheese
- 1 cup glazed pecans
- ½ cup chopped red onion
- ⅓ cup dried cranberries
- 5 bacon strips, cooked and crumbled, optional

DRESSING
- 2 tablespoons cider vinegar
- 1 tablespoon sugar
- ½ teaspoon Dijon mustard
- ⅛ teaspoon pepper
- ¼ cup canola oil

1. In a large bowl, combine the first six ingredients; stir in bacon if desired.
2. For dressing, in a small bowl, whisk vinegar, sugar, mustard and pepper until blended. Gradually whisk in oil. Pour over salad; toss to coat.

Per 1 cup: 109 cal., 8g fat (1g sat. fat), 4mg chol., 116mg sod., 9g carb. (6g sugars, 1g fiber), 2g pro.
Diabetic Exchanges: 1½ fat, 1 vegetable.

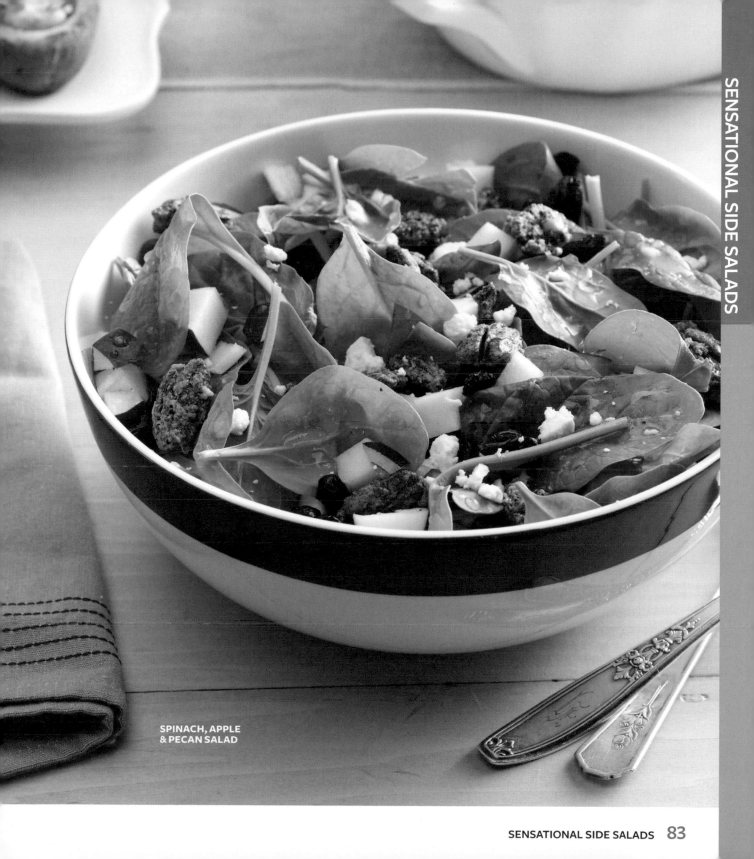

SPINACH, APPLE
& PECAN SALAD

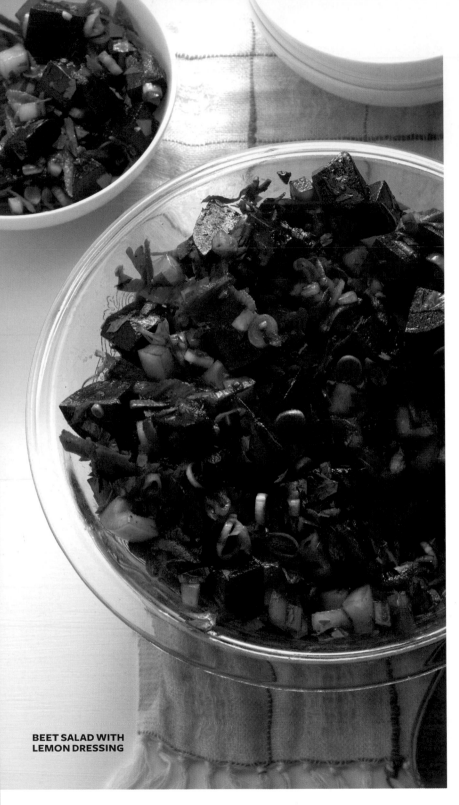

BEET SALAD WITH LEMON DRESSING

BEET SALAD WITH LEMON DRESSING

I was looking for a recipe for pickled beets and saw one with lemon instead of vinegar. I immediately thought of making a tabbouleh-inspired salad with beets instead of tomatoes.

—ANN SHEEHY LAWRENCE, MA

PREP: 10 MIN. • **BAKE:** 1¼ HOURS
MAKES: 6 SERVINGS

- 3 medium fresh beets (about 1 pound)
- 1 cup finely chopped English cucumber
- 6 green onions, thinly sliced
- ½ cup shredded carrot
- ½ cup chopped sweet yellow or red pepper
- ¼ cup finely chopped red onion
- ¼ cup finely chopped radish
- ¾ cup minced fresh parsley

DRESSING

- 3 tablespoons olive oil
- 2 teaspoons grated lemon peel
- 3 tablespoons lemon juice
- 1 garlic clove, minced
- ¼ teaspoon salt
- ¼ teaspoon pepper

1. Preheat oven to 400°. Scrub beets and trim tops. Wrap beets in foil; place on a baking sheet. Bake until tender, 1¼-1½ hours. Cool slightly. Peel beets and cut into cubes.

2. Place remaining vegetables and parsley in a large bowl. Whisk together the dressing ingredients; toss with cucumber mixture. Gently stir in beets.

Per ⅔ cup: 116 cal., 7g fat (1g sat. fat), 0 chol., 173mg sod., 13g carb. (8g sugars, 3g fiber), 2g pro.
Diabetic Exchanges: 1½ fat, 1 vegetable.

VIBRANT BLACK-EYED PEA SALAD

My black-eyed pea salad reminds me of a southern cooking class my husband and I took while visiting Savannah. People go nuts for it at picnics and potlucks.
—DANIELLE ULAM HOOKSTOWN, PA

PREP: 25 MIN. + CHILLING
MAKES: 10 SERVINGS

- 2 cans (15½ ounces each) black-eyed peas, rinsed and drained
- 2 cups grape tomatoes, halved
- 1 each small green, yellow and red peppers, finely chopped
- 1 small red onion, chopped
- 1 celery rib, chopped
- 2 tablespoons minced fresh basil

DRESSING

- ¼ cup red wine vinegar or balsamic vinegar
- 1 tablespoon stone-ground mustard
- 1 teaspoon minced fresh oregano or ¼ teaspoon dried oregano
- ¾ teaspoon salt
- ½ teaspoon freshly ground pepper
- ¼ cup olive oil

1. In a large bowl, combine the peas, grape tomatoes, peppers, onion, celery and basil.

2. For dressing, in a small bowl, whisk vinegar, mustard, oregano, salt and pepper. Gradually whisk in oil until blended. Drizzle over salad; toss to coat. Refrigerate, covered, at least 3 hours before serving.

Per ¾ cup: 130 cal., 6g fat (1g sat. fat), 0 chol., 319mg sod., 15g carb. (3g sugars, 3g fiber), 5g pro.
Diabetic Exchanges: 1 starch, 1 fat.

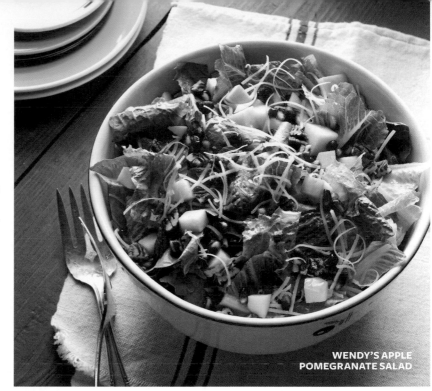

WENDY'S APPLE POMEGRANATE SALAD

FAST FIX ▶

WENDY'S APPLE POMEGRANATE SALAD

My grandparents grew pomegranates, pecans and walnuts and would send us some each year. Some of my best memories are the days I used to spend with my grandmother learning how to cook with her. Whenever I make this it's like having lunch with her again.
—WENDY G. BALL BATTLE CREEK, MI

START TO FINISH: 20 MIN.
MAKES: 8 SERVINGS

- 1 bunch romaine, torn (about 8 cups)
- ½ cup pomegranate seeds
- ½ cup chopped pecans or walnuts, toasted
- ½ cup shredded Parmesan cheese
- 1 large Granny Smith apple, chopped
- 1 tablespoon lemon juice
- ¼ cup olive oil
- ¼ cup white wine vinegar
- 2 tablespoons sugar
- ¼ teaspoon salt

1. In a large bowl, combine romaine, pomegranate seeds, pecans and cheese. Toss apple with lemon juice and add to salad.

2. In a small bowl, whisk remaining ingredients until blended. Drizzle over salad; toss to coat. Serve immediately.
Note: To toast nuts, bake in a shallow pan in a 350° oven for 5-10 minutes or cook in a skillet over low heat until lightly browned, stirring occasionally.

Per 1 cup: 165 cal., 13g fat (2g sat. fat), 4mg chol., 163mg sod., 10g carb. (8g sugars, 2g fiber), 3g pro.
Diabetic Exchanges: 2½ fat, 1 vegetable.

PESTO QUINOA SALAD

My daughter-in-law got me hooked on quinoa, and I'm so glad she did! I've been substituting quinoa in some of my favorite pasta recipes, and this dish is the happy result of one of those delicious experiments.

—SUE GRONHOLZ BEAVER DAM, WI

PREP: 25 MIN. + CHILLING
MAKES: 4 SERVINGS

- ⅔ cup water
- ⅓ cup quinoa, rinsed
- 2 tablespoons prepared pesto
- 1 tablespoon finely chopped sweet onion
- 1 tablespoon olive oil
- 1 teaspoon balsamic vinegar
- ¼ teaspoon salt
- 1 medium sweet red pepper, chopped
- 1 cup cherry tomatoes, quartered
- ⅔ cup fresh mozzarella cheese pearls (about 4 ounces)
- 2 tablespoons minced fresh basil, optional

1. In a small saucepan, bring water to a boil; stir in quinoa. Reduce heat; simmer, covered, until the iquid is absorbed, 10-12 minutes. Cool slightly.
2. Mix pesto, onion, oil, vinegar and salt; stir in pepper, tomatoes, cheese and quinoa. Refrigerate, covered, to allow flavors to blend, 1-2 hours. If desired, stir in basil.

Per ¾ cup: 183 cal., 11g fat (4g sat. fat), 15mg chol., 268mg sod., 14g carb. (3g sugars, 2g fiber), 6g pro.
Diabetic Exchanges: 1 starch, 1 medium-fat meat, ½ fat.

FAST FIX

MIXED GREENS WITH ORANGE-GINGER VINAIGRETTE

Zingy vinaigrette starts with orange juice, ginger and a flick of cayenne. Just whisk, toss with greens and top the salad your way.

—JOY ZACHARIA CLEARWATER, FL

START TO FINISH: 20 MIN.
MAKES: 8 SERVINGS

- ¼ cup orange juice
- ¼ cup canola oil
- 2 tablespoons white vinegar
- 2 tablespoons honey
- 2 teaspoons grated fresh gingerroot
- ½ teaspoon salt
- ¼ teaspoon cayenne pepper

SALAD

- 12 cups torn mixed salad greens
- 2 medium navel oranges, peeled and sliced crosswise
- 1 cup thinly sliced red onion

In a small bowl, whisk the first seven ingredients until blended. In a large bowl, toss the mixed greens with ¼ cup vinaigrette; transfer to a serving dish. Top with oranges and onion. Serve immediately with remaining vinaigrette.
Per 1½ cups: 119 cal., 7g fat (1g sat. fat), 0 chol., 202mg sod., 15g carb. (9g sugars, 3g fiber), 2g pro.
Diabetic Exchanges: 1½ fat, 1 vegetable, ½ starch.

✱

TEST KITCHEN TIP
Many fruit juices and nectars—orange, grapefruit, apple, lemon, pomegranate, mango—can be made into light and flavorful vinaigrettes to dress salad greens.

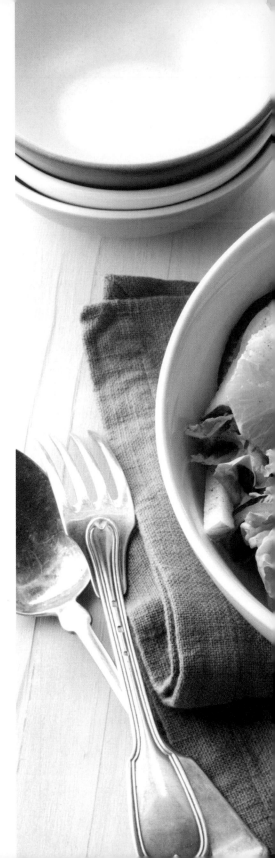

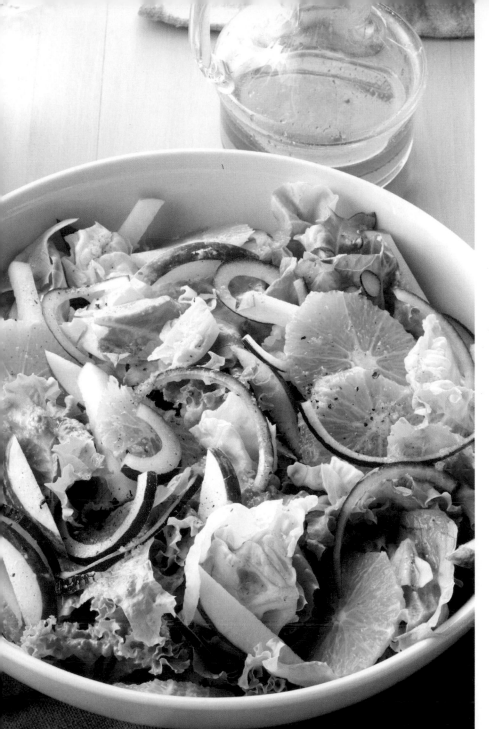

**MIXED GREENS WITH
ORANGE-GINGER VINAIGRETTE**

GARDEN BOUNTY POTATO SALAD

A parent from a school where I previously taught gave me this recipe, and I think of that parent and child every time I make this potato salad. The salad looks beautiful, and the basil vinaigrette keeps it light.

—DEE DEE CALOW WARREN, IL

PREP: 35 MIN. **COOK:** 25 MIN. + CHILLING
MAKES: 20 SERVINGS

   3 pounds small red potatoes, quartered
   1 pound fresh green beans, trimmed and cut in half
   ⅓ cup olive oil
   ¼ cup red wine vinegar
   ¼ cup minced fresh basil
   2 tablespoons minced fresh parsley
   1½ teaspoons salt
   ½ teaspoon pepper
   6 hard-cooked large eggs, sliced
   1 cup grape tomatoes

1. Place potatoes in a large saucepan and cover with water. Bring to a boil. Reduce heat; cover and cook for 10-15 minutes or until tender, adding beans during the last 4 minutes of cooking. Drain. Transfer to a large bowl.
2. In a small bowl, whisk oil, vinegar, basil, parsley, salt and pepper. Pour over potato mixture; toss to coat. Cover and refrigerate for at least 1 hour.
3. Stir before serving; top with eggs and tomatoes.
Per ¾ cup: 113 cal., 5g fat (1g sat. fat), 64mg chol., 202mg sod., 13g carb. (2g sugars, 2g fiber), 4g pro.
Diabetic Exchanges: 1 starch, 1 fat.

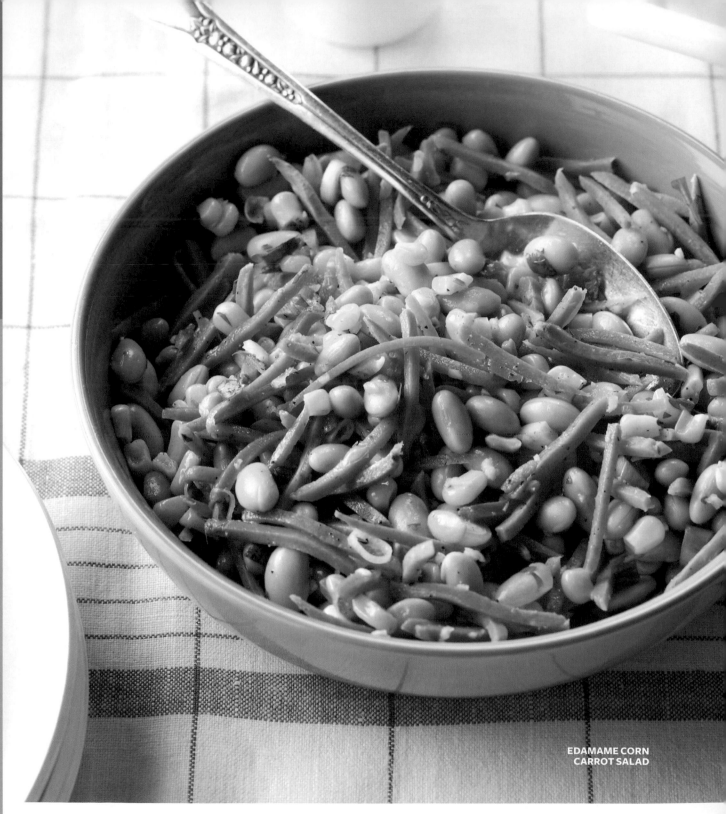

EDAMAME CORN CARROT SALAD

FAST FIX

SPRING GREEK PASTA SALAD

For a light meal, we toss rotini pasta with cucumber, zucchini and sweet peppers. Make it into a main dish by adding some grilled chicken.

—**CHRISTINE SCHENHER** EXETER, CA

START TO FINISH: 30 MIN.
MAKES: 16 SERVINGS

- 4 cups veggie rotini or other spiral pasta (about 12 ounces)

VINAIGRETTE

- ¼ cup olive oil
- 3 tablespoons lemon juice
- 2 tablespoons balsamic vinegar
- 1 tablespoon water
- 3 garlic cloves, minced
- 1 teaspoon salt
- ¼ teaspoon pepper
- 3 tablespoons minced fresh oregano or 1 tablespoon dried oregano

SALAD

- 3 large tomatoes, seeded and chopped
- 1 medium sweet red pepper, chopped
- 1 small cucumber, seeded and chopped
- 1 small zucchini, chopped
- 1 small red onion, halved and thinly sliced
- ⅓ cup sliced pitted Greek olives, optional
- 1 cup (4 ounces) crumbled feta cheese

1. Cook pasta according to package directions. Drain; rinse with cold water and drain well.

2. In a small bowl, whisk oil, lemon juice, vinegar, water, garlic, salt and pepper until blended. Stir in oregano.

3. In a large bowl, combine pasta, vegetables and, if desired, olives. Add vinaigrette and cheese; toss to combine. Refrigerate, covered, until ready to serve.

Per ¾ cup without olives: 142 cal., 5g fat (1g sat. fat), 4mg chol., 219mg sod., 20g carb. (3g sugars, 2g fiber), 5g pro.
Diabetic Exchanges: 1 starch, 1 fat.

EDAMAME CORN CARROT SALAD

I created my salad recipe by trying to think of a protein-filled, nutritious and light dish. It was easy and appealing.

—**MAIAH MILLER** MONTEREY, CA

PREP: 25 MIN + CHILLING
MAKES: 8 SERVINGS

- 2½ cups frozen shelled edamame
- 3 cups julienned carrots
- 1½ cups frozen corn, thawed
- 4 green onions, chopped
- 2 tablespoons minced fresh cilantro

VINAIGRETTE

- 3 tablespoons rice vinegar
- 3 tablespoons lemon juice
- 4 teaspoons canola oil
- 2 garlic cloves, minced
- ½ teaspoon salt
- ½ teaspoon pepper

1. Place edamame in a small saucepan; add water to cover. Bring to a boil; cook 4-5 minutes or until tender. Drain and place in a large bowl; cool slightly.

2. Add carrots, corn, green onions and cilantro. Whisk together vinaigrette ingredients; toss with salad. Refrigerate, covered, at least 2 hours before serving.

Per ⅔ cup: 111 cal., 5g fat (0 sat. fat), 0 chol., 135mg sod., 14g carb. (4g sugars, 3g fiber), 5g pro.
Diabetic Exchanges: 1 starch, ½ fat.

FAST FIX

BASIL & HEIRLOOM TOMATO TOSS

I came up with this garden-fresh salad to showcase the heirloom tomatoes and peppers we raised for our stall at the farmers market. Try out other types of basil, such as lemon, lime, licorice and even cinnamon.

—**SUE GRONHOLZ** BEAVER DAM, WI

START TO FINISH: 15 MIN.
MAKES: 4 SERVINGS

- ¼ cup olive oil
- 3 tablespoons red wine vinegar
- 2 teaspoons sugar
- 1 garlic clove, minced
- ¾ teaspoon salt
- ¼ teaspoon ground mustard
- ¼ teaspoon pepper
- 2 large heirloom tomatoes, cut into ½-inch pieces
- 1 medium sweet yellow pepper, cut into ½-inch pieces
- ½ small red onion, thinly sliced
- 1 tablespoon chopped fresh basil

In a large bowl, whisk the first seven ingredients until blended. Add the remaining ingredients; toss gently to combine.

Per 1 cup: 162 cal., 14g fat (2g sat. fat), 0 chol., 449mg sod., 10g carb. (5g sugars, 2g fiber), 1g pro.
Diabetic Exchanges: 3 fat, 1 vegetable.

✱

DID YOU KNOW?
Heirloom tomatoes are generally considered to be any variety that has been passed down for several generations for its unique qualities. From large green zebra-striped fruits to small cherries almost black in color, try a new one in your next salad.

FAST FIX ▶

RIBBON SALAD WITH ORANGE VINAIGRETTE

Zucchini, cucumbers and carrots are peeled into ribbons for this citrusy salad. We like to serve it for parties and special occasions throughout the year.

—**NANCY HEISHMAN** LAS VEGAS, NV

START TO FINISH: 30 MIN.
MAKES: 8 SERVINGS

- 1   medium zucchini
- 1   medium cucumber
- 1   medium carrot
- 3   medium oranges
- 3   cups fresh baby spinach
- 4   green onions, finely chopped
- ½   cup chopped walnuts
- ½   teaspoon salt
- ½   teaspoon pepper
- ½   cup golden raisins, optional

VINAIGRETTE

- ¼   cup olive oil
- 4   teaspoons white wine vinegar
- 1   tablespoon finely chopped green onion
- 2   teaspoons honey
- ¼   teaspoon salt
- ¼   teaspoon pepper

1. Using a vegetable peeler, shave the zucchini, cucumber and carrot lengthwise into very thin strips.

2. Finely grate enough peel from oranges to measure 2 tablespoons. Cut one orange crosswise in half; squeeze juice from orange to measure ½ cup. Reserve peel and juice for vinaigrette. Cut a thin slice from both the top and bottom of remaining oranges; stand oranges upright on a cutting board. With a knife, cut off peel and outer membrane from orange. Cut along the membrane of each segment to remove the fruit.

3. In a large bowl, combine spinach, orange sections, green onions, walnuts, salt, pepper and, if desired, raisins. Add vegetable ribbons; gently toss to combine. In a small bowl, combine vinaigrette ingredients. Add reserved orange peel and juice; whisk until blended. Drizzle half of the vinaigrette over salad; toss to coat. Serve with remaining vinaigrette.

Per 1½ cups: 162 cal., 12g fat (1g sat. fat), 0 chol., 240mg sod., 14g carb. (9g sugars, 2g fiber), 3g pro.
Diabetic Exchanges: 2 fat, 1 vegetable, ½ starch.

⑤INGREDIENTS

DILL-MARINATED BROCCOLI

A co-worker tipped me off to this splashy marinade for broccoli. The longer you wait, the better it gets.

—**TIFFONY BUSH** HUNTINGDON, PA

PREP: 15 MIN.+ MARINATING
MAKES: 8 SERVINGS

- 6   cups fresh broccoli florets
- 1   cup canola oil
- 1   cup cider vinegar
- 2   tablespoons snipped fresh dill
- 2   teaspoons sugar
- 1   teaspoon garlic salt
- 1   teaspoon salt

1. Place broccoli in a large resealable plastic bag. Whisk together remaining ingredients; add to broccoli. Seal bag and turn to coat; refrigerate 4 hours or overnight. To serve, drain broccoli, discarding marinade.

Per serving: 79 cal., 7g fat (1g sat. fat), 0 chol., 119mg sod., 3g carb. (0 sugars, 2g fiber), 2g pro.
Diabetic Exchanges: 1½ fat, 1 vegetable.

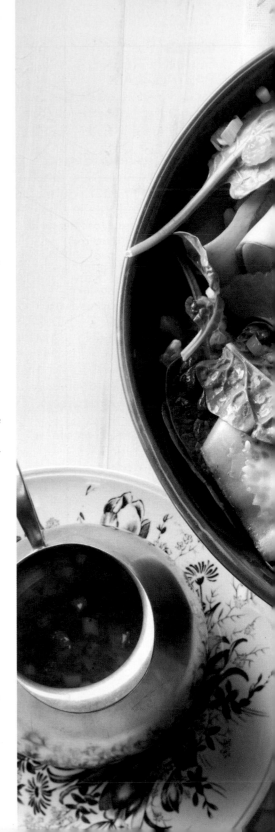

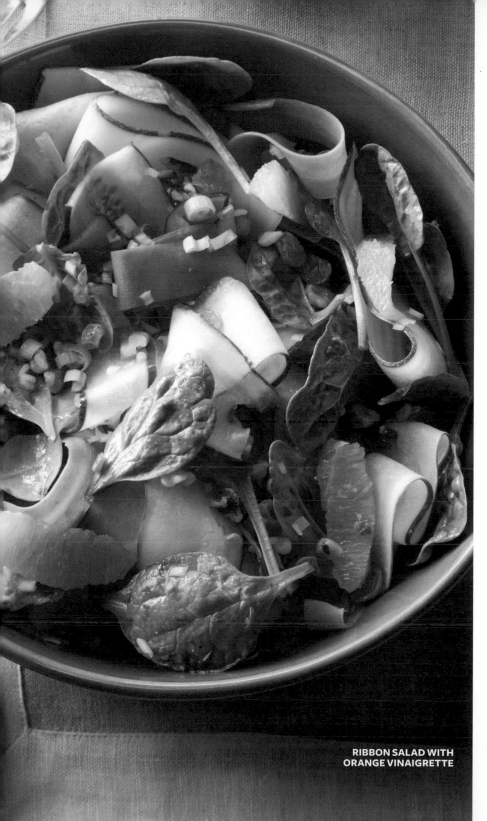

RIBBON SALAD WITH ORANGE VINAIGRETTE

SUMMER MACARONI SALAD

When we grill out, my mother asks me to make the family macaroni salad. To make it extra-creamy, I like to keep a small amount of dressing separate and stir it in just before serving.

—**CARLY CURTIN** ELLICOTT CITY, MD

PREP: 20 MIN. + CHILLING • **COOK:** 15 MIN.
MAKES: 16 SERVINGS

- 1 package (16 ounces) elbow macaroni
- 1 cup reduced-fat mayonnaise
- 3 to 4 tablespoons water or 2% milk
- 2 tablespoons red wine vinegar
- 1 tablespoon sugar
- 1½ teaspoons salt
- ¼ teaspoon garlic powder
- ¼ teaspoon pepper
- 1 small sweet yellow, orange or red pepper, finely chopped
- 1 small green pepper, finely chopped
- 1 small onion, finely chopped
- 1 celery rib, finely chopped
- 2 tablespoons minced fresh parsley

1. Cook macaroni according to package directions. Drain; rinse with cold water and drain again.
2. In a small bowl, mix mayonnaise, water, vinegar, sugar and seasonings until blended. In a large bowl, combine macaroni, peppers, onion and celery. Add 1 cup dressing; toss gently to coat. Refrigerate, covered, 2 hours or until cold. Cover and refrigerate remaining dressing to add just before serving.
3. To serve, stir in reserved dressing. Sprinkle with parsley.
Per ¾ cup: 160 cal., 6g fat (1g sat. fat), 5mg chol., 320mg sod., 24g carb. (3g sugars, 1g fiber), 4g pro.
Diabetic Exchanges: 1½ starch, 1 fat.

SPECIAL OCCASION BEEF
BOURGUIGNON, PAGE 113

Beef Entrees

· ·

Beef lovers rejoice! These recipes—sometimes hearty,
sometimes light—will win over the whole family and
leave you feeling satisfied. Beef is chockful of protein,
iron and B vitamins, and can certainly be part
of a healthy diet.

SPINACH & FETA BURGERS

Turkey burgers have their fans, but we prefer burgers of ground beef, spinach and feta. We serve them on toasted buns with lettuce, tomato and tzatziki.

—SUSAN STETZEL GAINESVILLE, NY

PREP: 25 MIN. • **GRILL:** 15 MIN.
MAKES: 8 SERVINGS

- 1 tablespoon olive oil
- 2 shallots, chopped
- 2½ cups fresh baby spinach, coarsely chopped
- 3 garlic cloves, minced
- ⅔ cup crumbled feta cheese
- ¾ teaspoon Greek seasoning
- ½ teaspoon salt
- ¼ teaspoon pepper
- 2 pounds lean ground beef (90% lean)
- 8 whole wheat hamburger buns, split
  Optional toppings: refrigerated tzatziki sauce, fresh baby spinach and tomato slices

1. In a large skillet, heat the oil over medium-high heat. Add shallots; cook and stir 1-2 minutes or until tender. Add spinach and garlic; cook 30-45 seconds longer or until the spinach is wilted. Transfer to a large bowl; cool slightly.
2. Stir feta cheese and seasonings into spinach mixture. Add beef; mix lightly but thoroughly. Shape the mixture into eight ½-in.-thick patties.
3. Grill burgers, covered, over medium heat 6-8 minutes on each side or until a thermometer reads 160°. Grill buns over medium heat, cut side down, for 30-60 seconds or until toasted. Serve burgers on buns with the toppings if desired.

To freeze: Place patties on a plastic wrap-lined baking sheet; wrap and freeze until firm. Remove from pan and transfer to a resealable plastic freezer bag; return to freezer. To use, cook frozen patties as directed, increasing time as necessary for a thermometer to read 160°.

Per 1 burger without toppings: 343 cal., 15g fat (5g sat. fat), 76mg chol., 636mg sod., 25g carb. (4g sugars, 4g fiber), 28g pro.
Diabetic Exchanges: 3 lean meat, 2 fat, 1½ starch.

ASPARAGUS BEEF STIR-FRY ON POTATOES

I created my light and quick version of a steak dinner when I had leftover grilled steak and asparagus.

—FRANCES PIETSCH FLOWER MOUND, TX

PREP: 25 MIN. • **COOK:** 15 MIN.
MAKES: 4 SERVINGS

- 2 large baking potatoes (about 12 ounces each)
- 2 tablespoons butter
- ¼ cup reduced-sodium soy sauce
- 2 teaspoons balsamic vinegar
- 2 teaspoons canola oil, divided
- 1 pound beef top sirloin steak, cut into thin strips
- 1½ cups cut fresh asparagus (1 inch)
- 1½ cups sliced fresh mushrooms
- ¼ teaspoon salt
- ⅛ teaspoon pepper

1. Scrub potatoes; pierce several times with a fork. Place on a microwave-safe plate. Microwave, uncovered, on high until tender, 12-16 minutes, turning once. Cool slightly.
2. In a small saucepan, melt butter over medium heat. Heat until the butter is golden brown, 3-4 minutes, stirring constantly. Remove from heat; stir in soy sauce and vinegar. Keep warm.
3. In a large skillet, heat 1 teaspoon oil over medium-high heat; stir-fry beef until browned, 2-3 minutes. Remove from pan.
4. In same pan, stir-fry asparagus and mushrooms in remaining oil until the asparagus is crisp-tender, 2-3 minutes. Stir in beef, salt and pepper; heat the mixture through.
5. Cut potatoes lengthwise in half; fluff pulp with a fork. Top with beef mixture; drizzle with sauce.

Note: This recipe was tested in a 1,100-watt microwave.

Per ½ baked potato with 1 cup beef mixture and 1 tablespoon sauce: 387 cal., 13g fat (6g sat. fat), 61mg chol., 832mg sod., 37g carb. (4g sugars, 5g fiber), 31g pro.
Diabetic Exchanges: 4 lean meat, 2 starch, 1½ fat.

✳

DID YOU KNOW?
When preparing a stir-fry, cut the veggies and meats a uniform size to help them cook more evenly. Bite-size pieces work best. Also, always start with hot oil so the ingredients saute instead of steam.

**SPINACH & FETA
BURGERS**

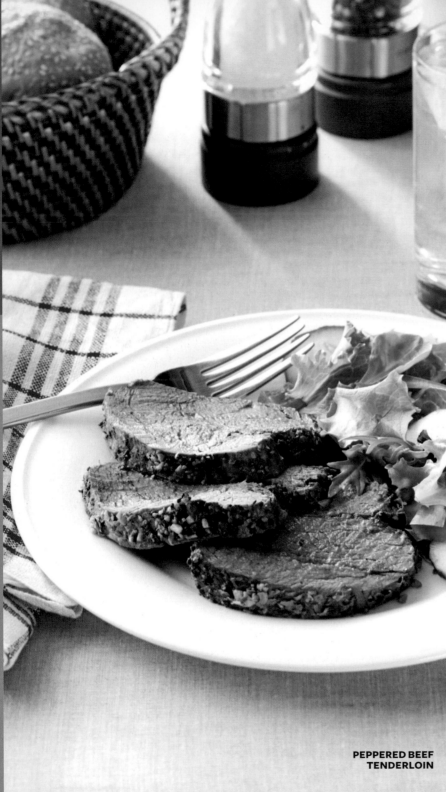

PEPPERED BEEF
TENDERLOIN

(5)INGREDIENTS

PEPPERED BEEF TENDERLOIN

A pepper rub gives beef tenderloin rich, bold flavor. It takes just minutes to prepare, and lining the pan with foil makes cleanup a breeze, too.

—DENISE BITNER REEDSVILLE, PA

PREP: 10 MIN.
BAKE: 40 MIN. + STANDING
MAKES: 12 SERVINGS

- 3 tablespoons coarsely ground pepper
- 2 tablespoons olive oil
- 1 tablespoon grated lemon peel
- 2 garlic cloves, minced
- 1 teaspoon salt
- 1 beef tenderloin roast (3 to 4 pounds)

1. Preheat oven to 400°. Mix the first five ingredients.

2. Place roast on a rack in a roasting pan; rub with pepper mixture. Roast until desired doneness (for medium-rare, a thermometer should read 145°; medium, 160°; well-done, 170°), 40-60 minutes. Remove roast from oven; tent with foil. Let roast stand 15 minutes before slicing.

Per 3 ounces cooked beef: 188 cal., 9g fat (3g sat. fat), 49mg chol., 197mg sod., 1g carb. (0 sugars, 1g fiber), 24g pro.
Diabetic Exchanges: 3 lean meat, ½ fat.

✳

DID YOU KNOW?
Beef tenderloin is a lean cut of beef and a good source of protein. Eating protein increases the feeling of being satisfied and may help curb cravings for carbs and fats.

FAST FIX ▶
MOM'S SPANISH RICE

My mom is famous for her Spanish rice. When I want a taste of home, I pull out this recipe and prepare it for my family.

—JOAN HALLFORD
NORTH RICHLAND HILLS, TX

START TO FINISH: 20 MIN.
MAKES: 4 SERVINGS

- 1 **pound lean ground beef (90% lean)**
- 1 **large onion, chopped**
- 1 **medium green pepper, chopped**
- 1 **can (15 ounces) tomato sauce**
- 1 **can (14½ ounces) no-salt-added diced tomatoes, drained**
- 1 **teaspoon ground cumin**
- 1 **teaspoon chili powder**
- ½ **teaspoon garlic powder**
- ¼ **teaspoon salt**
- 2⅔ **cups cooked brown rice**

1. In a large skillet, cook beef, onion and pepper over medium heat 6-8 minutes or until beef is no longer pink and onion is tender, breaking up the beef into crumbles; drain.
2. Stir in tomato sauce, tomatoes and seasonings; bring to a boil. Add rice; heat through, stirring occasionally.
Per 1½ cups: 395 cal., 11g fat (4g sat. fat), 71mg chol., 757mg sod., 46g carb. (8g sugars, 6g fiber), 29g pro.
Diabetic Exchanges: 3 lean meat, 2 starch, 2 vegetable.

SASSY SALSA MEAT LOAVES

Here's a twist on classic meat loaf that can be made ahead to last for a few days afterward. Leftovers reheat easily in the microwave. I top loaves with Monterey Jack cheese for tasty sandwiches.

—TASHA TULLY OWINGS MILLS, MD

PREP: 25 MIN.
BAKE: 1 HOUR 5 MIN. + STANDING
MAKES: 2 LOAVES (6 SERVINGS EACH)

- ¾ **cup uncooked instant brown rice**
- 1 **can (8 ounces) tomato sauce**
- 1½ **cups salsa, divided**
- 1 **large onion, chopped**
- 1 **large egg, lightly beaten**
- 1 **celery rib, finely chopped**
- ¼ **cup minced fresh parsley**
- 2 **tablespoons minced fresh cilantro**
- 2 **garlic cloves, minced**
- 1 **tablespoon chili powder**
- 1½ **teaspoons salt**
- ½ **teaspoon pepper**
- 2 **pounds lean ground beef (90% lean)**
- 1 **pound ground turkey**
- ½ **cup shredded reduced-fat Monterey Jack cheese or Mexican cheese blend**

1. Preheat oven to 350°. Cook rice according to package directions; cool slightly. In a large bowl, combine tomato sauce, ½ cup salsa, onion, egg, celery, parsley, cilantro, garlic and seasonings; stir in rice. Add beef and turkey; mix lightly but thoroughly.
2. Shape into two 8x4-in. loaves on a greased rack in a broiler pan. Bake 1 to 1¼ hours or until a meat thermometer reads 165°.
3. Spread with remaining salsa; sprinkle with cheese; bake 5 minutes or until cheese is melted. Let stand 10 minutes before slicing.
To freeze: Bake meat loaves without topping. Cool; securely wrap in plastic wrap, then foil. To use, partially thaw in refrigerator overnight. Unwrap meat loaves; place in a greased 15x10x1-in. baking pan. Reheat in a preheated 350° oven for 40-45 minutes or until a thermometer inserted in center reads 165°; top and bake as directed.
Per slice: 237 cal., 11g fat (4g sat. fat), 91mg chol., 634mg sod., 9g carb. (2g sugars, 1g fiber), 25g pro.
Diabetic Exchanges: 3 lean meat, ½ starch, ½ fat.

★ ★ ★ ★ ★ **READER REVIEW**

"I made this delicious and super-fast rice recipe to serve to company. I used tri-color bell peppers and added a touch of crushed red pepper."

ANNRMS TASTEOFHOME.COM

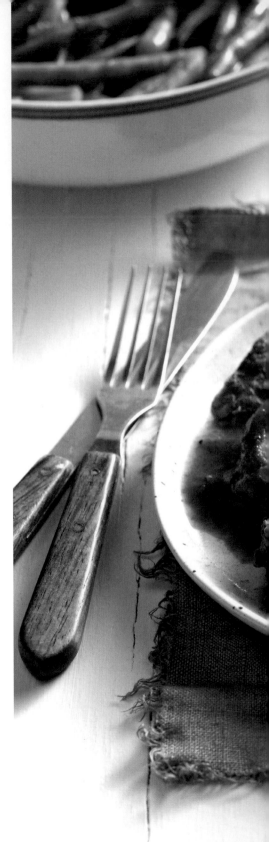

(5)INGREDIENTS
ITALIAN CRUMB-CRUSTED BEEF ROAST

Panko crumbs and seasoning give this roast a special touch. It's a wonderful, effortless weeknight meal, so you can put your energy into relaxing.

—**MARIA REGAKIS** SAUGUS, MA

PREP: 10 MIN.
BAKE: 1¾ HOURS + STANDING
MAKES: 8 SERVINGS

- 1 beef sirloin tip roast (3 pounds)
- ¼ teaspoon salt
- ¾ cup Italian-style panko (Japanese) bread crumbs
- ¼ cup mayonnaise
- 3 tablespoons dried minced onion
- ½ teaspoon Italian seasoning
- ¼ teaspoon pepper

1. Preheat oven to 325°. Place roast on a rack in a shallow roasting pan; sprinkle with salt. In a small bowl, mix remaining ingredients; press onto top and sides of roast.
2. Roast 1¾-2¼ hours or until meat reaches desired doneness (for medium-rare, a thermometer should read 145°; medium, 160°; well-done, 170°). Remove roast from oven; tent with foil. Let roast stand 10 minutes before slicing.
Per 5 ounces cooked beef: 319 cal., 15g fat (3g sat. fat), 111mg chol., 311mg sod., 7g carb. (0 sugars, 0 fiber), 35g pro.
Diabetic Exchanges: 5 lean meat, 1 fat, ½ starch.

EASY MARINATED FLANK STEAK

I got this recipe from a friend 15 years ago. Even now, when my family makes steak on the grill, this is the recipe we use. It's a must when we're inviting company for dinner.

—**DEBBIE BONCZEK** TARIFFVILLE, CT

PREP: 10 MIN. + MARINATING
GRILL: 15 MIN. • **MAKES:** 8 SERVINGS

- 3 tablespoons ketchup
- 1 tablespoon chopped onion
- 1 tablespoon canola oil
- 1 teaspoon brown sugar
- 1 teaspoon Worcestershire sauce
- 1 garlic clove, minced
- ⅛ teaspoon pepper
- 1 beef flank steak (about 2 pounds)

1. In a large resealable plastic bag, combine the first seven ingredients. Add beef; seal bag and turn to coat. Refrigerate 8 hours or overnight.
2. Drain beef, discarding marinade. Lightly coat grill rack with cooking oil.
3. Grill beef, covered, over medium heat or broil 4 in. from heat 6-8 minutes on each side or until meat reaches desired doneness (for medium-rare, a thermometer should read 145°; medium, 160°; well-done, 170°). To serve, thinly slice across the grain.
To freeze: Freeze beef with marinade in a resealable plastic freezer bag. To use, thaw in refrigerator overnight. Drain beef, discarding marinade. Grill as directed above.
Per 3 ounces cooked beef: 192 cal., 10g fat (4g sat. fat), 54mg chol., 145mg sod., 2g carb. (2g sugars, 0 fiber), 22g pro.
Diabetic Exchanges: 3 lean meat.

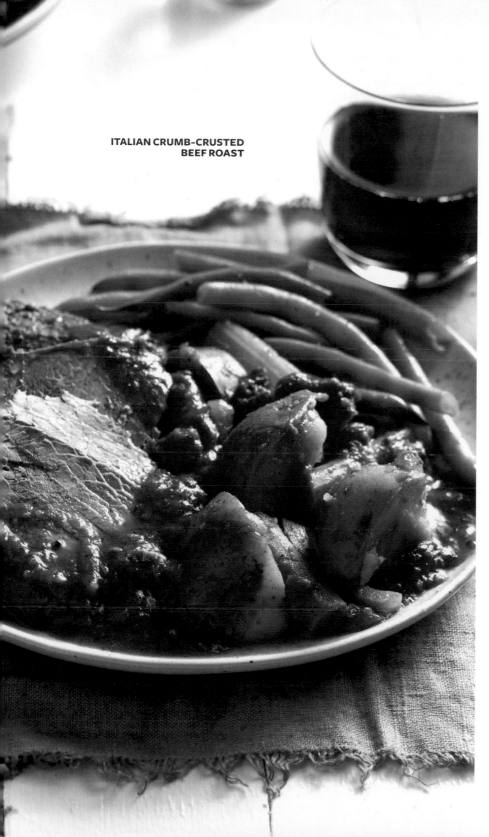

**ITALIAN CRUMB-CRUSTED
BEEF ROAST**

FAST FIX ▶

GREEK-STYLE RAVIOLI

I gave an Italian dish a Greek twist with spinach, olives and feta. Serve this easy weeknight ravioli dinner with garlic cheese toast.

—HETTI WILLIAMS RAPID CITY, SD

START TO FINISH: 25 MIN.
MAKES: 2 SERVINGS

- 12 frozen cheese ravioli
- ⅓ pound lean ground beef (90% lean)
- 1 cup canned diced tomatoes with basil, oregano and garlic
- 1 cup fresh baby spinach
- ¼ cup sliced ripe olives
- ¼ cup crumbled feta cheese

1. Cook ravioli according to package directions; drain. Meanwhile, in a skillet, cook beef over medium heat for 4-6 minutes or until no longer pink; drain. Stir in tomatoes; bring to a boil. Reduce heat; simmer, uncovered, 10 minutes, stirring occasionally.
2. Add ravioli, spinach and olives; heat through, stirring gently to combine. Sprinkle with cheese.
Per serving: 333 cal., 12g fat (5g sat. fat), 61mg chol., 851mg sod., 28g carb. (5g sugars, 4g fiber), 23g pro.
Diabetic Exchanges: 3 lean meat, starch, ½ fat.

★ ★ ★ ★ ★ **READER REVIEW**

"My husband is very picky, and he loves this recipe, so we make it once a month."

CHRISTAKS TASTEOFHOME.COM

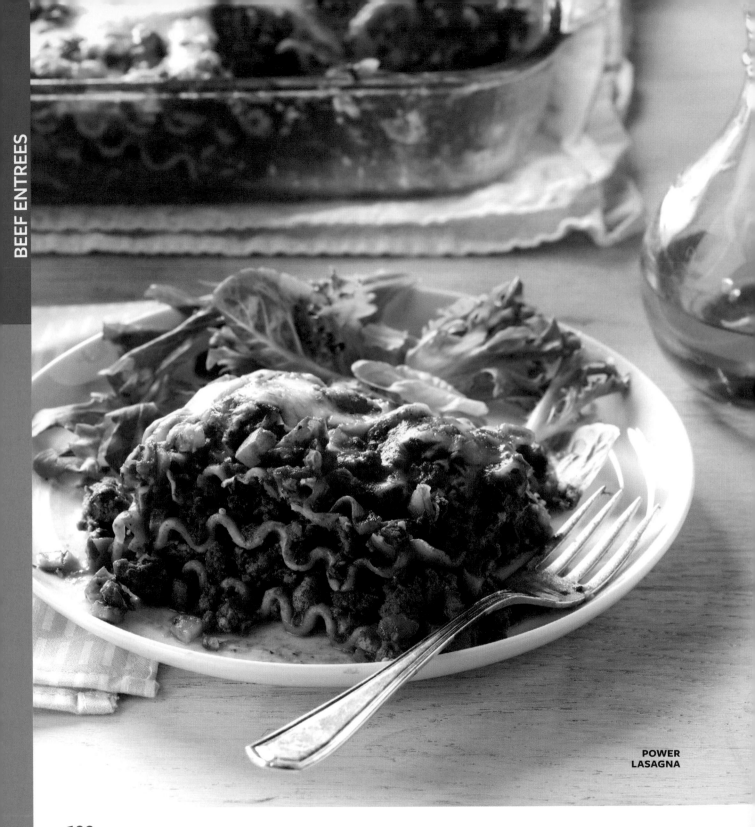

POWER
LASAGNA

POWER LASAGNA

When my husband and I wanted to live healthier, our first step was to eat more power foods, such as whole grains, fresh veggies and protein. This tasty lasagna is the result of using more nutritious ingredients in the Italian food we love.

—JENNIFER YADEN RICHMOND, KY

PREP: 30 MIN.
BAKE: 40 MIN. + STANDING
MAKES: 8 SERVINGS

- 9 whole wheat lasagna noodles
- 1 pound lean ground beef (90% lean)
- 1 medium zucchini, finely chopped
- 1 medium onion, finely chopped
- 1 medium green pepper, finely chopped
- 3 garlic cloves, minced
- 1 jar (24 ounces) meatless pasta sauce
- 1 can (14½ ounces) no-salt-added diced tomatoes, drained
- ½ cup loosely packed basil leaves, chopped
- 2 tablespoons ground flaxseed
- 5 teaspoons Italian seasoning
- ¼ teaspoon pepper
- 1 carton (15 ounces) fat-free ricotta cheese
- 1 package (10 ounces) frozen chopped spinach, thawed and squeezed dry
- 1 large egg, lightly beaten
- 2 tablespoons white balsamic vinegar
- 2 cups (8 ounces) shredded part-skim mozzarella cheese
- ¼ cup grated Parmesan cheese

1. Preheat oven to 350°. Cook noodles according to the package directions. Meanwhile, in a 6-qt. stockpot, cook beef, zucchini, onion and green pepper over medium heat until beef is no longer pink, breaking up beef into crumbles. Add garlic; cook 1 minute longer. Drain.

2. Stir in pasta sauce, diced tomatoes, basil, flax, Italian seasoning and pepper; heat though. Drain noodles and rinse in cold water.

3. In a small bowl, mix ricotta cheese, spinach, egg and vinegar. Spread 1 cup meat mixture into a 13x9-in. baking dish coated with cooking spray. Layer with three noodles, 2 cups meat mixture, 1¼ cups ricotta cheese mixture and ⅔ cup mozzarella cheese. Repeat layers. Top with the remaining noodles, meat mixture and the mozzarella cheese; sprinkle with Parmesan cheese.

4. Bake, covered, 30 minutes. Bake, uncovered, 10-15 minutes longer or until cheese is melted. Let the lasagna stand 10 minutes before serving.

Per piece: 392 cal., 12g fat (5g sat. fat), 89mg chol., 691mg sod., 39g carb. (13g sugars, 8g fiber), 32g pro.
Diabetic Exchanges: 3 lean meat, 2 starch, 1 vegetable, 1 fat.

FAST FIX
BBQ YUMBURGERS

We can't resist these barbecued delights. I freeze patties ahead of time so I'm ready whenever a craving hits.

—DONNA HOYE WHITMORE LAKE, MI

START TO FINISH: 30 MIN.
MAKES: 4 SERVINGS

- 2 teaspoons canola oil
- 1 large onion, halved and sliced
- 1 pound lean ground beef (90% lean)
- 2 tablespoons finely chopped onion
- 2 tablespoons barbecue sauce
- 2 garlic cloves, minced
- 1 teaspoon onion powder
- ½ teaspoon salt
- ¼ teaspoon pepper
- 4 whole wheat hamburger buns, split
  Optional toppings: tomato slices, lettuce leaves and additional barbecue sauce

1. In a skillet, heat oil over medium-high heat. Add the sliced onion; cook and stir 4-6 minutes or until tender.

2. In a large bowl, combine the beef, chopped onion, barbecue sauce, garlic, onion powder, salt and pepper, mixing lightly but thoroughly. Shape into four ½-in.-thick patties.

3. Grill burgers, covered, over medium heat or broil 4 in. from heat 4-6 minutes on each side or until a thermometer reads 160°. Serve on buns with the cooked onions and, if desired, optional toppings and sauce.

To freeze: Do not cook onion slices. Place patties on a plastic wrap-lined baking sheet; wrap and freeze until firm. Remove from pan and transfer to a resealable plastic freezer bag; return to freezer. To use, prepare sliced onions. Grill the frozen patties as directed, increasing time as necessary for a thermometer to read 160°. Serve on buns with onions and desired toppings.

Per burger without toppings: 341 cal., 14g fat (4g sat. fat), 71mg chol., 634mg sod., 28g carb. (7g sugars, 4g fiber), 26g pro.
Diabetic Exchanges: 3 lean meat, 2 starch, ½ fat.

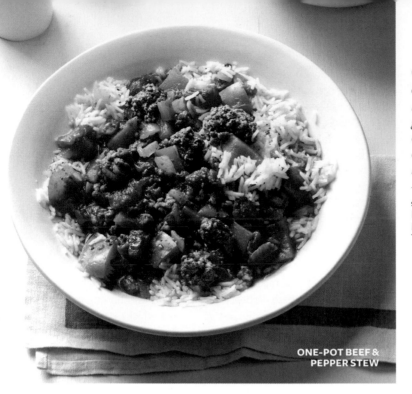

ONE-POT BEEF &
PEPPER STEW

ONE-POT BEEF & PEPPER STEW

I love most things that are made with green peppers, tomatoes or green chilies. Wanting a quick and satisfying dish one evening, I came up with this recipe using what I had on hand.
—**SANDRA CLARK** SIERRA VISTA, AZ

PREP: 10 MIN. • **COOK:** 30 MIN.
MAKES: 8 SERVINGS

- 1 **pound lean ground beef (90% lean)**
- 3 **cans (14½ ounces each) diced tomatoes, undrained**
- 4 **large green peppers, coarsely chopped**
- 1 **large onion, chopped**
- 2 **cans (4 ounces each) chopped green chilies**
- 3 **teaspoons garlic powder**
- 1 **teaspoon pepper**
- ¼ **teaspoon salt**
- 2 **cups uncooked instant rice**
  Hot pepper sauce, optional

1. In a 6-qt. stockpot, cook beef over medium heat 6-8 minutes or until no longer pink, breaking into crumbles; drain. Add tomatoes, green peppers, onion, chilies and seasonings; bring to a boil. Reduce heat; simmer, covered, for 20-25 minutes or until vegetables are tender.
2. Prepare rice according to package directions. Serve with the stew and, if desired, pepper sauce.
Per 1½ cups: 244 cal., 5g fat (2g sat. fat), 35mg chol., 467mg sod., 35g carb. (8g sugars, 5g fiber), 15g pro.
Diabetic Exchanges: 2 lean meat, 2 vegetable, 1½ starch.

PHILLY CHEESESTEAK ROLLS

My light take on cheesesteak skips the bread and gets straight to the tender meat, creamy cheese and sweet-and-tangy veggies.
—**PAIGE DAY** NORTH AUGUSTA, SC

PREP: 30 MIN. • **BAKE:** 15 MIN.
MAKES: 4 SERVINGS

- ½ **pound sliced fresh mushrooms**
- 1 **medium onion, halved and sliced**
- 1 **small green pepper, cut into thin strips**
- 1 **beef top round steak (1 pound)**
- 4 **wedges The Laughing Cow light Swiss cheese**
- ¼ **teaspoon pepper**
- 3 **cups hot mashed potatoes (made with fat-free milk)**

1. Preheat oven to 450°. Place a large nonstick skillet coated with cooking spray over medium-high heat. Add mushrooms, onion and green pepper; cook and stir until tender, 8-10 minutes. Remove from pan; cool slightly.
2. Cut steak into four pieces; pound with a meat mallet to ¼-in. thickness. Spread wedges with cheese. Sprinkle with pepper; top with the mushroom mixture. Roll up from a short side; secure with toothpicks. Place rolls in a foil-lined 15x10x1-in. baking pan.
3. Bake until meat reaches desired doneness (for medium-rare, a thermometer should read 145°; medium, 160°), for 12-17 minutes. Let stand 5 minutes before serving. Serve with mashed potatoes.
Per 1 roll with ¾ cup mashed potatoes: 364 cal., 10g fat (3g sat. fat), 68mg chol., 822mg sod., 34g carb. (5g sugars, 4g fiber), 33g pro.
Diabetic Exchanges: 4 lean meat, 2 starch, 1 vegetable.

(5) INGREDIENTS **FAST FIX**

CHILI-RUBBED STEAK WITH BLACK BEAN SALAD

Busy weeknights don't stop my husband from firing up the grill. This meal in one comes together fast. Add chimichurri sauce and cotija cheese to make it even better.

—**NAYLET LAROCHELLE** MIAMI, FL

START TO FINISH: 30 MIN.
MAKES: 4 SERVINGS

- 1 beef flank steak (1 pound)
- 4 teaspoons chili powder
- ½ teaspoon salt
- 1 package (8.8 ounces) ready-to-serve brown rice
- 1 can (15 ounces) black beans, rinsed and drained
- ½ cup salsa verde
  Minced fresh cilantro, optional

1. Rub steak with chili powder and salt. Grill, covered, over medium heat or broil 4 in. from heat 6-8 minutes on each side or until meat reaches desired doneness (for medium-rare, a thermometer should read 145°; medium, 160°).

2. Heat rice according to package directions. Transfer rice to a small bowl; stir in beans and salsa. Slice steak thinly across the grain; serve with bean salad. If desired, sprinkle with cilantro.

Per 3 ounces cooked beef with ¾ cup bean salad: 367 cal., 10g fat (4g sat. fat), 54mg chol., 762mg sod., 35g carb. (2g sugars, 6g fiber), 29g pro.
Diabetic Exchanges: 3 lean meat, 2 starch.

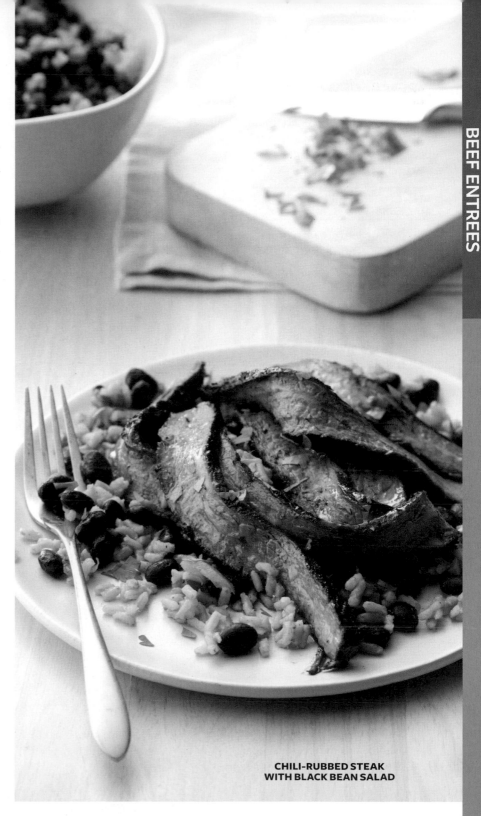

CHILI-RUBBED STEAK WITH BLACK BEAN SALAD

FAST FIX

OPEN-FACED ROAST BEEF SANDWICHES

Arugula brings the zing to this sandwich. I usually make extras because most people who taste them want seconds.

—MARY PRICE YOUNGSTOWN, OH

START TO FINISH: 15 MIN.
MAKES: 8 SERVINGS

- 1 pound sliced deli roast beef
- 8 slices ciabatta bread (½ inch thick)
- 2 cups fresh arugula
- 2 cups torn romaine
- 4 teaspoons olive oil
- 1 tablespoon lemon juice
- 1 tablespoon white wine vinegar
- 1½ teaspoons prepared horseradish

Place roast beef on ciabatta slices. In a large bowl, combine the arugula and romaine. In a small bowl, whisk the remaining ingredients until blended. Drizzle over greens; toss to coat. Arrange over beef; serve immediately.

Per sandwich: 150 cal., 5g fat (1g sat. fat), 32mg chol., 422mg sod., 14g carb. (1g sugars, 1g fiber), 14g pro.
Diabetic Exchanges: 2 lean meat, 1 starch, ½ fat.

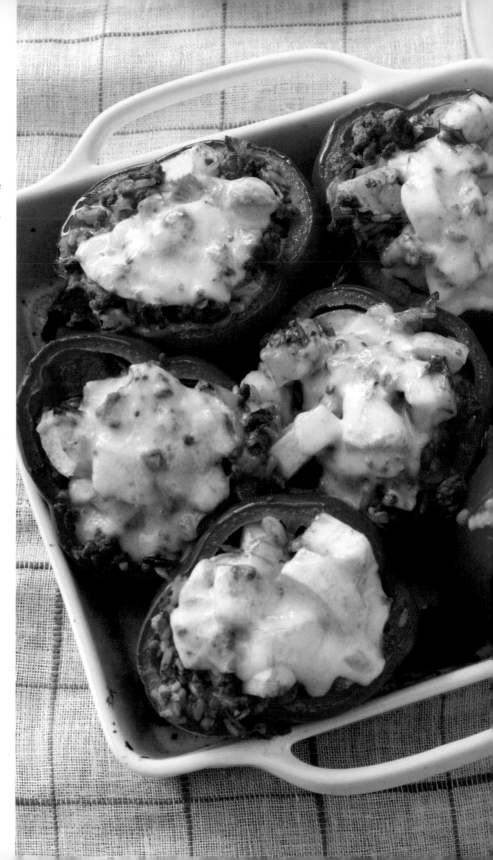

VEGETABLE & BEEF STUFFED RED PEPPERS

I love this recipe because it's one of the few ways my husband will eat veggies! For a meatless version, replace the beef with eggplant and add more vegetables, such as mushrooms or squash. You can replace the rice with couscous, barley, or even orzo if you like it better.

—JENNIFER ZIMMERMAN AVONDALE, AZ

PREP: 35 MIN. • **BAKE:** 40 MIN.
MAKES: 6 SERVINGS

- 6 medium sweet red peppers
- 1 pound lean ground beef (90% lean)
- 1 tablespoon olive oil
- 1 medium zucchini, chopped
- 1 medium yellow summer squash, chopped
- 1 medium onion, finely chopped
- 1/3 cup finely chopped green pepper
- 2 cups coarsely chopped fresh spinach
- 4 garlic cloves, minced
- 1 cup ready-to-serve long grain and wild rice
- 1 can (8 ounces) tomato sauce
- 1/2 cup shredded part-skim mozzarella cheese
- 1/4 teaspoon salt
- 3 slices reduced-fat provolone cheese, halved

1. Preheat oven to 350°. Cut and discard tops from red peppers; remove seeds. In a 6-qt. stockpot, cook peppers in boiling water about 3-5 minutes or until crisp-tender; drain and rinse in cold water.

2. In a large skillet, cook beef over medium heat 6-8 minutes or until no longer pink, breaking into crumbles. Remove with a slotted spoon; pour off drippings.

3. In same pan, heat oil over medium heat; saute zucchini, yellow squash, onion and green pepper 4-5 minutes or until tender. Add spinach and garlic; cook and stir 1 minute or until wilted. Stir in cooked beef, rice, tomato sauce, mozzarella cheese and salt.

4. Place red peppers in a greased 8-in. square baking dish. Fill with the meat mixture. Bake, covered, 35-40 minutes or until peppers are tender. Top with provolone cheese; bake, uncovered, 5 minutes or until cheese is melted.

Per stuffed pepper: 287 cal., 13g fat (5g sat. fat), 57mg chol., 555mg sod., 21g carb. (8g sugars, 5g fiber), 23g pro.
Diabetic Exchanges: 3 lean meat, 2 vegetable, 1 fat, 1/2 starch.

✳
TEST KITCHEN TIP
Pressed for time? Make the filling for the peppers a day or two beforehand and store in the refrigerator until you're ready to use it. Make a little extra to stuff into wraps for lunch!

VEGETABLE & BEEF STUFFED RED PEPPERS

WEEKNIGHT PASTA

Lovely herb accents enhance this easy gluten-free spaghetti and sauce.

—MARV SALTER WEST HILLS, CA

PREP: 15 MIN. • **COOK:** 20 MIN.
MAKES: 2 SERVINGS

- ½ pound lean ground beef (90% lean)
- 1 cup sliced fresh mushrooms
- ⅓ cup chopped onion
- 1 garlic clove, minced
- 1 cup gluten-free reduced-sodium beef broth
- ⅔ cup water
- ⅓ cup tomato paste
- ½ teaspoon dried basil
- ½ teaspoon dried oregano
- ⅛ teaspoon pepper
- 3 ounces uncooked gluten-free spaghetti, broken in half
- 2 teaspoons grated Parmesan cheese

1. In a large skillet, cook the beef, mushrooms, onion and garlic over medium heat until meat is no longer pink and vegetables are tender; drain.
2. Stir in broth, water, tomato paste, seasonings and spaghetti. Bring to a boil. Reduce heat; cover and simmer for 15-20 minutes or until spaghetti is tender. Sprinkle with cheese.
Note: Read all ingredient labels for possible gluten content prior to use. Ingredient formulas can change, and production facilities vary among brands. If you're concerned that your brand may contain gluten, contact the company.
Per serving: 412 cal., 11g fat (4g sat. fat), 75mg chol., 335mg sod., 46g carb. (6g sugars, 4g fiber), 31g pro.
Diabetic Exchanges: 3 lean meat, 2½ starch, 2 vegetable.

---

⑤INGREDIENTS FAST FIX ▶

SPINACH STEAK PINWHEELS

Bacon and spinach bring plenty of flavor to these spirals of sirloin steak, and they are perfect for backyard cookouts.

—HELEN VAIL GLENSIDE, PA

START TO FINISH: 25 MIN.
MAKES: 6 SERVINGS

- 1½ pounds beef top sirloin steak
- 8 bacon strips, cooked
- 1 package (10 ounces) frozen chopped spinach, thawed and squeezed dry
- ¼ cup grated Parmesan cheese
- ½ teaspoon salt
- ⅛ teaspoon cayenne pepper

1. Lightly score the steak by making shallow diagonal cuts at 1-in. intervals into top of steak; repeat cuts in the opposite direction. Cover steak with plastic wrap; pound with a meat mallet to ½-in. thickness. Remove plastic.
2. Place bacon widthwise at center of steak. In a bowl, mix the remaining ingredients; spoon over bacon. Starting at a short side, roll up steak jelly-roll style; secure with toothpicks. Cut into six slices.
3. Lightly coat grill rack with cooking oil. Grill pinwheels, covered, over medium heat 5-6 minutes on each side or until beef reaches desired doneness (for medium-rare, a thermometer should read 145°; medium, 160°). Discard toothpicks before serving.
Per pinwheel: 227 cal., 10g fat (4g sat. fat), 60mg chol., 536mg sod., 3g carb. (0 sugars, 1g fiber), 31g pro.
Diabetic Exchanges: 4 lean meat, 1 fat.

FAST FIX ▶

SUBLIME LIME BEEF

It's fun to watch the happy reactions of others when they try my lime beef kabobs for the first time. They're so good it's hard not to smile.

—DIEP NGUYEN HANFORD, CA

START TO FINISH: 25 MIN.
MAKES: 4 SERVINGS

- ⅓ cup lime juice
- 2 teaspoons sugar
- 2 garlic cloves, minced
- 1 beef top sirloin steak (1 inch thick and 1 pound)
- 1½ teaspoons pepper
- ¾ teaspoon salt
- 2 tablespoons unsalted dry roasted peanuts, chopped
- 3 cups hot cooked brown rice

1. In a small bowl, mix lime juice, sugar and garlic until blended; set aside. Cut steak into 2x1x¾-in. pieces; toss with pepper and salt. Thread beef onto four metal or soaked wooden skewers.
2. Grill kabobs, covered, over medium heat or broil 4 in. from heat 2-4 minutes on each side or until the beef reaches the desired doneness. Add peanuts to sauce; serve with kabobs and rice.
Per 1 kabob with ¾ cup rice and 1 tablespoon sauce: 352 cal., 8g fat (2g sat. fat), 46mg chol., 502mg sod., 39g carb. (3g sugars, 3g fiber), 29g pro.
Diabetic Exchanges: 3 lean meat, 2½ starch.

SUBLIME LIME BEEF

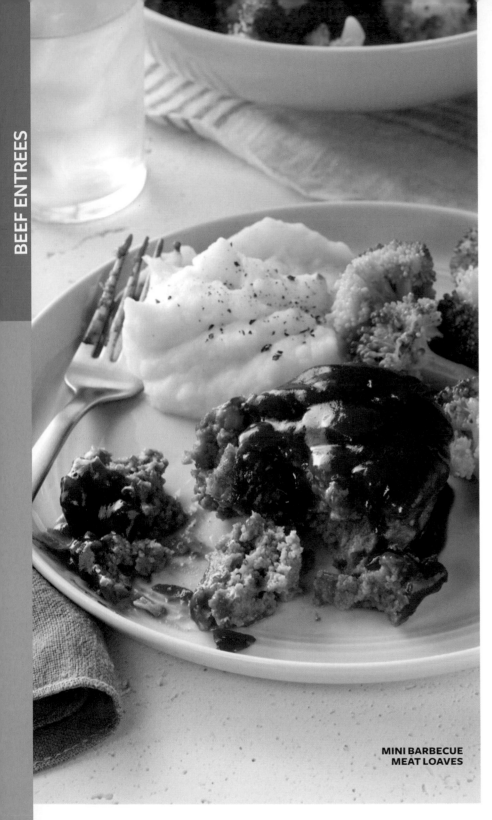

MINI BARBECUE MEAT LOAVES

I gave classic meat loaf a tasty twist by adding barbecue sauce. My kids usually get bored with beef entrees, but they keep asking for this dish. It's become a dinner staple at my house.

—VICKI SMITH OKEECHOBEE, FL

PREP: 15 MIN. • **BAKE:** 20 MIN.
MAKES: 1 DOZEN

- ⅔ cup barbecue sauce
- ⅓ cup salsa
- 2 teaspoons Worcestershire sauce
- 1 cup dry bread crumbs
- 1 small onion, finely chopped
- 1 small green pepper, finely chopped
- 1 large egg, lightly beaten
- 2 tablespoons Montreal steak seasoning
- 1½ pounds lean ground beef (90% lean)

1. Preheat oven to 400°. In a large bowl, mix barbecue sauce, salsa and Worcestershire sauce; reserve ½ cup mixture for topping. Add bread crumbs, onion, pepper, egg and steak seasoning to remaining sauce mixture. Add beef; mix lightly but thoroughly.

2. Place ⅓ cup beef mixture into each of 12 greased muffin cups. Spoon the reserved sauce mixture over tops.

3. Bake for 20-25 minutes or until a thermometer reads 160°. Let stand 5 minutes before removing from pan.

Per mini meat loaf: 163 cal., 6g fat (2g sat. fat), 51mg chol., 633mg sod., 14g carb. (6g sugars, 1g fiber), 13g pro. **Diabetic Exchanges:** 2 lean meat, 1 starch.

MINI BARBECUE MEAT LOAVES

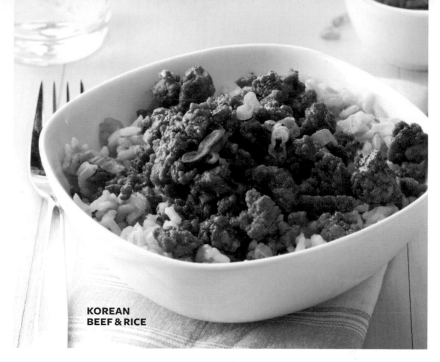

KOREAN BEEF & RICE

FAST FIX
KOREAN BEEF & RICE

A friend raved about beef cooked in soy sauce and ginger, so I gave it a try. It's delicious and ideal for busy nights!
—BETSY KING DULUTH, MN

START TO FINISH: 15 MIN.
MAKES: 4 SERVINGS

- 1 **pound lean ground beef (90% lean)**
- 3 **garlic cloves, minced**
- ¼ **cup packed brown sugar**
- ¼ **cup reduced-sodium soy sauce**
- 2 **teaspoons sesame oil**
- ¼ **teaspoon ground ginger**
- ¼ **teaspoon crushed red pepper flakes**
- ¼ **teaspoon pepper**
- 2⅔ **cups hot cooked brown rice**
- 3 **green onions, thinly sliced**

1. In a large skillet, cook beef and garlic over medium heat 6-8 minutes or until beef is no longer pink, breaking up beef into crumbles. Meanwhile, in a small bowl, mix brown sugar, soy sauce, oil and seasonings.
2. Stir sauce into the beef; heat through. Serve with rice. Sprinkle with green onions.
To freeze: Freeze the cooled meat mixture in freezer containers. To use, partially thaw in refrigerator overnight. Heat through in a saucepan, stirring occasionally.
Per ½ cup beef mixture with ⅔ cup rice: 413 cal., 13g fat (4g sat. fat), 71mg chol., 647mg sod., 46g carb. (14g sugars, 3g fiber), 27g pro.
Diabetic Exchanges: 3 starch, 3 lean meat, ½ fat.

CHILI SLOPPY JOES

Kids of all ages will love this zesty take on the classic loose-meat sandwich, and if there are any leftovers, they freeze well.
—BRITTANY ALLYN MESA, AZ

PREP: 15 MIN. • **COOK:** 20 MIN.
MAKES: 6 SERVINGS

- 1 **pound lean ground beef (90% lean)**
- 1 **cup finely chopped sweet onion**
- ½ **cup finely chopped green pepper**
- 1 **jalapeno pepper, seeded and finely chopped, optional**
- ½ **cup chili sauce**
- ½ **cup water**
- 1 **to 2 chipotle peppers in adobo sauce, finely chopped**
- 1 **tablespoon packed brown sugar**
- 1 **teaspoon yellow mustard**
- 6 **kaiser rolls or hamburger buns, split**
- 2 **tablespoons butter, softened**
  Pickle slices, optional

1. Preheat broiler. In a large skillet, cook beef, onion, green pepper and if desired, jalapeno, over medium heat 5-7 minutes or until beef is no longer pink, breaking up beef into crumbles; drain.
2. Stir in chili sauce, water, chipotle peppers, brown sugar and mustard; bring to a boil. Simmer, uncovered, 8-10 minutes or until slightly thickened, stirring occasionally.
3. Spread cut sides of rolls with butter; arrange on a baking sheet, buttered side up. Broil 3-4 in. from heat until lightly toasted, about 30 seconds. Fill with beef mixture and, if desired, pickles.
To freeze: Freeze cooled meat mixture in freezer containers. To use, partially thaw in refrigerator overnight. Heat through in a saucepan, stirring meat occasionally and adding a little water if necessary.
Per sandwich: 313 cal., 12g fat (5g sat. fat), 57mg chol., 615mg sod., 32g carb. (11g sugars, 2g fiber), 19g pro.
Diabetic Exchanges: 2 starch, 2 lean meat, 1 fat.

VEGETABLE STEAK KABOBS

The marinade for these skewers is the best I've ever found. Try it on chicken!
—**NORMA HARDER** WEYAKWIN, SK

PREP: 20 MIN. + MARINATING
GRILL: 10 MIN. • **MAKES:** 6 SERVINGS

- ½ cup olive oil
- ⅓ cup red wine vinegar
- 2 tablespoons ketchup
- 2 to 3 garlic cloves, minced
- 1 teaspoon Worcestershire sauce
- ½ teaspoon each dried marjoram, basil and oregano
- ½ teaspoon dried rosemary, crushed
- 1 beef top sirloin steak (1½ pounds), cut into 1-inch cubes
- ½ pound whole fresh mushrooms
- 2 medium onions, cut into wedges
- 1½ cups cherry tomatoes
- 2 small green peppers, cut into 1-inch pieces

1. In a small bowl, whisk oil, vinegar, ketchup, garlic, Worcestershire sauce and seasonings. Pour ½ cup marinade into a large resealable plastic bag. Add beef; seal bag and turn to coat. Pour remaining marinade into another large resealable plastic bag. Add mushrooms, onions, tomatoes and peppers; seal bag and turn to coat. Refrigerate beef and vegetables 8 hours or overnight.
2. Drain beef, discarding marinade. Drain vegetables, reserving marinade. On six metal or soaked wooden skewers, thread beef and vegetables.
3. Grill kabobs, covered, over medium heat or broil 4 in. from heat 10-15 minutes or until beef reaches desired doneness and vegetables are crisp-tender, turning occasionally. Baste with reserved marinade the last 5 minutes.

Per kabob: 234 cal., 10g fat (2g sat. fat), 69mg chol., 99mg sod., 10g carb. (0 sugars, 2g fiber), 26g pro.
Diabetic Exchanges: 3 lean meat, 2 vegetable.

FAST FIX
SMOKY ESPRESSO STEAK

This juicy steak, rubbed with espresso, cocoa and pumpkin pie spice, is one of my husband's favorites. We usually grill it, but broiling works in chilly months. What a hearty dinner!
—**DEBORAH BIGGS** OMAHA, NE

START TO FINISH: 30 MIN.
MAKES: 4 SERVINGS

- 3 teaspoons instant espresso powder
- 2 teaspoons brown sugar
- 1½ teaspoons smoked or regular paprika
- 1 teaspoon salt
- 1 teaspoon baking cocoa
- ¼ teaspoon pumpkin pie spice
- ¼ teaspoon pepper
- 1 pound beef flat iron or top sirloin steak (¾ inch thick)

1. Preheat broiler. Mix first seven ingredients; rub over both sides of steak. Place steak on a broiler pan; let stand 10 minutes.
2. Broil steak 3-4 in. from heat 4-6 minutes on each side or until meat reaches desired doneness (for medium-rare, a thermometer should read 145°; medium, 160°). Let stand 5 minutes before slicing.
Per 3 ounces cooked beef: 216 cal., 12g fat (5g sat. fat), 73mg chol., 661mg sod., 4g carb. (2g sugars, 0 fiber), 22g pro.
Diabetic Exchanges: 3 lean meat.

FAST FIX
SUMMER SALAD WITH CITRUS VINAIGRETTE

I live in Orange County, named for its beautiful orange groves. This salad is one of my favorite ways to use the fresh fruit. It makes a nice light supper on a hot day.
—**CAROLYN WILLIAMS** COSTA MESA, CA

START TO FINISH: 20 MIN.
MAKES: 4 SERVINGS

- 3 tablespoons red wine vinegar
- 3 tablespoons orange juice
- 2 teaspoons honey
- 1½ teaspoons Dijon mustard
- 1 teaspoon olive oil

SALAD

- 1 tablespoon canola oil
- 1 pound beef top sirloin steak, cut into thin strips
- ½ teaspoon salt, optional
- 4 cups torn romaine
- 2 large oranges, peeled and sectioned
- ½ cup sliced fresh strawberries
- ¼ cup chopped walnuts, toasted, optional

1. Whisk together first five ingredients.
2. For salad, in a large skillet, heat oil over medium-high heat; stir-fry beef until browned, 1-3 minutes. Remove from heat. If desired, sprinkle with salt.
3. Place romaine, fruit and beef in a serving dish. Toss with the vinaigrette. If desired, top with the walnuts. Serve salad immediately.
Per 1½ cups: 265 cal., 10g fat (2g sat. fat), 46mg chol., 101mg sod., 19g carb. (14g sugars, 4g fiber), 26g pro.
Diabetic Exchanges: 3 lean meat, 1 vegetable, 1 fat, ½ starch, ½ fruit.

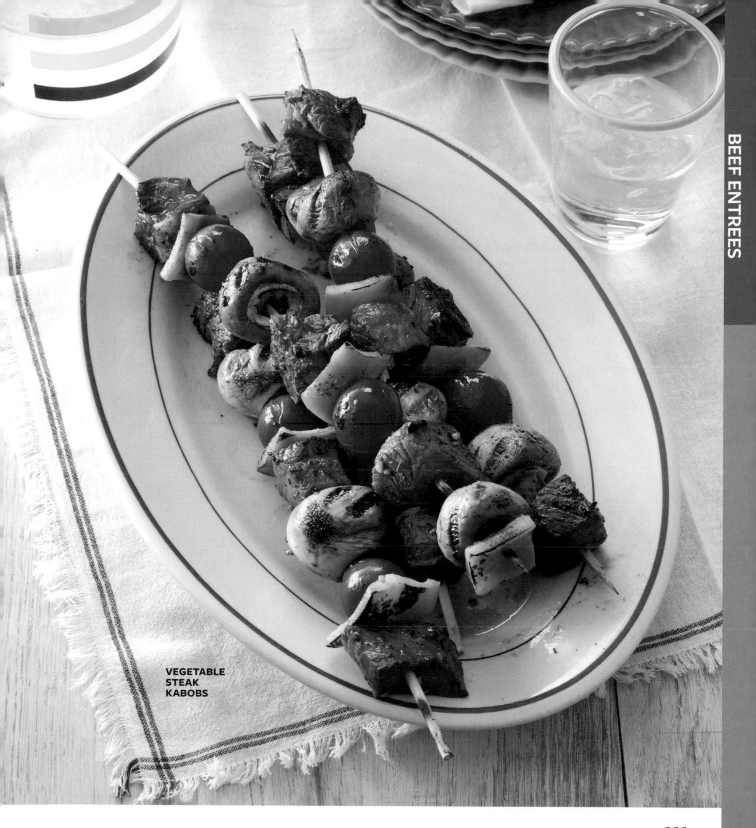

VEGETABLE
STEAK
KABOBS

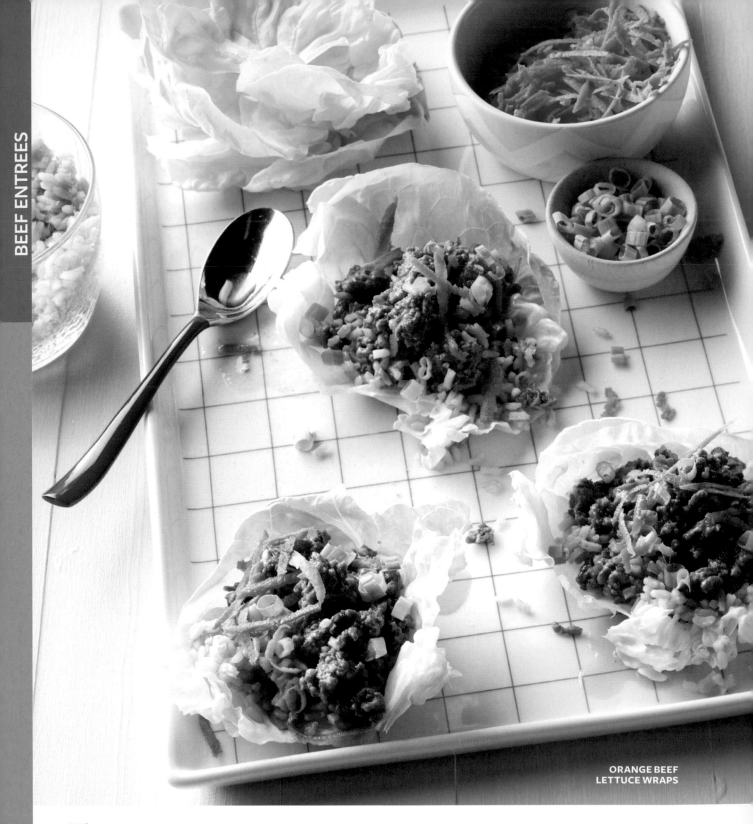

ORANGE BEEF
LETTUCE WRAPS

ORANGE BEEF LETTUCE WRAPS

This is a lighter version of a restaurant favorite. I also recommend trying these wraps with ground chicken or turkey.

—ROBIN HAAS CRANSTON, RI

PREP: 20 MIN. • **COOK:** 15 MIN.
MAKES: 8 SERVINGS

SAUCE

- ¼ cup rice vinegar
- 3 tablespoons water
- 3 tablespoons orange marmalade
- 1 tablespoon sugar
- 1 tablespoon reduced-sodium soy sauce
- 2 garlic cloves, minced
- 1 teaspoon Sriracha Asian hot chili sauce

WRAPS

- 1½ pounds lean ground beef (90% lean)
- 2 garlic cloves, minced
- 2 teaspoons minced fresh gingerroot
- ¼ cup reduced-sodium soy sauce
- 2 tablespoons orange juice
- 1 tablespoon sugar
- 1 tablespoon orange marmalade
- ¼ teaspoon crushed red pepper flakes
- 2 teaspoons cornstarch
- ¼ cup cold water
- 8 Bibb or Boston lettuce leaves
- 2 cups cooked brown rice
- 1 cup shredded carrots
- 3 green onions, thinly sliced

1. In a small bowl, combine the sauce ingredients.
2. In a large skillet, cook beef, garlic and ginger over medium heat 8-10 minutes or until no longer pink, breaking into crumbles; drain. Stir in the soy sauce, orange juice, sugar, marmalade and pepper flakes. In a small bowl, mix the cornstarch and water; stir into pan. Cook and stir 1-2 minutes or until sauce is thickened.
3. Serve in lettuce leaves with rice. Top with carrots and green onions; drizzle with sauce.

Per wrap: 250 cal., 8g fat (3g sat. fat), 53mg chol., 462mg sod., 26g carb. (11g sugars, 2g fiber), 19g pro.
Diabetic Exchanges: 2 starch, 2 lean meat.

SPECIAL OCCASION BEEF BOURGUIGNON

I've found many satisfying variations of beef bourguignon, including a classic version that used beef cheeks for the meat and a rustic table wine. To make it gluten-free, swap white rice flour for all-purpose and potatoes for noodles.

—LEO COTNOIR JOHNSON CITY, NY

PREP: 50 MIN. • **BAKE:** 2 HOURS
MAKES: 8 SERVINGS

- 4 bacon strips, chopped
- 1 beef sirloin tip roast (2 pounds), cut into 1½-inch cubes and patted dry
- ¼ cup all-purpose flour
- ½ teaspoon salt
- ½ teaspoon pepper
- 1 tablespoon canola oil
- 2 medium onions, chopped
- 2 medium carrots, coarsely chopped
- ½ pound medium fresh mushrooms, quartered
- 4 garlic cloves, minced
- 1 tablespoon tomato paste
- 2 cups dry red wine
- 1 cup beef stock
- 2 bay leaves
- ½ teaspoon dried thyme
- 8 ounces uncooked egg noodles
  Minced fresh parsley

1. Preheat oven to 325°. In a Dutch oven, cook bacon over medium-low heat until crisp, stirring occasionally. Remove with a slotted spoon, reserving drippings; drain on paper towels.
2. In batches, brown beef in drippings over medium-high heat; remove from pan. Toss with flour, salt and pepper.
3. In same pan, heat 1 tablespoon oil over medium heat; saute the onions, carrots and mushrooms until onions are tender, 4-5 minutes. Add garlic and tomato paste; cook and stir 1 minute. Add wine and stock, stirring to loosen browned bits from pan. Add herbs, bacon and beef; bring to a boil.
4. Transfer to oven; bake, covered, until meat is tender, 2 to 2¼ hours. Remove bay leaves.
5. To serve, cook noodles according to package directions; drain. Serve stew with noodles; sprinkle with parsley.
To freeze: Freeze the cooled stew in freezer containers. To use, partially thaw in refrigerator overnight. Heat through in a saucepan, stirring occasionally and adding extra stock or broth if necessary.
Per ⅔ cup stew with ⅔ cup noodles: 422 cal., 14g fat (4g sat. fat), 105mg chol., 357mg sod., 31g carb. (4g sugars, 2g fiber), 31g pro.
Diabetic Exchanges: 4 lean meat, 2 fat, 1½ starch, 1 vegetable.

✳

DID YOU KNOW?
Beef bourguignon may be famous around the world, but its culinary roots are in the Burgundy region in France, which is known for its excellent red wines.

BEEF & BULGUR-STUFFED ZUCCHINI BOATS

I adapted this recipe from my mother's favorite weeknight meals.

—SUSAN PETERSON BLAINE, MN

PREP: 35 MIN. • **BAKE:** 30 MIN.
MAKES: 4 SERVINGS

- 4 medium zucchini
- 1 pound lean ground beef (90% lean)
- 1 large onion, finely chopped
- 1 small sweet red pepper, chopped
- 1½ cups tomato sauce
- ½ cup bulgur
- ¼ teaspoon pepper
- ½ cup salsa
- ½ cup shredded reduced-fat cheddar cheese

1. Preheat oven to 350°. Cut each zucchini lengthwise in half. Scoop out pulp, leaving a ¼-in. shell; chop pulp.
2. In a large skillet, cook beef, onion and red pepper over medium heat 6-8 minutes or until meat is no longer pink, breaking into crumbles; drain. Stir in tomato sauce, bulgur, pepper and zucchini pulp. Bring to a boil. Reduce heat; simmer, uncovered, for 12-15 minutes or until bulgur is tender. Stir in salsa. Spoon into zucchini shells.
3. Place in a 13x9-in. baking dish coated with cooking spray. Bake, covered, 20 minutes. Sprinkle with the cheese. Bake, uncovered, for 10-15 minutes longer or until the zucchini is tender and filling is heated through.
Per 2 stuffed zucchini halves: 361 cal., 13g fat (6g sat. fat), 81mg chol., 714mg sod., 31g carb. (9g sugars, 7g fiber), 32g pro.
Diabetic Exchanges: 4 lean meat, 2 vegetable, 1 starch.

CABBAGE ROLL SKILLET

Have a nice big helping of this lighter, quicker take on something our grandmothers would make. We serve it over brown rice.

—SUSAN CHICKNESS PICTOU COUNTY, NS

PREP: 15 MIN. • **COOK:** 20 MIN.
MAKES: 6 SERVINGS

- 1 can (28 ounces) whole plum tomatoes, undrained
- 1 pound extra-lean ground beef (95% lean)
- 1 large onion, chopped
- 1 can (8 ounces) tomato sauce
- 2 tablespoons cider vinegar
- 1 tablespoon brown sugar
- 1 teaspoon dried oregano
- 1 teaspoon dried thyme
- ½ teaspoon pepper
- 1 small head cabbage, thinly sliced (about 6 cups)
- 1 medium green pepper, cut into thin strips
- 4 cups hot cooked brown rice

1. Drain tomatoes, reserving liquid; coarsely chop tomatoes. In a large nonstick skillet, cook beef and onion over medium-high heat 6-8 minutes or until beef is no longer pink, breaking up beef into crumbles. Stir in the tomato sauce, vinegar, brown sugar, seasonings, chopped tomatoes and reserved liquid.
2. Add cabbage and pepper; cook, covered, 6 minutes, stirring mixture occasionally. Cook, uncovered, 6-8 minutes or until cabbage is tender. Serve with rice.
Per 1⅓ cups with ⅔ cup rice: 332 cal., 5g fat (2g sat. fat), 43mg chol., 439mg sod., 50g carb. (12g sugars, 9g fiber), 22g pro.
Diabetic Exchanges: 3 starch, 3 lean meat.

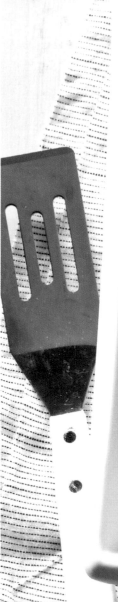

BEEF & BULGUR-STUFFED ZUCCHINI BOATS

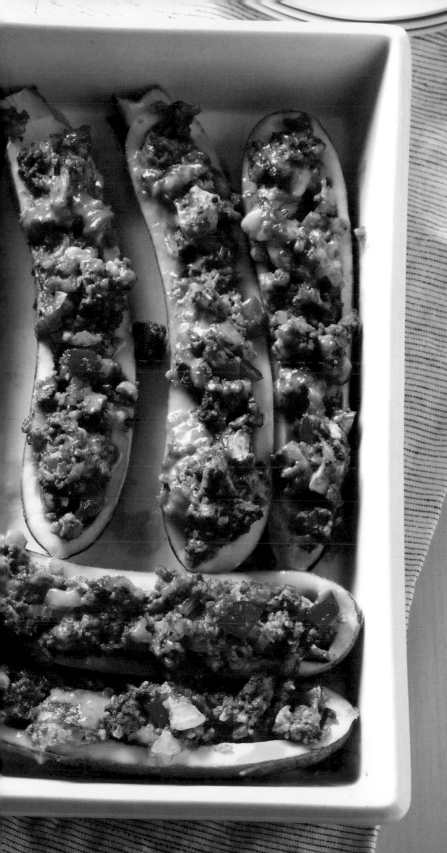

BALSAMIC BEEF KABOB SANDWICHES

This dish is popular wherever it goes. The flavorful sandwiches will surely be the highlight of your summer barbecue.
—**PEGGY LABOR** LOUISVILLE, KY

PREP: 15 MIN. + MARINATING
GRILL: 10 MIN. • **MAKES:** 8 SERVINGS

- ¼ cup balsamic vinegar
- ¼ cup olive oil
- 2 garlic cloves, minced
- 1 teaspoon dried rosemary, crushed
- ½ teaspoon pepper, divided
- ¼ teaspoon salt, divided
- 1½ pounds beef top sirloin steak, cut into ¼-inch-thick strips
- 2 medium onions
- 8 naan flatbreads
- 2 cups chopped heirloom tomatoes

1. Mix first four ingredients; stir in ¼ teaspoon pepper and ⅛ teaspoon salt. Toss with the beef; let stand for 20 minutes.
2. Cut each onion into eight wedges; thread onto metal or soaked wooden skewers. Thread beef strips, weaving back and forth, onto separate skewers.
3. Grill onions, covered, over medium heat until tender, 5-7 minutes per side. Grill beef, covered, over medium heat until desired doneness, 3-4 minutes per side. Grill the flatbreads until lightly browned, 1-2 minutes per side.
4. Toss tomatoes with the remaining pepper and salt. Remove onion and beef from skewers; serve on flatbreads. Top with tomatoes.
Per sandwich: 353 cal., 14g fat (3g sat. fat), 39mg chol., 595mg sod., 34g carb. (7g sugars, 2g fiber), 23g pro.
Diabetic Exchanges: 3 lean meat, 2 starch, 1½ fat.

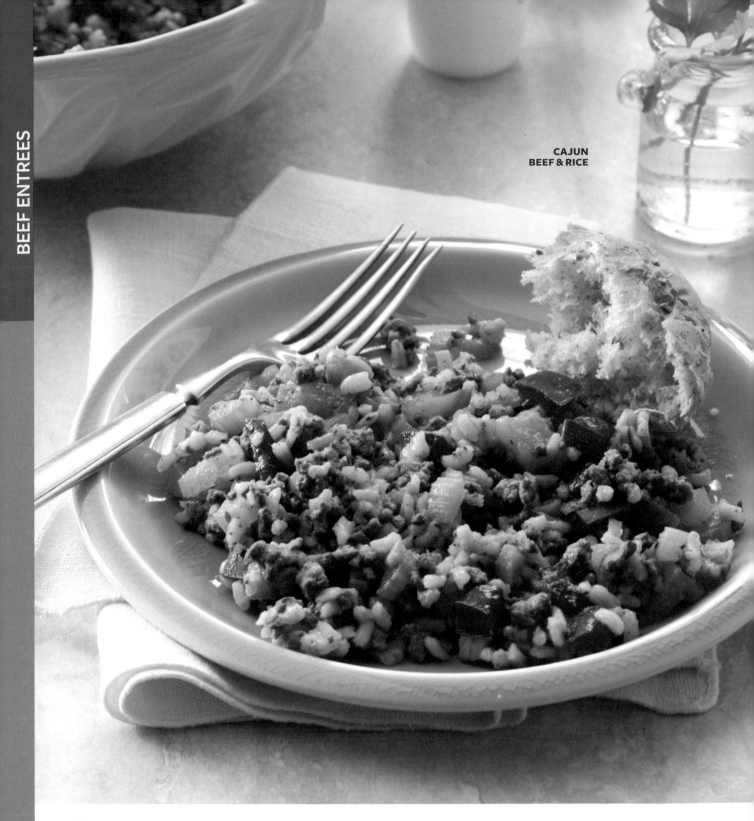

CAJUN
BEEF & RICE

CAJUN BEEF & RICE

Dirty rice from a restaurant or box can have a lot of sodium and fat. Here's a hearty, healthy way I like to trim it.
—RAQUEL HAGGARD EDMOND, OK

START TO FINISH: 30 MIN.
MAKES: 4 SERVINGS

- 1 pound lean ground beef (90% lean)
- 3 celery ribs, chopped
- 1 small green pepper, chopped
- 1 small sweet red pepper, chopped
- ¼ cup chopped onion
- 2 cups water
- 1 cup instant brown rice
- 1 tablespoon minced fresh parsley
- 1 tablespoon Worcestershire sauce
- 2 teaspoons reduced-sodium beef bouillon granules
- 1 teaspoon Cajun seasoning
- ¼ teaspoon crushed red pepper flakes
- ¼ teaspoon pepper
- ⅛ teaspoon garlic powder

1. In a large skillet, cook beef, celery, green and red peppers, and onion over medium heat 8-10 minutes or until beef is no longer pink, breaking up beef into crumbles; drain.
2. Stir in remaining ingredients. Bring to a boil. Reduce heat; simmer, covered, 12-15 minutes or until rice is tender.
Per 1½ cups: 291 cal., 10g fat (4g sat. fat), 71mg chol., 422mg sod., 23g carb. (3g sugars, 2g fiber), 25g pro.
Diabetic Exchanges: 3 lean meat, 1 starch, 1 vegetable.

TASTY TACOS

I make taco seasoning from scratch, then use pantry staples to turn my dinners into all-out fiestas. Add your favorite toppings, and dinner is served!
—REBECCA LEVESQUE ST. GEORGE, NB

START TO FINISH: 30 MIN.
MAKES: 4 SERVINGS

- 1 pound lean ground beef (90% lean)
- 1 medium onion, finely chopped
- 1 garlic clove, minced
- ½ cup water
- 1 tablespoon chili powder
- 1½ teaspoons ground cumin
- ½ teaspoon salt
- ½ teaspoon paprika
- ½ teaspoon pepper
- ¼ teaspoon dried oregano
- ¼ teaspoon crushed red pepper flakes
- 8 taco shells, warmed
  Optional toppings: shredded lettuce, chopped tomatoes, sliced green onions and shredded cheddar cheese

1. In a large skillet, cook the beef, onion and garlic over medium heat until meat is no longer pink; drain. Stir in the water and seasonings. Bring to a boil. Reduce heat; simmer mixture, uncovered, for 5-10 minutes or until thickened.
2. Spoon beef mixture into taco shells. Serve with toppings of your choice.
Per 2 tacos without toppings: 306 cal., 15g fat (5g sat. fat), 71mg chol., 468mg sod., 19g carb. (2g sugars, 3g fiber), 24g pro.
Diabetic Exchanges: 3 lean meat, 1 starch, 1 fat.

HEARTY GARDEN SPAGHETTI

My husband and I wanted a pleasing dish that didn't leave a ton of leftovers, and spaghetti with beef and fresh veggies is perfectly filling for four.
—WANDA QUIST LOVELAND, CO

PREP: 15 MIN. • **COOK:** 30 MIN.
MAKES: 4 SERVINGS

- 1 pound lean ground beef (90% lean)
- 1 small onion, finely chopped
- 1 medium sweet red pepper, finely chopped
- 1 medium zucchini, finely chopped
- ½ pound sliced fresh mushrooms
- 1 can (8 ounces) tomato sauce
- 2 teaspoons Italian seasoning
- ½ teaspoon salt
- ¼ teaspoon pepper
- 8 ounces uncooked multigrain spaghetti
  Grated Parmesan cheese, optional

1. In a Dutch oven coated with cooking spray, cook beef, onion and red pepper over medium-high heat 5-7 minutes or until beef is no longer pink, breaking up beef into crumbles; drain.
2. Add zucchini and mushrooms; cook 3-5 minutes longer or until tender. Stir in tomato sauce and seasonings; bring to a boil. Reduce heat; simmer, covered, 15 minutes to allow the flavors to blend. Meanwhile, cook spaghetti according to package directions.
3. Serve spaghetti with sauce and, if desired, cheese.
Per 1¼ cups sauce with 1 cup spaghetti: 432 cal., 11g fat (4g sat. fat), 71mg chol., 649mg sod., 48g carb. (6g sugars, 7g fiber), 36g pro.
Diabetic Exchanges: 3 lean meat, 2½ starch, 2 vegetable.

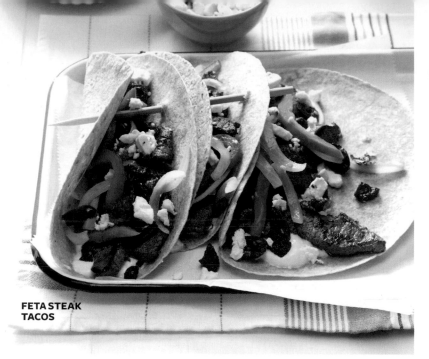

FETA STEAK TACOS

(5) INGREDIENTS

EASY & ELEGANT TENDERLOIN ROAST

A friend of mine served this tenderloin several years ago and passed along the recipe. It's simple, but don't skimp on the seasonings and you'll get perfect results every time.

—MARY KANDELL HURON, OH

PREP: 10 MIN.
BAKE: 50 MIN. + STANDING
MAKES: 12 SERVINGS

- 1 beef tenderloin (5 pounds)
- 2 tablespoons olive oil
- 4 garlic cloves, minced
- 2 teaspoons sea salt
- 1½ teaspoons coarsely ground pepper

FAST FIX

FETA STEAK TACOS

These tacos combine Mediterranean and Mexican flavors. They're a big hit with my family. Best of all, they're ready in just half an hour!

—DEBBIE REID CLEARWATER, FL

START TO FINISH: 30 MIN.
MAKES: 8 SERVINGS

- 1 beef flat iron steak or top sirloin steak (1¼ pounds), cut into thin strips
- ¼ cup Greek vinaigrette
- ½ cup fat-free plain Greek yogurt
- 2 teaspoons lime juice
- 1 tablespoon oil from sun-dried tomatoes
- 1 small green pepper, cut into thin strips
- 1 small onion, cut into thin strips
- ¼ cup chopped oil-packed sun-dried tomatoes
- ¼ cup sliced Greek olives
- 8 whole wheat tortillas (8 inches), warmed
- ¼ cup crumbled garlic and herb feta cheese
    Lime wedges

1. In a large bowl, toss beef with the vinaigrette; let stand 15 minutes. In a small bowl, mix yogurt and lime juice.
2. In a large skillet, heat oil from the sun-dried tomatoes over medium-high heat. Add pepper and onion; cook and stir 3-4 minutes or until crisp-tender. Remove to a small bowl; stir in sun-dried tomatoes and olives.
3. Place same skillet over medium-high heat. Add beef; cook and stir for 2-3 minutes or until no longer pink. Remove from pan.
4. Serve steak and pepper mixture in tortillas; top with cheese. Serve with yogurt mixture and lime wedges.
Per 1 taco with 1 tablespoon yogurt mixture: 317 cal., 15g fat (4g sat. fat), 48mg chol., 372mg sod., 25g carb. (2g sugars, 3g fiber), 20g pro.
Diabetic Exchanges: 3 lean meat, 2 fat, 1½ starch.

1. Preheat oven to 425°. Place roast on a rack in a shallow roasting pan. In a small bowl, mix the oil, garlic, salt and pepper; rub over roast.
2. Roast 50-70 minutes or until meat reaches desired doneness (for medium-rare, a thermometer should read 145°; medium, 160°). Remove from oven; tent with foil. Let stand 15 minutes before slicing.
Per 5 ounces cooked beef: 294 cal., 13g fat (5g sat. fat), 82mg chol., 394mg sod., 1g carb. (0 sugars, 0 fiber), 40g pro.
Diabetic Exchanges: 5 lean meat, ½ fat.

✳

DID YOU KNOW?
You can use this mouthwatering seasoning mix for pork and chicken, too. Just put the oil, garlic, salt and pepper in a food processor and pulse a few times to create a quick rub that's ideal for grilling.

GRILLED BEEF CHIMICHANGAS

After making this dish, it instantly became my new go-to meal!

—JACKIE BURNS KETTLE FALLS, WA

PREP: 25 MIN. **GRILL:** 10 MIN.
MAKES: 6 SERVINGS

- 1 pound lean ground beef (90% lean)
- 1 small onion, chopped
- 2 garlic cloves, minced
- 1 can (4 ounces) chopped green chilies
- ¼ cup salsa
- ¼ teaspoon ground cumin
- 6 whole wheat tortillas (8 inches)
- ¾ cup shredded Monterey Jack cheese
  Reduced-fat sour cream and guacamole, optional

1. In a large skillet, cook beef, onion and garlic over medium heat for 6-8 minutes or until beef is no longer pink and onion is tender, breaking up beef into crumbles; drain. Stir in chilies, salsa and cumin.

2. Spoon ½ cup beef mixture across center of each tortilla; top with 2 tablespoons cheese. Fold bottom and sides of tortilla over filling and roll up.

3. Place chimichangas on grill rack, seam side down. Grill, covered, over medium-low heat 10-12 minutes or until crisp and browned, turning once. If desired, serve with sour cream and guacamole.

Per chimichanga without sour cream and guacamole: 295 cal., 12g fat (5g sat. fat), 60mg chol., 370mg sod., 25g carb. (1g sugars, 4g fiber), 22g pro.
Diabetic Exchanges: 2 lean meat, 1½ starch, 1 fat.

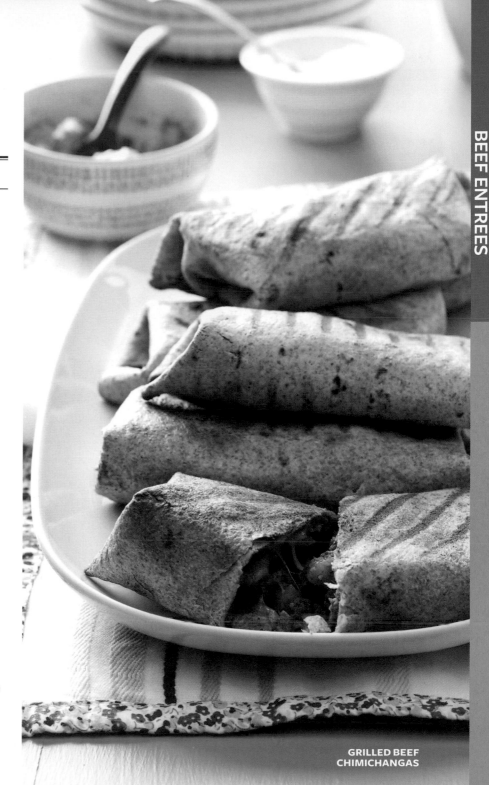

GRILLED BEEF CHIMICHANGAS

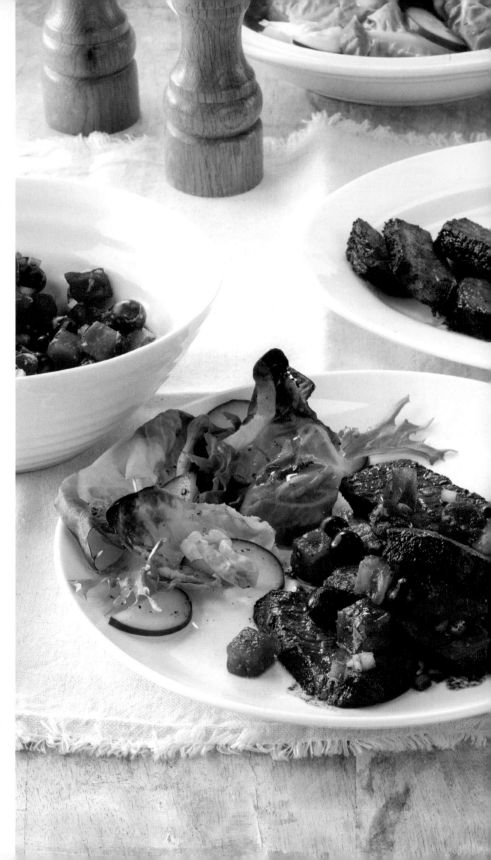

FAST FIX ▶

ANCHO GARLIC STEAKS WITH SUMMER SALSA

The first time I tasted this, I was amazed how well the berries and watermelon go with the peppery steak.

—VERONICA CALLAGHAN
GLASTONBURY, CT

START TO FINISH: 30 MIN.
MAKES: 4 SERVINGS

- 2 boneless beef top loin steaks (1¼ inches thick and 8 ounces each)
- 2 teaspoons ground ancho chili pepper
- 1 teaspoon garlic salt

SALSA

- 1 cup seeded diced watermelon
- 1 cup fresh blueberries
- 1 medium tomato, chopped
- ¼ cup finely chopped red onion
- 1 tablespoon minced fresh mint
- 1½ teaspoons grated fresh gingerroot
- ¼ teaspoon salt

1. Rub steaks with chili pepper and garlic salt. Grill, covered, over medium heat or broil 4 in. from heat 7-9 minutes on each side or until meat reaches desired doneness (for medium-rare, a thermometer should read 145°; medium, 160°).

2. In a bowl, combine salsa ingredients. Cut steak into slices; serve with salsa.

Notes: Top loin steak may be labeled as strip steak, Kansas City steak, New York strip steak, ambassador steak or boneless club steak in your region.

Per 3 ounces cooked beef with ½ cup salsa: 195 cal., 5g fat (2g sat. fat), 50mg chol., 442mg sod., 10g carb. (7g sugars, 2g fiber), 25g pro.

Diabetic Exchanges: 3 lean meat, ½ fruit.

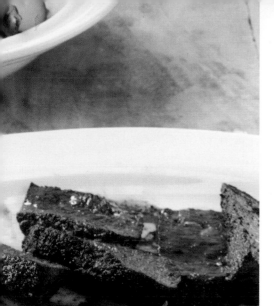

ANCHO GARLIC STEAKS WITH SUMMER SALSA

FAST FIX ▶

BARLEY BEEF BURGERS

I stirred cooked barley and barbecue sauce into hamburger patties to make them moist and flavorful. It's a smart way to work grains into a meal.

—**ROSELLA PETERS** GULL LAKE, SK

START TO FINISH: 30 MIN.
MAKES: 2 SERVINGS

- ½ cup water
- ¼ cup quick-cooking barley
- ½ small onion, halved
- 1 tablespoon barbecue sauce
- 1½ teaspoons all-purpose flour
- ¼ teaspoon salt
- ⅛ teaspoon pepper
- ½ pound lean ground beef
- 2 hamburger buns, split
    Optional toppings: lettuce leaves, tomato slices and onion slices

1. In a small saucepan, bring water to a boil. Stir in barley. Reduce heat; simmer, covered, 8-10 minutes or until barley is tender. Remove from heat; let stand 5 minutes. Cool slightly.
2. Place onion and barley in a food processor; process until finely chopped. Remove to a bowl; stir in the barbecue sauce, flour, salt and pepper. Add beef; mix lightly but thoroughly. Shape into two ½-in. thick patties.
3. Grill, covered, over medium heat for 4 5 minutes on each side or until a thermometer reads 160°. Serve on buns with toppings as desired.
Per burger without toppings: 395 cal., 12g fat (4g sat. fat), 69mg chol., 625mg sod., 42g carb. (5g sugars, 5g fiber), 29g pro.
Diabetic Exchanges: 3 lean meat, 2½ starch, 2 fat.

FAST FIX ▶

ITALIAN BEEF & SHELLS

I fix this supper when I'm pressed for time. It's as tasty as it is fast. Team it with salad, bread and fresh fruit for a healthy meal that really satisfies.

—**MIKE TCHOU** PEPPER PIKE, OH

START TO FINISH: 30 MIN.
MAKES: 4 SERVINGS

- 1½ cups uncooked medium pasta shells
- 1 pound lean ground beef (90% lean)
- 1 small onion, chopped
- 1 garlic clove, minced
- 1 jar (24 ounces) marinara sauce
- 1 small yellow summer squash, quartered and sliced
- 1 small zucchini, quartered and sliced
- ¼ cup dry red wine or reduced-sodium beef broth
- ½ teaspoon salt
- ½ teaspoon Italian seasoning
- ½ teaspoon pepper

1. Cook pasta according to package directions.
2. Meanwhile, in a Dutch oven, cook beef, onion and garlic over medium heat until meat is no longer pink; drain. Stir in the marinara sauce, squash, zucchini, wine and seasonings. Bring to a boil. Reduce heat; simmer, uncovered, for 10-15 minutes or until thickened. Drain pasta; stir into beef mixture and heat through.
Per 1¾ cups: 396 cal., 10g fat (4g sat. fat), 71mg chol., 644mg sod., 45g carb. (16g sugars, 5g fiber), 29g pro.
Diabetic Exchanges: 3 starch, 3 lean meat.

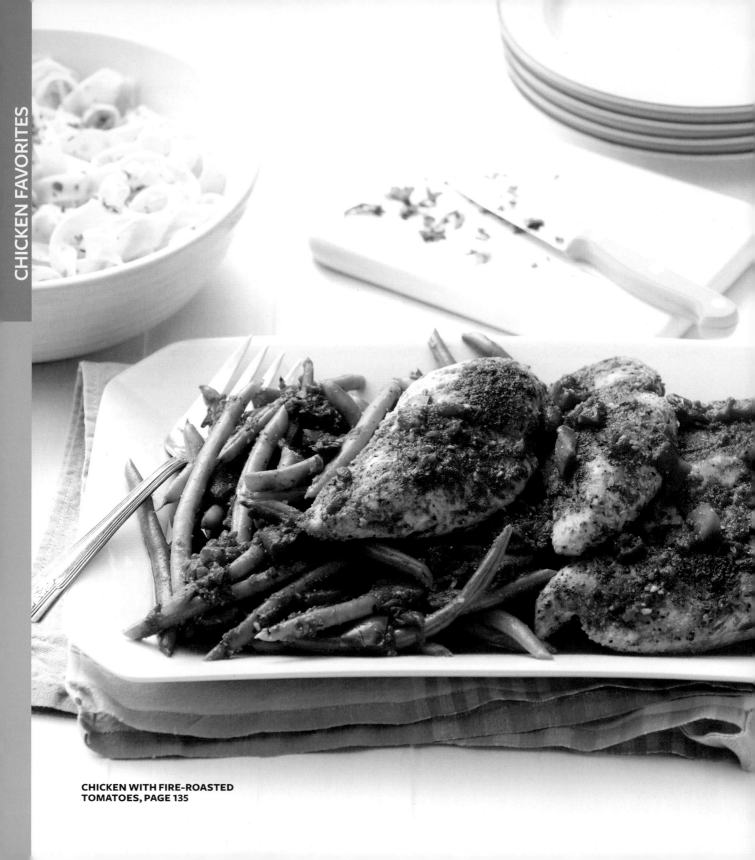

**CHICKEN WITH FIRE-ROASTED
TOMATOES, PAGE 135**

Chicken Favorites

Bird is the word when it comes to these recipes featuring everyone's favorite white meat. Tossed in a skillet with pasta or tucked in an enchilada, chicken is the basis for creations that are anything but ordinary.

FAST FIX
TAPENADE-STUFFED CHICKEN BREASTS

I created this recipe for my husband, who absolutely loves olives. Make a double batch of the olive tapenade and serve it with crackers as an appetizer.
—JESSICA LEVINSON NYACK, NY

START TO FINISH: 30 MIN.
MAKES: 4 SERVINGS

- 4 oil-packed sun-dried tomatoes
- 4 pitted Greek olives
- 4 pitted Spanish olives
- 4 pitted ripe olives
- ¼ cup roasted sweet red peppers, drained
- 4 garlic cloves, minced
- 1 tablespoon olive oil
- 2 teaspoons balsamic vinegar
- 4 boneless skinless chicken breast halves (6 ounces each)
  Grated Parmesan cheese

1. Place the first eight ingredients in a food processor; pulse until tomatoes and olives are coarsely chopped. Cut a pocket horizontally in the thickest part of each chicken breast. Fill with olive mixture; secure with toothpicks.

2. Lightly coat grill rack with cooking oil. Grill chicken, covered, over medium heat or broil 4 in. from heat for 8-10 minutes on each side or until a thermometer inserted in stuffing reads 165°. Sprinkle with cheese. Discard toothpicks before serving.

Per 1 stuffed chicken breast half without cheese: 264 cal., 11g fat (2g sat. fat), 94mg chol., 367mg sod., 5g carb. (1g sugars, 1g fiber), 35g pro.
Diabetic Exchanges: 5 lean meat, 1 fat.

ITALIAN SPAGHETTI WITH CHICKEN & ROASTED VEGETABLES

When I get a craving for homemade tomato sauce, I make a zesty batch to toss with chicken and veggies. The flavors do wonders for penne, too.
—CARLY CURTIN ELLICOTT CITY, MD

PREP: 25 MIN. • **COOK:** 25 MIN.
MAKES: 6 SERVINGS

- 3 plum tomatoes, seeded and chopped
- 2 medium zucchini, cubed
- 1 medium yellow summer squash, cubed
- 2 tablespoons olive oil, divided
- 2 teaspoons Italian seasoning, divided
- 8 ounces uncooked whole wheat spaghetti
- 1 pound boneless skinless chicken breasts, cubed
- ½ teaspoon garlic powder
- ½ cup reduced-sodium chicken broth
- ⅓ cup dry red wine or additional reduced-sodium chicken broth
- 4 cans (8 ounces each) no-salt-added tomato sauce
- 1 can (6 ounces) tomato paste
- ¼ cup minced fresh basil
- 2 tablespoons minced fresh oregano
- ¼ teaspoon salt
- 6 tablespoons shredded Parmesan cheese

1. Preheat oven to 425°. In a large bowl, combine tomatoes, zucchini and squash. Add 1 tablespoon oil and 1 teaspoon Italian seasoning. Transfer to a 15x10x1-in. baking pan coated with cooking spray. Bake 15-20 minutes or until tender.

2. Meanwhile, cook the spaghetti according to package directions. Sprinkle chicken with garlic powder and remaining Italian seasoning. In a large nonstick skillet, heat remaining oil over medium heat. Add chicken; cook until no longer pink. Remove from skillet.

3. Add broth and wine to skillet, stirring to loosen browned bits from pan. Stir in the tomato sauce, tomato paste, basil, oregano and salt. Bring to a boil. Return chicken to skillet. Reduce heat; simmer, covered, 4-6 minutes or until sauce is slightly thickened.

4. Drain spaghetti. Add spaghetti and vegetables to the tomato mixture; heat through. Sprinkle with cheese.

Per 1⅔ cups with 1 tablespoon cheese: 379 cal., 9g fat (2g sat. fat), 45mg chol., 345mg sod., 49g carb. (14g sugars, 8g fiber), 26g pro.
Diabetic Exchanges: 2½ starch, 2 lean meat, 2 vegetable, 1 fat.

✳

TEST KITCHEN TIP
Don't wash that pan! The sticky stuff left on the bottom after browning meat is called "fond," and it's a cook's best friend. Add a little liquid—water, juice, vinegar, stock, wine, brandy—and heat, scraping as it comes to a boil. Use this deglazed pan sauce to add deeper flavor and dimension to your cooking.

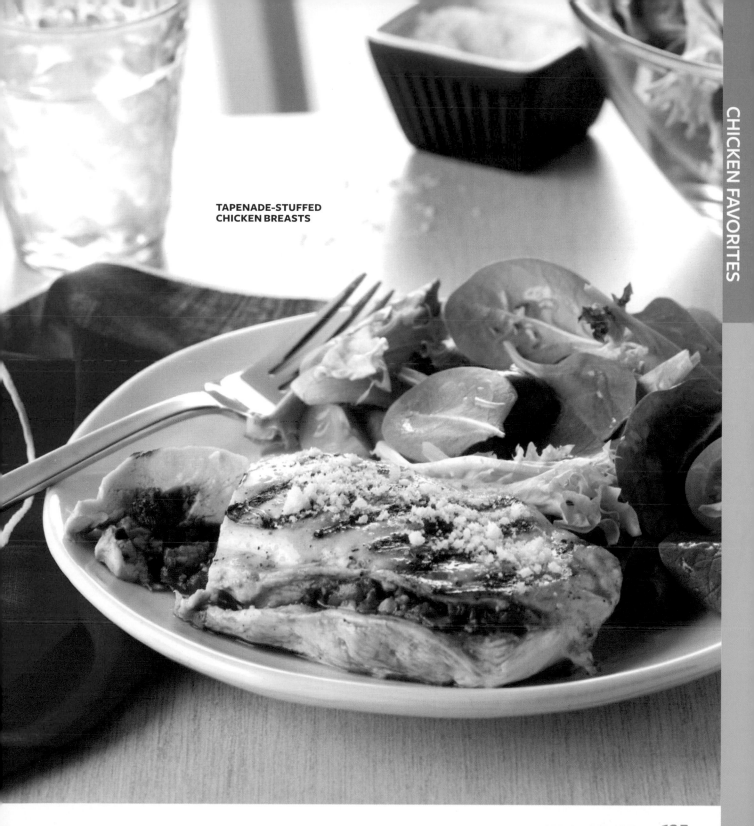

**TAPENADE-STUFFED
CHICKEN BREASTS**

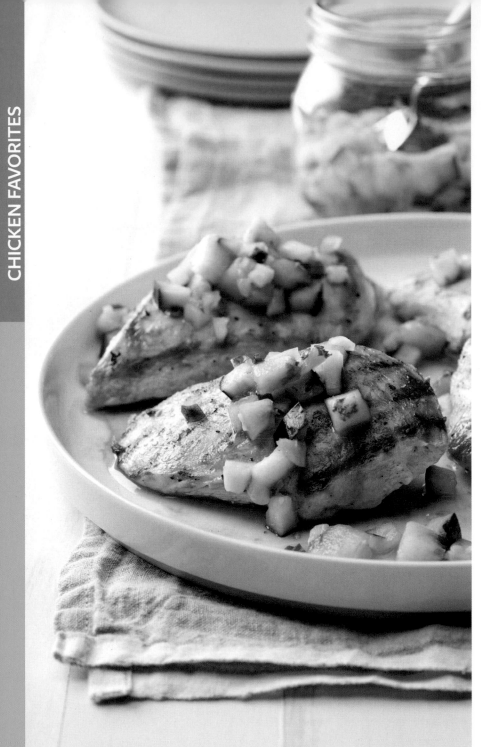

FAST FIX ▶

CHICKEN WITH PEACH-CUCUMBER SALSA

To keep our kitchen cool in summer, we grill chicken outdoors and then top it with a minty peach salsa that can easily be made ahead of time.

—JANIE COLLE HUTCHINSON, KS

START TO FINISH: 25 MIN.
MAKES: 4 SERVINGS

- 1½ cups chopped peeled fresh peaches (about 2 medium)
- ¾ cup chopped cucumber
- 4 tablespoons peach preserves, divided
- 3 tablespoons finely chopped red onion
- 1 teaspoon minced fresh mint
- ¾ teaspoon salt, divided
- 4 boneless skinless chicken breast halves (6 ounces each)
- ¼ teaspoon pepper

1. In a bowl, combine the peaches, cucumber, 2 tablespoons preserves, onion, mint and ¼ teaspoon salt.

2. Sprinkle chicken with pepper and remaining salt. On a lightly greased grill rack, grill chicken, covered, over medium heat 5 minutes. Turn; grill 7-9 minutes longer or until a thermometer reads 165°, brushing tops occasionally with remaining preserves. Serve with the salsa.

Per 1 chicken breast half with ½ cup salsa: 261 cal., 4g fat (1g sat. fat), 94mg chol., 525mg sod., 20g carb. (17g sugars, 1g fiber), 35g pro.
Diabetic Exchanges: 5 lean meat, ½ starch, ½ fruit.

CHICKEN WITH PEACH-CUCUMBER SALSA

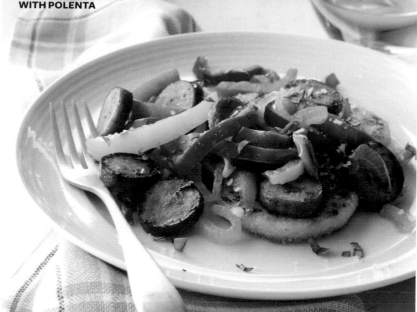

CHICKEN SAUSAGES
WITH POLENTA

FAST FIX

SPICY BARBECUED CHICKEN

I serve this zesty chicken with corn on the cob, grilled and basil-buttered.

—RITA WINTRODE CORRYTON, TN

START TO FINISH: 30 MIN.
MAKES: 8 SERVINGS

- 1 tablespoon canola oil
- 2 garlic cloves, minced
- ½ cup chili sauce
- 3 tablespoons brown sugar
- 2 teaspoons salt-free seasoning blend, divided
- ¾ teaspoon cayenne pepper, divided
- 2 teaspoons ground mustard
- 2 teaspoons chili powder
- 8 boneless skinless chicken breast halves (4 ounces each)

1. In a small saucepan, heat oil over medium heat. Add garlic; cook and stir 1 minute. Add chili sauce, brown sugar, 1 teaspoon seasoning blend and ¼ teaspoon cayenne. Bring to a boil; cook and stir for 1 minute. Remove from the heat.
2. In a small bowl, mix mustard, chili powder and remaining seasoning blend and cayenne; rub over chicken. Lightly coat grill rack with cooking oil.
3. Grill chicken, covered, over medium heat for 4 minutes. Turn; grill about 4-6 minutes longer or until a meat thermometer reads 165°, brushing chicken tops occasionally with the chili sauce mixture.

Per 1 chicken breast half : 179 cal., 5g fat (1g sat. fat), 63mg chol., 293mg sod., 10g carb. (8g sugars, 0 fiber), 23g pro.
Diabetic Exchanges: 3 lean meat, ½ starch, ½ fat.

FAST FIX

CHICKEN SAUSAGES WITH POLENTA

I get a kick out of serving this dish—everyone's always on time for dinner when they know it's on the menu.

—ANGELA SPENGLER TAMPA, FL

START TO FINISH: 30 MIN.
MAKES: 6 SERVINGS

- 4 teaspoons olive oil, divided
- 1 tube (1 pound) polenta, cut into ½-inch slices
- 1 each medium green, sweet red and yellow peppers, thinly sliced
- 1 medium onion, thinly sliced
- 1 package (12 ounces) fully cooked Italian chicken sausage links, thinly sliced
- ¼ cup grated Parmesan cheese
- 1 tablespoon minced fresh basil

1. In a large nonstick skillet, heat 2 teaspoons oil over medium heat. Add the polenta; cook 9-11 minutes on each side or until golden brown. Keep warm.
2. Meanwhile, in another large skillet, heat remaining oil over medium-high heat. Add peppers and onion; cook and stir until tender. Remove from pan.
3. Add sausages to same pan; cook and stir for 4-5 minutes or until browned. Return pepper mixture to pan; heat through. Serve with polenta; sprinkle with cheese and basil.

Per ⅔ cup sausage mixture with 2 slices polenta: 212 cal., 9g fat (2g sat. fat), 46mg chol., 628mg sod., 19g carb. (4g sugars, 2g fiber), 13g pro.
Diabetic Exchanges: 2 lean meat, 1 starch, 1 vegetable, ½ fat.

FAST FIX ▶

STRAWBERRY MINT CHICKEN

We love this with freshly picked strawberries and spring greens.
—**ALICIA DUERST** MENOMONIE, WI

START TO FINISH: 30 MIN.
MAKES: 4 SERVINGS

- 1 tablespoon cornstarch
- 1 tablespoon sugar
- ⅛ teaspoon ground nutmeg
- ⅛ teaspoon pepper
- ½ cup water
- 1 cup fresh strawberries, chopped
- ½ cup white wine or grape juice
- 2 teaspoons minced fresh mint

CHICKEN

- 4 boneless skinless chicken breast halves (6 ounces each)
- ½ teaspoon salt
- ¼ teaspoon pepper
  Sliced green onion

1. In a saucepan, mix the first five ingredients until smooth; stir in the strawberries and wine. Bring to a boil. Reduce heat; simmer, uncovered, 3-5 minutes or until thickened, stirring occasionally. Remove from heat; stir in the mint.

2. Sprinkle the chicken with salt and pepper. On a lightly greased grill rack, grill chicken, covered, over medium heat 5-7 minutes on each side or until a thermometer reads 165°; brush occasionally with ¼ cup sauce during the last 4 minutes. Serve with remaining sauce. Sprinkle with green onion.

Per 1 chicken breast half with ¼ cup sauce: 224 cal., 4g fat (1g sat. fat), 94mg chol., 378mg sod., 8g carb. (5g sugars, 1g fiber), 35g pro.
Diabetic Exchanges: 5 lean meat, ½ starch.

SAUSAGE CHICKEN JAMBALAYA

If you enjoy entertaining, this jambalaya is a terrific one-pot meal for feeding a hungry crowd. It has all the classic flavor but is easier on the waistline.
—**BETTY BENTHIN** GRASS VALLEY, CA

PREP: 20 MIN. • **COOK:** 30 MIN.
MAKES: 9 SERVINGS

- 6 fully cooked spicy chicken sausage links (3 ounces each), cut into ½-inch slices
- ½ pound chicken tenderloins, cut into ½-inch slices
- 1 tablespoon olive oil
- 3 celery ribs, chopped
- 1 large onion, chopped
- 2¾ cups chicken broth
- 1 can (14½ ounces) diced tomatoes, undrained
- 1½ cups uncooked long grain rice
- 1 teaspoon dried thyme
- 1 teaspoon Cajun seasoning

1. In a large saucepan, saute sausage and chicken in oil for 5 minutes. Add celery and onion; saute 6-8 minutes longer or until vegetables are tender. Stir in the broth, tomatoes, rice, thyme and Cajun seasoning.

2. Bring to a boil. Reduce heat; cover and simmer for 15-20 minutes or until rice is tender. Let stand for 5 minutes.

Per 1 cup: 259 cal., 7g fat (2g sat. fat), 60mg chol., 761mg sod., 31g carb. (3g sugars, 2g fiber), 19g pro.
Diabetic Exchanges: 2 lean meat, 1½ starch, 1 vegetable, ½ fat.

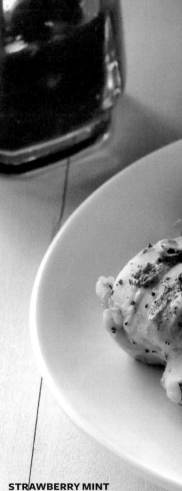

STRAWBERRY MINT CHICKEN

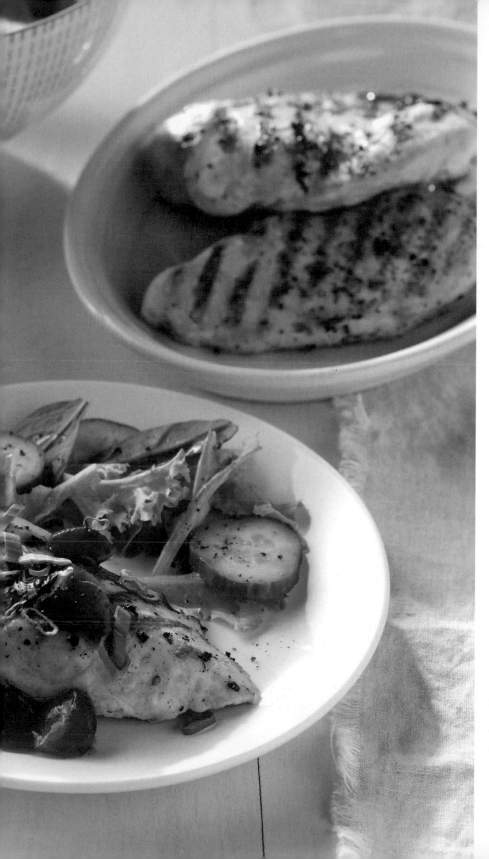

⑤INGREDIENTS

MARINATED CHICKEN & ZUCCHINI KABOBS

These tasty and healthy kabobs are a favorite in our family, and they're so easy to make! Change them up with turkey tenderloins and other veggies, such as summer squash or sweet bell peppers.

—**TAMMY SLADE** STANSBURY PARK, UT

PREP: 25 MIN. + MARINATING
GRILL: 10 MIN. • **MAKES:** 8 SERVINGS

- ¾ cup lemon-lime soda
- ½ cup reduced-sodium soy sauce
- ½ cup canola oil, divided
- 2 pounds boneless skinless chicken breasts or turkey breast tenderloins, cut into 1-inch cubes
- 3 medium zucchini, cut into 1-inch pieces
- 2 medium red onions, cut into 1-inch pieces
- ½ teaspoon salt
- ¼ teaspoon pepper

1. In a large resealable plastic bag, combine soda, soy sauce and ¼ cup oil. Add chicken; seal bag and turn to coat. Refrigerate 8 hours or overnight.

2. Drain chicken, discarding marinade. On eight metal or soaked wooden skewers, alternately thread chicken and vegetables. Brush vegetables with the remaining oil; sprinkle with salt and pepper. On a greased grill, cook kabobs, covered, over medium heat for 8-10 minutes or until chicken is no longer pink and vegetables are tender, turning occasionally.

Per kabob: 224 cal., 11g fat (1g sat. fat), 63mg chol., 344mg sod., 6g carb. (3g sugars, 1g fiber), 24g pro.

Diabetic Exchanges: 3 lean meat, 2 fat, 1 vegetable.

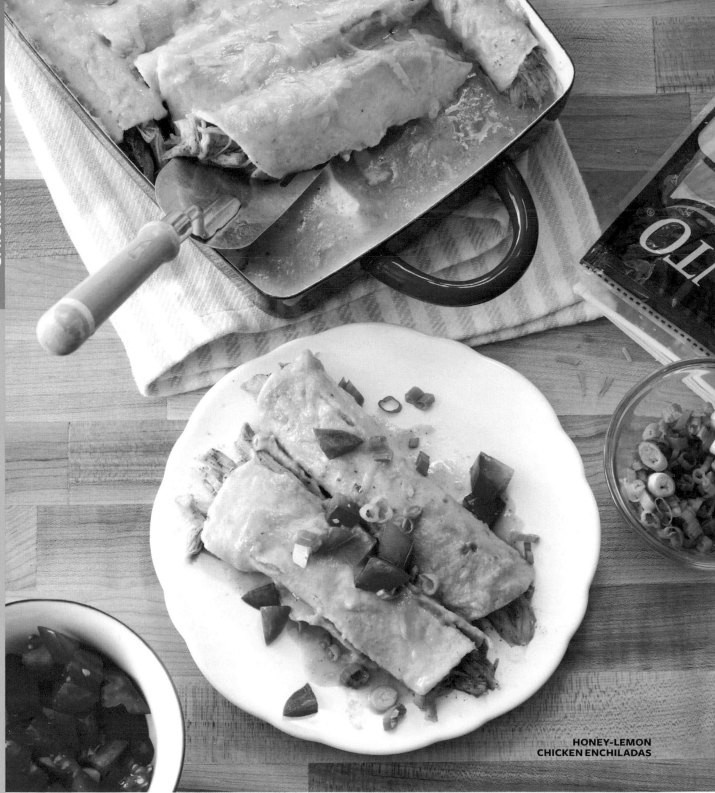

HONEY-LEMON CHICKEN ENCHILADAS

FAST FIX
HONEY-LEMON CHICKEN ENCHILADAS

The chicken filling works for soft tacos too: either way my family devours it.

—**KRISTI MOAK** GILBERT, AZ

START TO FINISH: 30 MIN.
MAKES: 6 SERVINGS

- ¼ cup honey
- 2 tablespoons lemon or lime juice
- 1 tablespoon canola oil
- 2 teaspoons chili powder
- ¼ teaspoon garlic powder
- 3 cups shredded cooked chicken breast
- 2 cans (10 ounces each) green enchilada sauce
- 12 corn tortillas (6 inches), warmed
- ¾ cup shredded reduced-fat cheddar cheese
  Sliced green onions and chopped tomatoes, optional

1. In a large bowl, whisk the first five ingredients. Add chicken and toss to coat. Pour 1 can enchilada sauce into a greased microwave-safe 11x7-in. dish. Place ¼ cup chicken mixture off center on each tortilla. Roll up and place in prepared dish, seam side down. Top with remaining enchilada sauce.

2. Microwave, covered, on high for 11-13 minutes or until heated through. Sprinkle with cheese. If desired, top with green onions and tomatoes.

Note: This recipe was tested in a full-size 1,100-watt microwave. If your microwave does not accommodate an 11x7-in. dish, bake casserole, covered, in a preheated 400° oven for 25-30 minutes or until heated through. Top as directed.

Per 2 enchiladas without toppings: 349 cal., 11g fat (3g sat. fat), 64mg chol., 698mg sod., 39g carb. (14g sugars, 3g fiber), 27g pro.
Diabetic Exchanges: 3 lean meat, 2½ starch.

⑤INGREDIENTS **FAST FIX**
APPLE-GLAZED CHICKEN THIGHS

My pickatarian child is choosy but willing to eat this chicken glazed with apple juice and thyme. I dish it up with mashed potatoes and green beans.

—**KERRY PICARD** SPOKANE, WA

START TO FINISH: 25 MIN.
MAKES: 6 SERVINGS

- 6 boneless skinless chicken thighs (1½ pounds)
- ¾ teaspoon seasoned salt
- ¼ teaspoon pepper
- 1 tablespoon canola oil
- 1 cup unsweetened apple juice
- 1 teaspoon minced fresh thyme or ¼ teaspoon dried thyme

1. Sprinkle chicken with seasoned salt and pepper. In a large skillet, heat oil over medium-high heat. Brown chicken on both sides. Remove from pan.

2. Add juice and thyme to skillet. Bring to a boil, stirring to loosen browned bits from pan; cook until liquid is reduced by half. Return chicken to the pan; cook, covered, over medium heat 3-4 minutes longer or until a thermometer inserted in chicken reads 170°.

Per 1 chicken thigh with about 1 tablespoon glaze: 204 cal., 11g fat (2g sat. fat), 76mg chol., 255mg sod., 5g carb. (4g sugars, 0 fiber), 21g pro.
Diabetic Exchanges: 3 lean meat, ½ fat.

FAST FIX
BACON & SWISS CHICKEN SANDWICHES

Dip your sandwich in the extra honey-mustard sauce—so good.

—**MARILYN MOBERG** PAPILLION, NE

START TO FINISH: 25 MIN.
MAKES: 4 SERVINGS

- ¼ cup reduced-fat mayonnaise
- 1 tablespoon Dijon mustard
- 1 tablespoon honey
- 4 boneless skinless chicken breast halves (4 ounces each)
- ½ teaspoon Montreal steak seasoning
- 4 slices Swiss cheese
- 4 whole wheat hamburger buns, split
- 2 bacon strips, cooked and crumbled
  Lettuce leaves and tomato slices, optional

1. In a small bowl, mix mayonnaise, mustard and honey. Pound chicken with a meat mallet to ½-in. thickness. Sprinkle chicken with steak seasoning. Grill chicken, covered, over medium heat or broil 4 in. from heat 4-6 minutes on each side or until a thermometer reads 165°. Top with cheese during the last 1 minute of cooking.

2. Grill buns over medium heat, cut side down, for 30-60 seconds or until toasted. Serve chicken on buns with bacon, mayonnaise mixture and, if desired, lettuce and tomato.

Per sandwich: 410 cal., 17g fat (6g sat. fat), 91mg chol., 667mg sod., 29g carb. (9g sugars, 3g fiber), 34g pro.
Diabetic Exchanges: 4 lean meat, 2 starch, 2 fat.

CARIBBEAN DELIGHT

When hot summer nights drive me out of the kitchen, I head for the grill with this recipe. Along with a salad, my family loves this not-so-subtle spicy chicken.
—LEIGH ANN GRADY MURRAY, KY

PREP: 5 MIN. + MARINATING
GRILL: 10 MIN. • **MAKES:** 6 SERVINGS

- 2 tablespoons finely chopped onion
- ¼ cup butter, cubed
- 2 garlic cloves, minced
- ⅓ cup white vinegar
- ⅓ cup lime juice
- ¼ cup sugar
- 2 tablespoons curry powder
- 1 teaspoon salt
- ¼ to ½ teaspoon cayenne pepper
- 6 boneless skinless chicken breast halves (4 ounces each)

1. In a small saucepan, saute onion in butter until tender. Add garlic; cook 1 minute longer. Stir in the vinegar, lime juice, sugar, curry, salt and cayenne. Place chicken in a large resealable plastic bag; add onion mixture. Seal bag and turn to coat. Refrigerate chicken for at least 2 hours.
2. Drain and discard marinade. Grill chicken, uncovered, over medium heat for 5-7 minutes on each side or until a thermometer reads 170°.

Per 1 chicken breast half : 162 cal., 5g fat (2g sat. fat), 70mg chol., 224mg sod., 4g carb. (3g sugars, 0 fiber), 23g pro.
Diabetic Exchanges: 3 lean meat, ½ fat.

FAST FIX ▶

ITALIAN SAUSAGE & PROVOLONE SKEWERS

My husband made sausage and veggie kabobs when we didn't have buns to make classic sausage bombers. Grill 'em up, then add cheese cubes.
—CINDY HILLIARD KENOSHA, WI

START TO FINISH: 30 MIN.
MAKES: 8 SERVINGS

- 1 large onion
- 1 large sweet red pepper
- 1 large green pepper
- 2 cups cherry tomatoes
- 1 tablespoon olive oil
- ½ teaspoon pepper
- ¼ teaspoon salt
- 2 packages (12 ounces each) fully cooked Italian chicken sausage links, cut into 1¼-inch slices
- 16 cubes provolone cheese (¾ inch each)

1. Cut onion and peppers into 1-in. pieces; place in a large bowl. Add the tomatoes, oil, pepper and salt; toss to coat. On 16 metal or soaked wooden skewers, alternately thread sausage and vegetables.
2. Grill, covered, over medium heat 8-10 minutes or until sausage is heated through and vegetables are tender, turning occasionally. Remove kabobs from grill; thread one cheese cube onto each kabob.

Per 2 kabobs: 220 cal., 13g fat (5g sat. fat), 75mg chol., 682mg sod., 7g carb. (3g sugars, 2g fiber), 20g pro.
Diabetic Exchanges: 3 medium-fat meat, 1 vegetable.

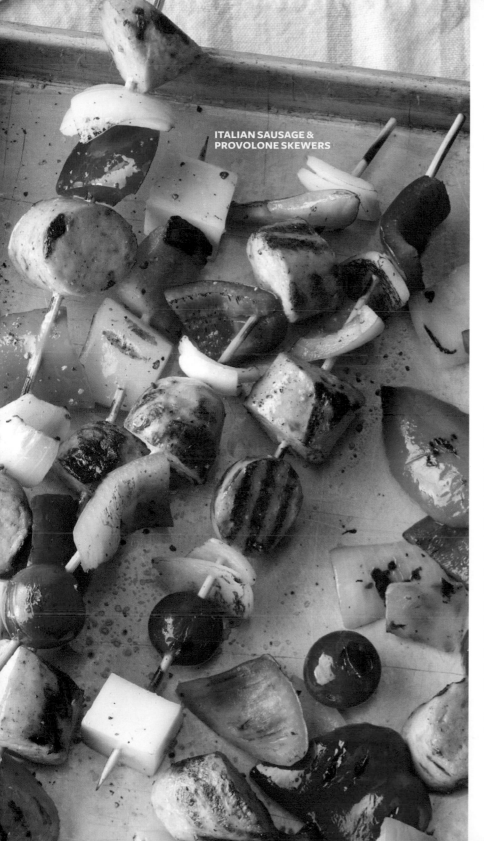

ITALIAN SAUSAGE &
PROVOLONE SKEWERS

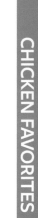

WILD RICE SALAD

I modified a recipe I received years ago and came up with this versatile salad.
—**ROBIN THOMPSON** ROSEVILLE, CA

PREP: 1¼ HOURS + CHILLING
MAKES: 4 SERVINGS

- 3 cups water
- 1 cup uncooked wild rice
- 2 chicken bouillon cubes
- 4½ teaspoons butter
- 1 cup cut fresh green beans
- 1 cup cubed cooked chicken breast
- 1 medium tomato, chopped
- 1 bunch green onions, sliced
- ¼ cup rice vinegar
- 1 tablespoon sesame oil
- 1 garlic clove, minced
- ½ teaspoon dried tarragon
- ¼ teaspoon pepper

1. In a large saucepan, bring water, rice, bouillon and butter to a boil. Reduce heat; cover and simmer for 45-60 minutes or until rice is tender. Drain if necessary; transfer to a large bowl and cool completely.
2. Place the green beans in a steamer basket; place in a small saucepan over 1 in. of water. Bring to a boil; cover and steam for 8-10 minutes or until beans are crisp-tender.
3. Add chicken, tomato, onions and green beans to the rice; stir until blended. Combine the remaining ingredients; drizzle over mixture and toss to coat. Refrigerate until chilled.
Per 1½ cups: 330 cal., 10g fat (4g sat. fat), 39mg chol., 618mg sod., 43g carb. (3g sugars, 4g fiber), 18g pro.
Diabetic Exchanges: 2 starch, 2 fat, 1 lean meat, 1 vegetable.

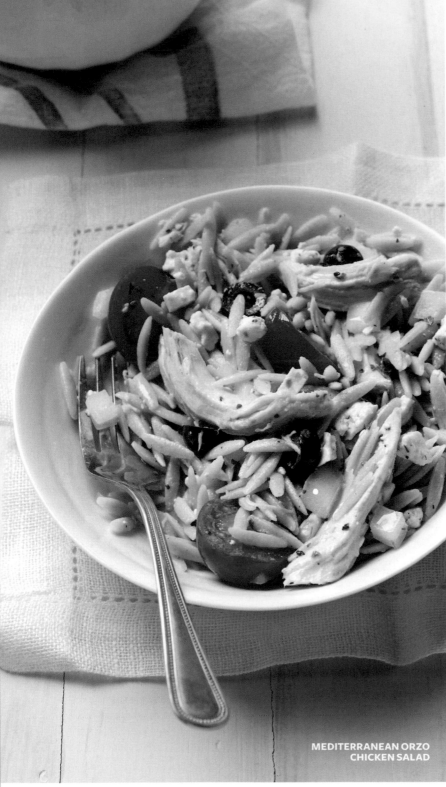

MEDITERRANEAN ORZO CHICKEN SALAD

MEDITERRANEAN ORZO CHICKEN SALAD

On hot days, I toss this together for a cool supper. The lemon dressing is so refreshing. Try it with grilled chicken.

—SUSAN KIEBOAM STREETSBORO, OH

START TO FINISH: 25 MIN.
MAKES: 6 SERVINGS

- 2 cups uncooked whole wheat orzo pasta
- 2 cups shredded rotisserie chicken
- 10 cherry tomatoes, halved
- ½ cup crumbled tomato and basil feta cheese
- 1 can (2¼ ounces) sliced ripe olives, drained
- ¼ cup chopped sweet onion
- ¼ cup olive oil
- 2 tablespoons lemon juice
- ½ teaspoon salt
- ¼ teaspoon dried oregano

1. Cook pasta according to package directions. Drain pasta; rinse with cold water and drain well.

2. In a large bowl, combine the pasta, chicken, tomatoes, cheese, olives and onion. In a small bowl, whisk remaining ingredients until blended. Drizzle over salad; toss to coat.

Per 1 cup: 397 cal., 16g fat (3g sat. fat), 47mg chol., 407mg sod., 40g carb. (1g sugars, 10g fiber), 22g pro.

Diabetic Exchanges: 3 lean meat, 2½ starch, 2 fat.

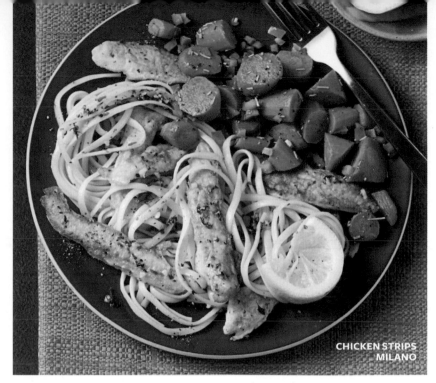

CHICKEN STRIPS MILANO

FAST FIX
CHICKEN STRIPS MILANO

A dear friend shared this recipe a few years ago. Since then, I've prepared it for both family dinners and get-togethers.
—**LARA PRIEST** GANSEVOORT, NY

START TO FINISH: 20 MIN.
MAKES: 6 SERVINGS

- 12 ounces linguine
- 1 tablespoon minced garlic
- 4½ teaspoons plus 2 tablespoons olive oil, divided
- ¾ teaspoon dried parsley flakes
- ¾ teaspoon pepper, divided
- ¼ cup all-purpose flour
- 1 teaspoon dried basil
- ½ teaspoon salt
- 2 large eggs
- 1½ pounds boneless skinless chicken breasts, cut into strips

1. Cook the linguine according to package directions.
2. Meanwhile, in a large skillet, saute garlic in 4½ teaspoons oil for 1 minute. Stir in parsley and ½ teaspoon pepper. Remove to a small bowl and set aside.
3. In a shallow bowl, combine the flour, basil, salt and remaining pepper. In another shallow bowl, whisk the eggs. Dredge chicken strips in flour mixture, then dip in eggs.
4. In the same skillet, cook and stir chicken in remaining oil over medium-high heat for 8-10 minutes or until no longer pink.
5. Drain linguine; place on a serving platter. Pour garlic mixture over linguine and toss to coat; top with chicken.
Per 3 ounces cooked chicken with ¾ cup linguine: 441 cal., 14g fat (3g sat. fat), 133mg chol., 278mg sod., 46g carb. (2g sugars, 2g fiber), 33g pro.
Diabetic Exchanges: 3 starch, 3 lean meat, 1½ fat.

FAST FIX
CHICKEN WITH FIRE-ROASTED TOMATOES

With the colors and flavors of Italy, my chicken is so easy and impressive!
—**MARGARET WILSON** SAN BERNARDINO, CA

START TO FINISH: 30 MIN.
MAKES: 4 SERVINGS

- 2 tablespoons salt-free garlic herb seasoning blend
- ½ teaspoon salt
- ¼ teaspoon Italian seasoning
- ¼ teaspoon pepper
- ⅛ teaspoon crushed red pepper flakes, optional
- 4 boneless skinless chicken breast halves (6 ounces each)
- 1 tablespoon olive oil
- 1 can (14½ ounces) fire-roasted diced tomatoes, undrained
- ¾ pound fresh green beans, trimmed
- 2 tablespoons water
- 1 tablespoon butter
  Hot cooked pasta, optional

1. Mix the first five ingredients; sprinkle over both sides of chicken breasts. In a large skillet, heat oil over medium heat. Brown the chicken on both sides. Add tomatoes; bring to a boil. Reduce heat; simmer, covered, 10-12 minutes or until a thermometer inserted in chicken reads 165°.
2. Meanwhile, in a 2-qt. microwave-safe dish, combine green beans and water; microwave, covered, on high for 3-4 minutes or just until tender. Drain.
3. Remove chicken from skillet; keep warm. Stir the butter and beans into tomato mixture. Serve with chicken and, if desired, pasta.
Per 1 chicken breast half with 1 cup bean mixture: 294 cal., 10g fat (3g sat. fat), 102mg chol., 681mg sod., 12g carb. (5g sugars, 4g fiber), 37g pro.
Diabetic Exchanges: 5 lean meat, 1 vegetable, 1 fat.

GRECIAN PASTA & CHICKEN SKILLET

Here's a Greek-inspired pasta that is lemony, herby and, thankfully, easy!
—ROXANNE CHAN ALBANY, CA

PREP: 30 MIN. • **COOK:** 10 MIN
MAKES: 4 SERVINGS

- 1 can (14½ ounces) reduced-sodium chicken broth
- 1 can (14½ ounces) no-salt-added diced tomatoes, undrained
- ¾ pound boneless skinless chicken breasts, cut into 1-inch pieces
- ½ cup white wine or water
- 1 garlic clove, minced
- ½ teaspoon dried oregano
- 4 ounces multigrain thin spaghetti
- 1 jar (7½ ounces) marinated quartered artichoke hearts, drained and coarsely chopped
- 2 cups fresh baby spinach
- ¼ cup roasted sweet red pepper strips
- ¼ cup sliced ripe olives
- 1 green onion, finely chopped
- 2 tablespoons minced fresh parsley
- ½ teaspoon grated lemon peel
- 2 tablespoons lemon juice
- 1 tablespoon olive oil
- ½ teaspoon pepper
  Crumbled reduced-fat feta cheese, optional

1. In a large skillet, combine the first six ingredients; add spaghetti. Bring to a boil. Cook 5-7 minutes or until chicken is no longer pink and spaghetti is tender.
2. Stir in artichoke hearts, spinach, red pepper, olives, green onion, parsley, lemon peel, lemon juice, oil and pepper. Cook and stir 2-3 minutes or until spinach is wilted. If desired, sprinkle with cheese.

Per 1½ cups: 373 cal., 15g fat (3g sat. fat), 47mg chol., 658mg sod., 30g carb. (8g sugars, 4g fiber), 25g pro.
Diabetic Exchanges: 2 starch, 2 lean meat, 2 fat, 1 vegetable.

FAST FIX
CHICKEN CUCUMBER BOATS

I've tended a garden for decades, and these colorful boats made from cucumbers hold my fresh tomatoes, peas and dill. It's absolute veggie-garden greatness for lunch or dinner.
—RONNA FARLEY ROCKVILLE, MD

START TO FINISH: 15 MIN.
MAKES: 2 SERVINGS

- 2 medium cucumbers
- ½ cup fat-free plain Greek yogurt
- 2 tablespoons mayonnaise
- ½ teaspoon garlic salt
- 3 teaspoons snipped fresh dill, divided
- 1 cup chopped cooked chicken breast
- 1 cup chopped seeded tomato (about 1 large), divided
- ½ cup fresh or frozen peas, thawed

1. Cut each cucumber lengthwise in half; scoop out pulp, leaving a ¼-in. shell. In a bowl, mix yogurt, mayonnaise, garlic salt and 1 teaspoon dill; gently stir in chicken, ¾ cup tomato and peas.
2. Spoon into cucumber shells. Top with the remaining tomato and dill.
Per 2 filled cucumber halves: 322 cal., 13g fat (2g sat. fat), 59mg chol.,398mg sod., 18g carb. (10g sugars, 6g fiber), 34g pro.
Diabetic Exchanges: 4 lean meat, 2 vegetable, 2 fat, ½ starch.

SPICY ROASTED SAUSAGE, POTATOES & PEPPERS

My hearty sheet-pan dinner has gotten a tasty reputation. People often ask for the recipe.
—LAURIE SLEDGE BRANDON, MS

PREP: 20 MIN. • **BAKE:** 30 MIN.
MAKES: 4 SERVINGS

- 1 pound potatoes (about 2 medium), peeled and cut into ½-inch cubes
- 1 package (12 ounces) fully cooked andouille chicken sausage links or flavor of your choice, cut into 1-inch pieces
- 1 medium red onion, cut into wedges
- 1 medium sweet red pepper, cut into 1-inch pieces
- 1 medium green pepper, cut into 1-inch pieces
- ½ cup pickled pepper rings
- 1 tablespoon olive oil
- ½ to 1 teaspoon Creole seasoning
- ¼ teaspoon pepper

1. Preheat oven to 400°. In a large bowl, combine the potatoes, sausage, onion, red pepper, green pepper and pepper rings. Mix oil, Creole seasoning and pepper; drizzle over the potato mixture and toss to coat.
2. Transfer to a 15x10x1-in. baking pan coated with cooking spray. Roast 30-35 minutes or until vegetables are tender, stirring occasionally.
Per 1½ cups: 257 cal., 11g fat (3g sat. fat), 65mg chol., 759mg sod., 24g carb. (5g sugars, 3g fiber), 17g pro.
Diabetic Exchanges: 3 lean meat, 1 starch, 1 vegetable, 1 fat.

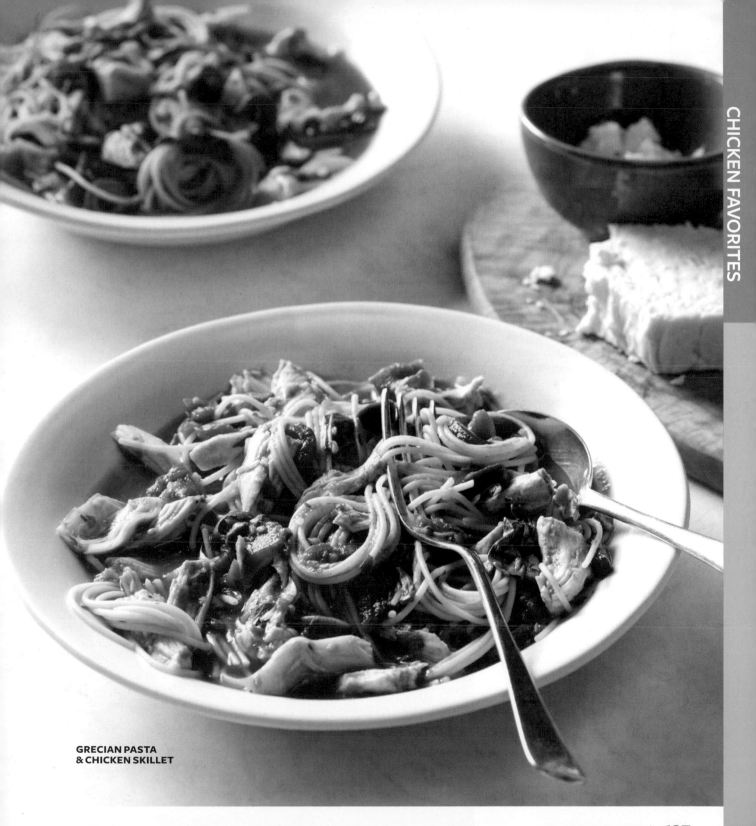

**GRECIAN PASTA
& CHICKEN SKILLET**

(5) INGREDIENTS

PESTO RICE-STUFFED CHICKEN

Juicy stuffed chicken is light, fresh and looks extra-special. The quick prep lets it fit right into your busy schedule. Substitute shredded cheese for the pesto if you have picky eaters.

—**RACHEL DION** PORT CHARLOTTE, FL

PREP: 20 MIN. • **BAKE:** 20 MIN.
MAKES: 8 SERVINGS

- ¾ cup uncooked instant rice
- ½ cup chopped seeded tomato
- ¼ cup prepared pesto
- ⅛ teaspoon salt
- 8 boneless skinless chicken breast halves (6 ounces each)
- 2 tablespoons canola oil, divided

1. Preheat oven to 375°. Cook rice according to package directions.

2. In a small bowl, combine tomato, pesto, salt and rice. Cut a pocket horizontally in the thickest part of each chicken breast. Fill each with 3 tablespoons rice mixture; secure with toothpicks.

3. In a large skillet, heat 1 tablespoon oil over medium-high heat. In batches, brown chicken breasts on each side, adding additional oil as needed. Transfer to a greased 15x10x1-in. baking pan.

4. Bake 18-22 minutes or until chicken is no longer pink. Discard toothpicks before serving.

Per 1 stuffed chicken breast half: 278 cal., 10g fat (2g sat. fat), 94mg chol., 210mg sod., 9g carb. (1g sugars, 0 fiber), 35g pro.

Diabetic Exchanges: 5 lean meat, 1 fat, ½ starch.

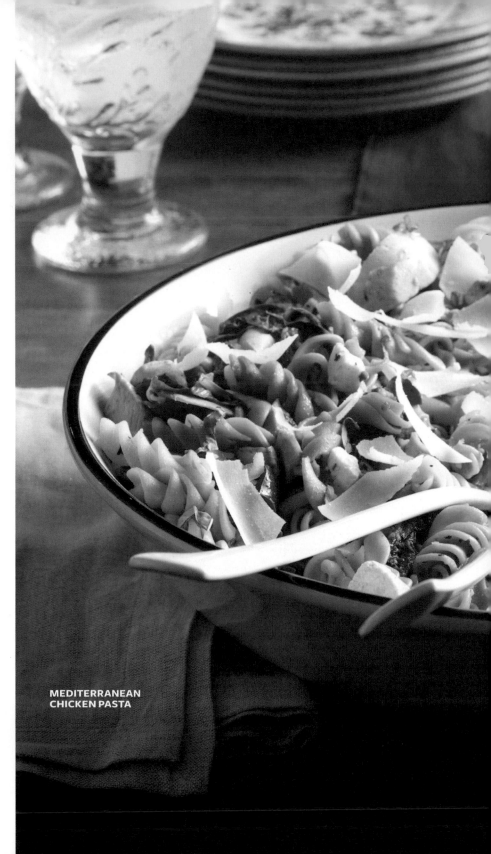

MEDITERRANEAN CHICKEN PASTA

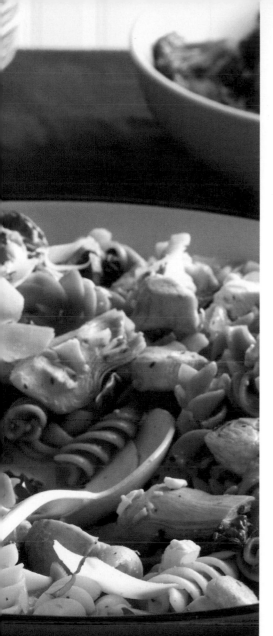

MEDITERRANEAN CHICKEN PASTA

On special days, I make this cheesy pasta bake loaded with chicken and all sorts of veggies. To go vegetarian, use veggie stock and instead of chicken, chickpeas.

—LIZ BELLVILLE JACKSONVILLE, NC

PREP: 25 MIN. • **COOK:** 20 MIN.
MAKES: 8 SERVINGS

- 1 package (12 ounces) uncooked tricolor spiral pasta
- 2 tablespoons olive oil, divided
- 1 pound boneless skinless chicken breasts, cut into ½-inch pieces
- 1 large sweet red pepper, chopped
- 1 medium onion, chopped
- 3 garlic cloves, peeled and thinly sliced
- 1 cup white wine or reduced-sodium chicken broth
- ¼ cup julienned soft sun-dried tomatoes (not packed in oil)
- 1 teaspoon dried basil
- 1 teaspoon Italian seasoning
- ½ teaspoon salt
- ¼ teaspoon crushed red pepper flakes
- ¼ teaspoon pepper
- 1 can (14½ ounces) reduced-sodium chicken broth
- 1 can (14 ounces) water-packed quartered artichoke hearts, drained
- 1 package (6 ounces) fresh baby spinach
- 1 cup (4 ounces) crumbled feta cheese
  Thinly sliced fresh basil leaves and shaved Parmesan cheese, optional

1. Cook pasta according to package directions. In a 6-qt. stockpot, heat 1 tablespoon oil over medium-high heat. Add chicken; cook and stir 4-6 minutes or until no longer pink. Remove from the pot.

2. In the same pot, heat remaining oil over medium heat. Add red pepper and onion; cook and stir for 4-5 minutes or until onion is tender. Add garlic; cook 1 minute longer. Add wine, sun-dried tomatoes and seasonings; bring to a boil. Reduce heat; simmer 5 minutes, stirring to loosen browned bits from the pot.

3. Add broth and artichoke hearts; return to a boil. Stir in spinach and chicken; cook just until spinach wilts.

4. Drain pasta; stir into the chicken mixture. Stir in feta cheese. If desired, top servings with the basil leaves and Parmesan cheese.

Note: This recipe was tested with sun-dried tomatoes that can be used without soaking. When using other sun-dried tomatoes that are not oil-packed, cover with boiling water and let stand until soft. Drain before using.

Per 1½ cups: 357 cal., 8g fat (2g sat. fat), 39mg chol., 609mg sod., 42g carb. (4g sugars, 4g fiber), 23g pro.
Diabetic Exchanges: 2 starch, 2 lean meat, 1½ fat, 1 vegetable.

★ ★ ★ ★ ★ **READER REVIEW**

"Outstanding! This is a fantastic meal that is easy to prepare. It's especially beautiful when it's served on white plates."

LAKOTAMOON1 TASTEOFHOME.COM

LEMON CHICKEN WITH ORZO

Summer calls for dishes that are light, bright and still filling. My kids love the veggies in this one—for real! If you like a lot of lemon, squeeze in an extra splash of juice just before serving.
—SHANNON HUMPHREY HAMPTON, VA

PREP: 20 MIN. • **COOK:** 20 MIN.
MAKES: 4 SERVINGS

- ⅓ cup all-purpose flour
- 1 teaspoon garlic powder
- 1 pound boneless skinless chicken breasts
- ¾ teaspoon salt, divided
- ½ teaspoon pepper
- 2 tablespoons olive oil
- 1 can (14½ ounces) reduced-sodium chicken broth
- 1¼ cups uncooked whole wheat orzo pasta
- 2 cups chopped fresh spinach
- 1 cup grape tomatoes, halved
- 3 tablespoons lemon juice
- 2 tablespoons minced fresh basil
  Lemon wedges, optional

1. In a shallow bowl, mix flour and garlic powder. Cut chicken into 1½-in. pieces; pound each with a meat mallet to ¼-in. thickness. Sprinkle with ½ teaspoon salt and pepper. Dip both sides of chicken in flour mixture to coat lightly; shake off any excess.
2. In a large skillet, heat the oil over medium heat. Add chicken; cook for 3-4 minutes on each side or until golden brown and chicken is no longer pink. Remove chicken from pan; keep warm. Wipe skillet clean.
3. In same pan, bring broth to a boil; stir in the orzo. Return to a boil. Reduce heat; simmer, covered, 8-10 minutes or until tender. Stir in the spinach, tomatoes, lemon juice, basil and remaining salt; remove from the heat. Return chicken to the pan. If desired, serve with lemon wedges.
Per 1¼ cups: 399 cal., 11g fat (2g sat. fat), 63mg chol., 807mg sod., 43g carb. (2g sugars, 9g fiber), 32g pro.
Diabetic Exchanges: 3 lean meat, 2 starch, 1½ fat, 1 vegetable.

SUNDAY ROAST CHICKEN

Here's proof that comfort food doesn't have to be full of unwanted calories.
—ROBIN HAAS CRANSTON, RI

PREP: 30 MIN.
BAKE: 1¾ HOURS + RESTING
MAKES: 6 SERVINGS

- 1 medium fennel bulb
- 5 large carrots, cut into 1½-inch pieces
- 1 large white onion, quartered, divided
- 1 medium lemon
- 3 garlic cloves, minced
- 1 tablespoon honey
- 1 teaspoon kosher salt
- 1 teaspoon crushed red pepper flakes
- 1 teaspoon pepper
- 1 broiler/fryer chicken (4 pounds)
- 2 garlic cloves
- 1 cup orange juice

1. Preheat oven to 350°. Using a sharp knife, trim stalks and root end of fennel bulb. Cut bulb lengthwise into quarters; cut and remove core. Cut fennel into 1-in. wedges. Place fennel, carrots and three of the onion quarters in a shallow roasting pan, spreading evenly.
2. Cut lemon in half; squeeze juice into a small bowl, reserving lemon halves. Stir minced garlic, honey, salt, pepper flakes and pepper into juice.
3. Place chicken on a work surface, neck side down. With fingers, carefully loosen skin from the tail end of the chicken breast. Spoon juice mixture under skin of breast; secure skin with toothpicks. Place garlic cloves, lemon halves and remaining onion inside the chicken cavity. Tuck wings underneath; tie drumsticks together. Place chicken over vegetables, breast side up.
4. Pour orange juice over chicken. Roast 1½ to 2 hours or until a thermometer inserted in thickest part of thigh reads 170°-175°. (Cover loosely with foil if the chicken browns too quickly.)
5. Remove roasting pan from oven; increase oven setting to 450°. Remove chicken from pan; tent with foil and let stand 15 minutes before carving.
6. Meanwhile, return roasting pan to oven; roast vegetables 10-15 minutes longer or until vegetables are tender and lightly browned. Using a slotted spoon, remove vegetables from pan. If desired, skim fat from pan juices and serve with chicken and vegetables.
Per 4 ounces cooked chicken (skin removed) with ½ cup vegetables: 292 cal., 8g fat (2g sat. fat), 98mg chol., 470mg sod., 20g carb. (12g sugars, 4g fiber), 34g pro.
Diabetic Exchanges: 4 lean meat, 1 starch, 1 vegetable.

✱

TEST KITCHEN TIP
Turn Sunday's roast chicken into leftover deliciousness during the week. Simply stir chopped chicken into soups or toss with salad greens. Or combine chicken, roasted red peppers and feta and roll inside a whole wheat tortilla.

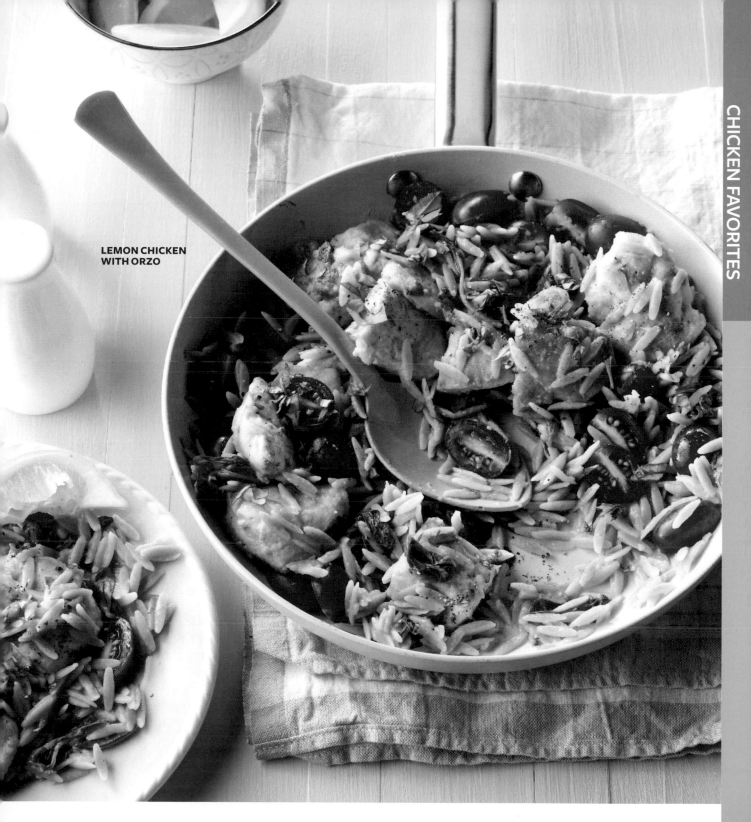

LEMON CHICKEN WITH ORZO

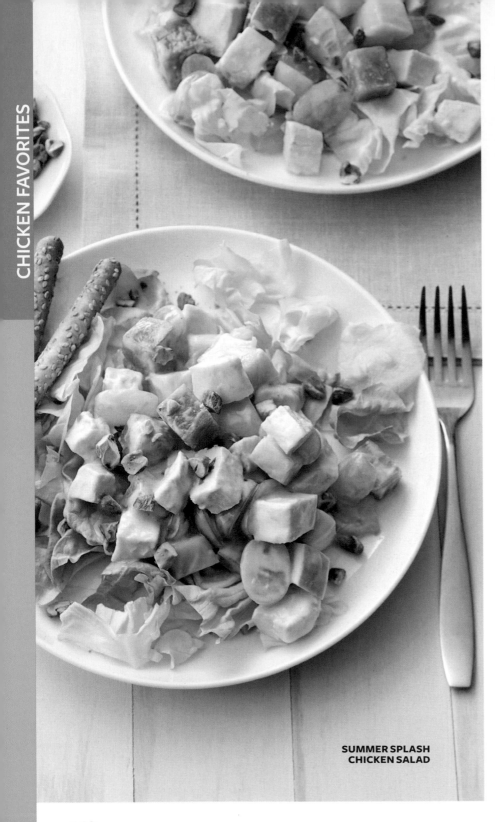

FAST FIX

SUMMER SPLASH CHICKEN SALAD

When it's too hot to eat inside, I head out to the patio. Cut up some rotisserie chicken and toss with mango, grapes and watermelon for a summer salad.
—BARBARA SPITZER LODI, CA

START TO FINISH: 20 MIN.
MAKES: 4 SERVINGS

- ½ cup plain yogurt
- 4½ teaspoons brown sugar
- ½ teaspoon grated lime peel
- 1 tablespoon lime juice
- ¼ teaspoon salt
- 2 cups cubed cooked chicken breast
- 1 cup green grapes, halved
- 1 cup chopped peeled mango
- 1 cup chopped seedless watermelon
- 4 cups torn Bibb or Boston lettuce
- ¼ cup chopped pistachios, toasted

1. In a bowl, mix first five ingredients until blended. Add chicken, grapes, mango and watermelon; toss gently to combine.

2. Divide lettuce among four plates; top with chicken mixture. Sprinkle with the pistachios.

Note: To toast nuts, bake in a shallow pan in a 350° oven for 5-10 minutes or cook in a skillet over low heat until lightly browned, stirring occasionally.

Per 1 cup chicken mixture with 1 cup lettuce and 1 tablespoon pistachios: 262 cal., 7g fat (2g sat. fat), 58mg chol., 249mg sod., 27g carb. (22g sugars, 3g fiber), 24g pro.

Diabetic Exchanges: 3 lean meat, 1 vegetable, 1 fruit, 1 fat, ½ starch.

SUMMER SPLASH CHICKEN SALAD

⑤INGREDIENTS FAST FIX

BALSAMIC CHICKEN WITH ROASTED TOMATOES

Savor some tomatoes, made sweeter by roasting, with your chicken. The tangy balsamic glaze makes both even better!

—**KAREN GEHRIG** CONCORD, NC

START TO FINISH: 25 MIN.
MAKES: 4 SERVINGS

- 2 **tablespoons honey**
- 2 **tablespoons olive oil, divided**
- 2 **cups grape tomatoes**
- 4 **boneless skinless chicken breast halves (6 ounces each)**
- ½ **teaspoon salt**
- ½ **teaspoon pepper**
- 2 **tablespoons balsamic glaze**

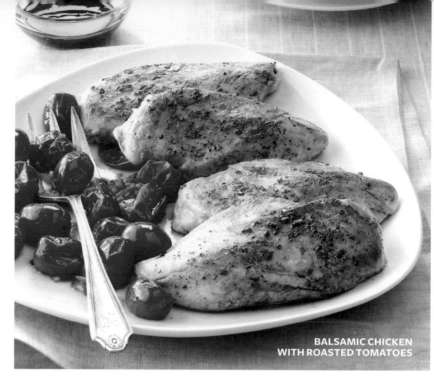

BALSAMIC CHICKEN WITH ROASTED TOMATOES

1. Preheat oven to 400°. In a small bowl, mix honey and 1 tablespoon oil. Add the tomatoes and toss to coat. Transfer to a greased 15x10x1-in. baking pan. Bake 5-7 minutes or until softened.
2. Pound chicken breasts with a meat mallet to ½-in. thickness; sprinkle with salt and pepper. In a large skillet, heat remaining oil over medium heat. Add chicken; cook 5-6 minutes on each side or until no longer pink. Serve with the roasted tomatoes; drizzle with glaze.
Note: To make your own balsamic glaze, bring ½ cup balsamic vinegar to a boil in a small saucepan. Reduce the heat to medium; simmer 10-12 minutes or until thickened to a glaze consistency.
Makes: about 2 tablespoons.
Per 1 chicken breast half with ½ cup tomatoes and 1½ teaspoons glaze: 306 cal., 11g fat (2g sat. fat), 94mg chol., 384mg sod., 16g carb. (14g sugars, 1g fiber), 35g pro.
Diabetic Exchanges: 5 lean meat, 1½ fat, 1 starch.

PARMESAN CHICKEN WITH ARTICHOKE HEARTS

With all the praise this dinner receives, it's so much fun for me to serve.

—**CARLY GILES** HOQUIAM, WA

PREP: 20 MIN. • **BAKE:** 20 MIN.
MAKES: 4 SERVINGS

- 4 **boneless skinless chicken breast halves (6 ounces each)**
- 3 **teaspoons olive oil, divided**
- 1 **teaspoon dried rosemary, crushed**
- ½ **teaspoon dried thyme**
- ⅓ **teaspoon pepper**
- 2 **cans (14 ounces each) water-packed artichoke hearts, drained and quartered**
- 1 **medium onion, coarsely chopped**
- ½ **cup white wine or reduced-sodium chicken broth**
- 2 **garlic cloves, chopped**
- ¼ **cup shredded Parmesan cheese**
- 1 **lemon, cut into 8 slices**
- 2 **green onions, thinly sliced**

1. Preheat oven to 375°. Place the breast halves in a 15x10x1-in. baking pan coated with cooking spray; drizzle with 1½ teaspoons oil. In a small bowl, mix the rosemary, thyme and pepper; sprinkle half over chicken.
2. In a large bowl, combine artichoke hearts, onion, wine, garlic, remaining oil and remaining herb mixture; toss to coat. Arrange around chicken. Sprinkle chicken with the cheese; top with the lemon slices.
3. Roast 20-25 minutes or until a thermometer inserted in chicken reads 165°. Sprinkle with green onions.
Per 1 chicken breast half with ¾ cup artichoke mixture: 339 cal., 9g fat (3g sat. fat), 98mg chol., 667mg sod., 18g carb. (2g sugars, 1g fiber), 42g pro.
Diabetic Exchanges: 5 lean meat, 1 vegetable, 1 fat, ½ starch.

PAN-ROASTED CHICKEN & VEGETABLES

My one-dish meal, so satisfying, tastes like it needs hours of hands-on time to put together. But it takes just minutes to prep the simple ingredients.
—SHERRI MELOTIK OAK CREEK, WI

PREP: 15 MIN. • **BAKE:** 45 MIN.
MAKES: 6 SERVINGS

- 2 pounds red potatoes (about 6 medium), cut into ¾-inch pieces
- 1 large onion, coarsely chopped
- 2 tablespoons olive oil
- 3 garlic cloves, minced
- 1¼ teaspoons salt, divided
- 1 teaspoon dried rosemary, crushed, divided
- ¾ teaspoon pepper, divided
- ½ teaspoon paprika
- 6 bone-in chicken thighs (about 2¼ pounds), skin removed
- 6 cups fresh baby spinach (about 6 ounces)

1. Preheat oven to 425°. In a large bowl, combine the potatoes, onion, oil, garlic, ¾ teaspoon salt, ½ teaspoon rosemary and ½ teaspoon pepper; toss to coat. Transfer to a 15x10x1-in. baking pan coated with cooking spray.
2. In a small bowl, mix paprika and the remaining salt, rosemary and pepper. Sprinkle chicken with paprika mixture; arrange over vegetables. Roast until a thermometer inserted in chicken reads 170°-175° and vegetables are just tender, 35-40 minutes.
3. Remove the chicken to a serving platter; keep warm. Top vegetables with spinach. Roast until the vegetables are tender and the spinach is wilted, 8-10 minutes longer. Stir the vegetables to combine; serve with chicken.

Per 1 chicken thigh with 1 cup vegetables: 357 cal., 14g fat (3g sat. fat), 87mg chol., 597mg sod., 28g carb. (3g sugars, 4g fiber), 28g pro.
Diabetic Exchanges: 4 lean meat, 1½ starch, 1 vegetable, 1 fat.

⑤ INGREDIENTS **FAST FIX**
IN-A-PINCH CHICKEN & SPINACH

I needed a fast supper while babysitting my grandchild. I used what my daughter-in-law had in the fridge and turned it into what's now one of our favorite recipes.
—SANDRA ELLIS STOCKBRIDGE, GA

START TO FINISH: 25 MIN.
MAKES: 4 SERVINGS

- 4 boneless skinless chicken breast halves (6 ounces each)
- 2 tablespoons olive oil
- 1 tablespoon butter
- 1 package (6 ounces) fresh baby spinach
- 1 cup salsa

1. Pound chicken with a meat mallet to ½-in. thickness. In a large skillet, heat oil and butter over medium heat. Cook the chicken for 5-6 minutes on each side or until no longer pink. Remove chicken and keep warm.
2. Add spinach and salsa to pan; cook and stir 3-4 minutes or just until spinach is wilted. Serve with chicken.

Per 1 chicken breast half with ⅓ cup spinach mixture: 297 cal., 14g fat (4g sat. fat), 102mg chol., 376mg sod., 6g carb. (2g sugars, 1g fiber), 36g pro.
Diabetic Exchanges: 5 lean meat, 2 fat, 1 vegetable.

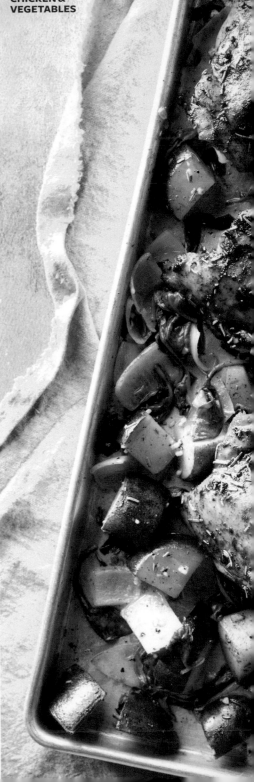

PAN-ROASTED
CHICKEN &
VEGETABLES

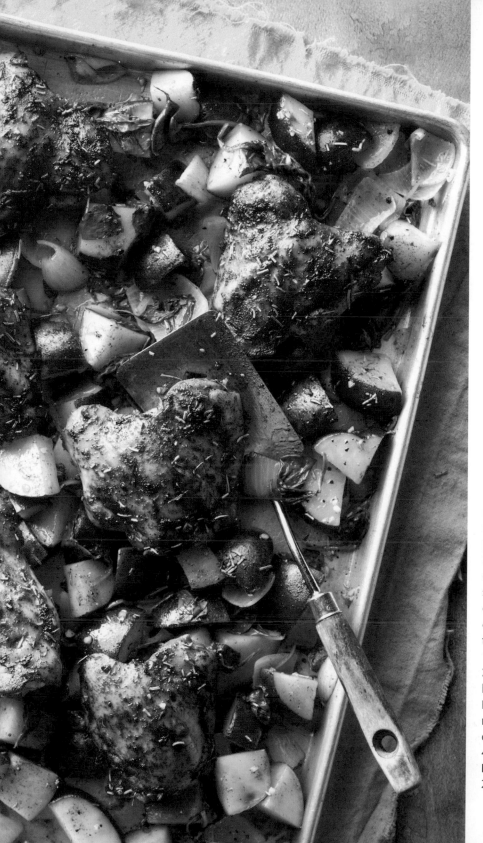

FAST FIX ▶
QUICK CHICKEN & BROCCOLI STIR-FRY

An Asian stir-fry is often a best bet; you add whatever veggies you have on hand.
—**KRISTIN RIMKUS** SNOHOMISH, WA

START TO FINISH: 25 MIN.
MAKES: 4 SERVINGS

- 2 tablespoons rice vinegar
- 2 tablespoons mirin (sweet rice wine)
- 2 tablespoons chili garlic sauce
- 1 tablespoon cornstarch
- 1 tablespoon reduced-sodium soy sauce
- 2 teaspoons fish sauce or additional soy sauce
- ½ cup reduced-sodium chicken broth, divided
- 2 cups instant brown rice
- 2 teaspoons sesame oil
- 4 cups fresh broccoli florets
- 2 cups cubed cooked chicken
- 2 green onions, sliced

1. In a small bowl, mix the first six ingredients and ¼ cup chicken broth until smooth. Cook rice according to package directions.
2. Meanwhile, in a large skillet, heat oil over medium-high heat. Add broccoli; stir-fry 2 minutes. Add remaining broth; cook 1-2 minutes or until broccoli is crisp-tender. Stir sauce mixture and add to pan. Bring to a boil; cook and stir 1-2 minutes or until sauce is thickened.
3. Stir in chicken and green onions; heat through. Serve with rice.
Per 1 cup chicken mixture with ½ cup rice: 387 cal., 9g fat (2g sat. fat), 62mg chol., 765mg sod., 45g carb. (6g sugars, 4g fiber), 28g pro.
Diabetic Exchanges: 3 lean meat, 2½ starch, 1 vegetable, ½ fat.

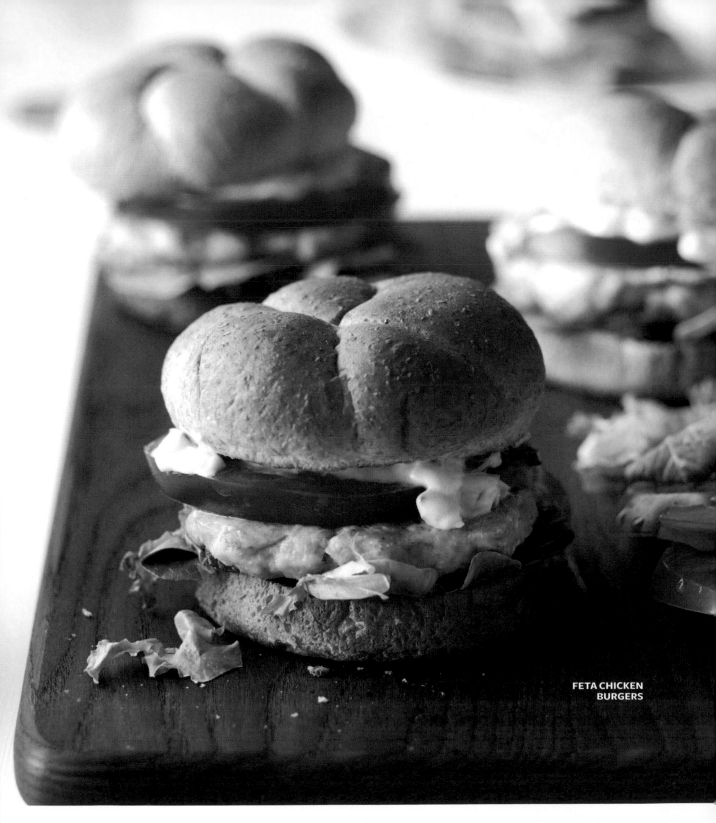

FETA CHICKEN
BURGERS

FAST FIX

FETA CHICKEN BURGERS

My friends always request these tasty chicken burgers on the grill. I sometimes add olives to punch up the flavor! Try them with the mayo topping.

—ANGELA ROBINSON FINDLAY, OH

START TO FINISH: 30 MIN.
MAKES: 6 SERVINGS

- ¼ cup finely chopped cucumber
- ¼ cup reduced-fat mayonnaise

BURGERS

- ½ cup chopped roasted sweet red pepper
- 1 teaspoon garlic powder
- ½ teaspoon Greek seasoning
- ¼ teaspoon pepper
- 1½ pounds lean ground chicken
- 1 cup crumbled feta cheese
- 6 whole wheat hamburger buns, split and toasted
  Lettuce leaves and tomato slices, optional

1. Preheat broiler. Mix cucumber and mayonnaise. For burgers, mix red pepper and seasonings. Add chicken and cheese; mix lightly but thoroughly (mixture will be sticky). Shape into six ½-in.-thick patties.
2. Broil burgers 4 in. from heat until a thermometer reads 165°, 3-4 minutes per side. Serve in buns with cucumber sauce. If desired, top with the lettuce and tomato.

Per 1 burger with 1 tablespoon sauce: 356 cal., 14g fat (5g sat. fat), 95mg chol., 703mg sod., 25g carb. (5g sugars, 4g fiber), 31g pro.
Diabetic Exchanges: 5 lean meat, 2 starch, ½ fat.

CHICKEN WITH THREE-CITRUS TOPPING

Honey sweetens up the citrusy fruit salad that makes this chicken such a pretty dish. Add bread and you have something delightful for company.

—MOLLY SLOSSON WESTPORT, WA

PREP: 30 MIN. • **BROIL:** 10 MIN.
MAKES: 8 SERVINGS

- ¼ cup lime juice
- 1 tablespoon honey
- 1 teaspoon grated lime peel
- ½ teaspoon cayenne pepper
- 4 cups sweet red grapefruit sections
- 2⅔ cups orange sections
- ⅔ cup lemon sections
- 1 tablespoon rotisserie chicken seasoning
- 8 boneless skinless chicken breast halves (4 ounces each)

1. Preheat broiler. In a large bowl, mix the lime juice, honey, lime peel and cayenne. Add citrus sections; toss to coat. Sprinkle seasoning over chicken.
2. Place chicken on greased rack of a broiler pan. Broil 4 in. from heat 5-6 minutes on each side or until a thermometer reads 165°. Serve with citrus topping.

Per 1 chicken breast half with about ¾ cup topping: 201 cal., 3g fat (1g sat. fat), 63mg chol., 446mg sod., 21g carb. (16g sugars, 3g fiber), 24g pro.
Diabetic Exchanges: 3 lean meat, 1½ fruit.

FAST FIX

LIME CHICKEN WITH SALSA VERDE SOUR CREAM

Whenever I'm in a time crunch, salsa verde and Mexican spices come to the rescue. They give broiled chicken a big pick-me-up. My friends always ask me for the recipe.

—ELLEN FOWLER SEATTLE, WA

START TO FINISH: 20 MIN.
MAKES: 4 SERVINGS

- ¾ teaspoon ground coriander
- ¼ teaspoon salt
- ¼ teaspoon ground cumin
- ¼ teaspoon pepper
- 4 boneless skinless chicken thighs (about 1 pound)
- ⅓ cup reduced-fat sour cream
- 2 tablespoons salsa verde
- 2 tablespoons minced fresh cilantro, divided
- 1 medium lime

1. Preheat broiler. Mix the seasonings; sprinkle over the chicken. Place chicken on a broiler pan. Broil 4 in. from the heat 6-8 minutes on each side or until a thermometer reads 170°.
2. Meanwhile, in a small bowl, mix sour cream, salsa and 1 tablespoon cilantro. Cut lime in half. Squeeze juice from one lime half into sour cream mixture; stir to combine. Cut remaining lime half into four wedges. Serve chicken with sauce and lime wedges. Sprinkle servings with remaining cilantro.

Per 1 thigh with 1½ tablespoons sour cream: 199 cal., 10g fat (3g sat. fat), 82mg chol., 267mg sod., 4g carb. (2g sugars, 1g fiber), 23g pro. **Diabetic Exchanges:** 3 lean meat, 1 fat.

THAI CHICKEN & SLAW

A bit of honey makes Thai chicken a hit with my gang!

—**KAREN NORRIS** PHILADELPHIA, PA

PREP: 25 MIN. + MARINATING
COOK: 30 MIN. • **MAKES:** 8 SERVINGS

- ½ cup canola oil
- ½ cup white wine vinegar
- ½ cup honey
- 2 tablespoons minced fresh gingerroot
- 2 tablespoons reduced-sodium soy sauce
- 2 garlic cloves, minced
- 1 teaspoon sesame oil
- 8 boneless skinless chicken thighs (about 2 pounds)

SLAW
- 6 cups coleslaw mix
- 1 cup frozen shelled edamame, thawed
- 1 medium sweet pepper, chopped
- 1 tablespoon creamy peanut butter
- ½ teaspoon salt
- 4 green onions, sliced

1. In a small bowl, whisk the first seven ingredients until blended. Pour 1 cup marinade into a large resealable plastic bag. Add chicken; seal bag and turn to coat. Refrigerate overnight. Cover and refrigerate remaining marinade.
2. Preheat oven to 350°. Drain chicken, discarding marinade in the bag. Place in a 13x9-in. baking dish coated with cooking spray. Bake, uncovered, for 30-40 minutes or until a thermometer reads 170°.
3. Meanwhile, place the coleslaw mix, edamame and pepper in a large bowl. Add peanut butter and salt to reserved marinade; whisk until blended. Pour over the coleslaw mixture; toss to coat. Refrigerate until serving.
4. Serve chicken with slaw. Sprinkle with green onions.

Per 3 ounces cooked chicken with ⅔ cup slaw: 326 cal., 18g fat (3g sat. fat), 76mg chol., 171mg sod., 16g carb. (12g sugars, 2g fiber), 24g pro.
Diabetic Exchanges: 3 lean meat, 2 fat, 1 vegetable, ½ starch.

SAUSAGE & PEPPER PIZZA

All pizza should satisfy a craving. This one easily beats delivery.

—**JAMES SCHEND** PLEASANT PRAIRIE, WI

PREP: 25 MIN. • **BAKE:** 20 MIN.
MAKES: 6 SERVINGS

- 1 package (6½ ounces) pizza crust mix
- 1 can (8 ounces) pizza sauce
- 1¼ cups (5 ounces) shredded pizza cheese blend
- 1 medium onion, sliced
- 1 medium green pepper, sliced
- 2 fully cooked Italian chicken sausage links, sliced
   Grated Parmesan cheese, optional

1. Preheat oven to 425°. Prepare pizza dough according to package directions. Press dough onto bottom and ½ in. up sides of a greased 13x9-in. baking pan.
2. Spread with pizza sauce. Top with 1 cup cheese blend, onion, pepper and sausage; sprinkle with remaining cheese blend.
3. Bake 17-20 minutes or until crust is golden brown. If desired, sprinkle with Parmesan cheese.

Per 1 piece without Parmesan cheese: 257 cal., 9g fat (5g sat. fat), 39mg chol., 565mg sod., 28g carb. (3g sugars, 2g fiber), 15g pro.
Diabetic Exchanges: 2 starch, 2 medium-fat meat.

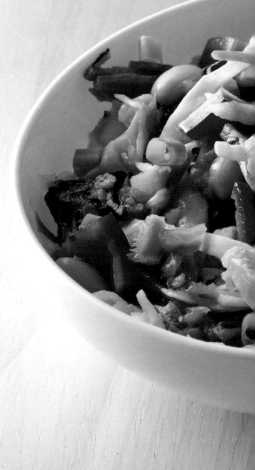

THAI CHICKEN & SLAW

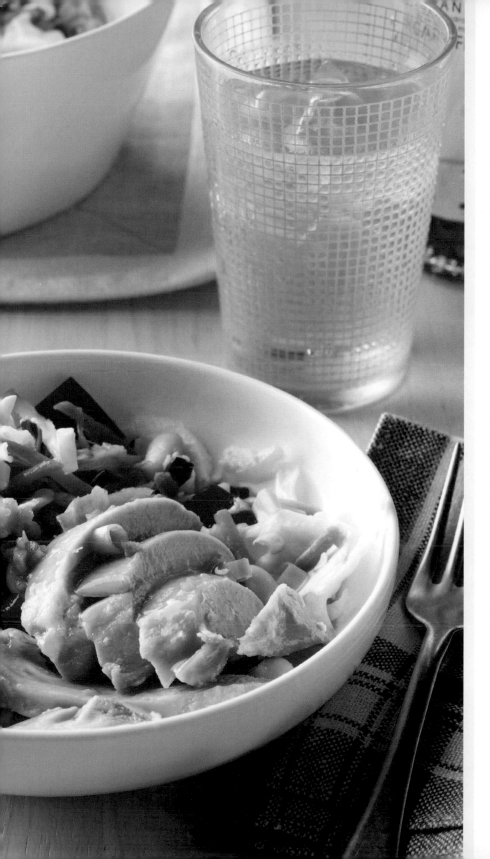

⑤INGREDIENTS

CITRUS-SPICED ROAST CHICKEN

I am the designated Thanksgiving host in my family because of my chipotle citrus roast turkey. Even finicky eaters love it. I use the same recipe for chicken so we can enjoy it year-round.

—**ROBIN HAAS** CRANSTON, RI

PREP: 20 MIN.
BAKE: 1 HOUR + STANDING
MAKES: 6 SERVINGS

- 3 tablespoons orange marmalade
- 4½ teaspoons chopped chipotle peppers in adobo sauce
- 3 garlic cloves, minced
- ¾ teaspoon salt, divided
- ½ teaspoon ground cumin
- 1 broiler/fryer chicken (4 pounds)

1. Preheat oven to 350°. Mix the marmalade, chipotle peppers, garlic, ½ teaspoon salt and cumin. With fingers, carefully loosen skin from chicken; rub mixture under the skin.

2. Place chicken on a rack in a shallow roasting pan, breast side up. Tuck wings under chicken; tie drumsticks together. Rub skin with remaining salt. Roast 1 to 1¼ hours or until a thermometer inserted in thickest part of thigh reads 170°-175°, covering chicken with foil halfway through cooking to prevent any overbrowning.

3. Remove chicken from the oven; let stand, loosely covered, for 15 minutes before carving. Remove and discard the skin before serving.

Per 4 ounces cooked chicken (skin removed): 239 cal., 8g fat (2g sat. fat), 98mg chol., 409mg sod., 8g carb. (6g sugars, 0 fiber), 32g pro.
Diabetic Exchanges: 4 lean meat.

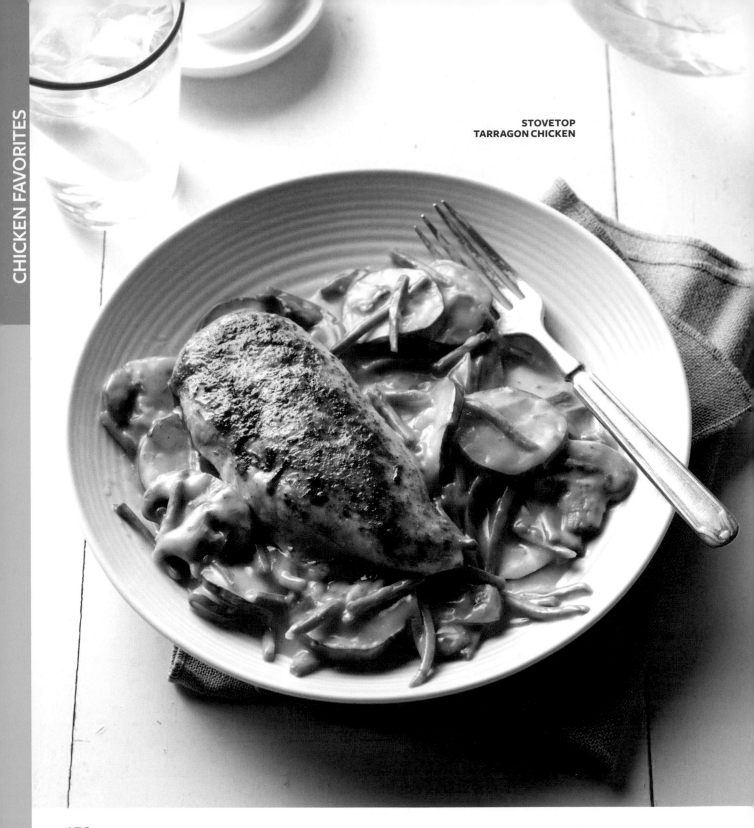

STOVETOP
TARRAGON CHICKEN

STOVETOP TARRAGON CHICKEN

My oldest daughter can't get enough of the tarragon sauce in this easy dish.

—TINA WESTOVER LA MESA, CA

PREP: 10 MIN. • **COOK:** 30 MIN.
MAKES: 4 SERVINGS

- 4 boneless skinless chicken breast halves (5 ounces each)
- 2 teaspoons paprika
- 1 tablespoon olive oil
- 1 package (10 ounces) julienned carrots
- ½ pound sliced fresh mushrooms
- 2 cans (10¾ ounces each) reduced-fat reduced-sodium condensed cream of chicken soup, undiluted
- 3 teaspoons dried tarragon
- 1 tablespoon lemon juice
- 3 small zucchini, thinly sliced

1. Sprinkle chicken with paprika. In a Dutch oven, heat oil over medium heat. Cook chicken 2 minutes on each side or until lightly browned; remove from pan.
2. Add carrots and mushrooms to the same pan; cook, covered, 6-8 minutes or until carrots are crisp-tender, stirring occasionally. In a small bowl, mix soup, tarragon and lemon juice until blended; pour over vegetables. Return chicken to pan. Bring to a boil; reduce heat to low. Cook, covered, 8 minutes. Top with zucchini; cook, covered, 6-8 minutes longer or until a thermometer inserted in chicken reads 165° and vegetables are tender.

Per 1 chicken breast with 1 cup vegetables: 345 cal., 11g fat (3g sat. fat), 85mg chol., 649mg sod., 28g carb. (16g sugars, 5g fiber), 35g pro.
Diabetic Exchanges: 4 lean meat, 2 vegetable, 1 starch, 1 fat.

---

⑤ INGREDIENTS

BASIL CHICKEN

Italian-style marinade gives chicken lots of flavor. Try slices on a ciabatta roll with lettuce, tomato and mozzarella cheese for a zesty sandwich.

—LISA MORIARTY WILTON, NH

PREP: 10 MIN. + MARINATING
GRILL: 10 MIN. • **MAKES:** 4 SERVINGS

- 3 tablespoons red wine vinegar
- 3 tablespoons olive oil
- 2 tablespoons chopped red onion
- 2 tablespoons minced fresh basil
- 1 garlic clove, minced
- ¼ teaspoon salt
- ¼ teaspoon pepper
- 4 boneless skinless chicken breast halves (6 ounces each)
  Grilled romaine, optional

1. In a large resealable plastic bag, combine the first seven ingredients. Add chicken; seal bag and turn to coat. Refrigerate 8 hours or overnight.
2. Drain chicken, discarding marinade. Grill chicken, covered, over medium heat or broil 4 in. from heat 5-7 minutes on each side or until a thermometer reads 165°. If desired, serve chicken over grilled romaine.
To freeze: Freeze chicken with marinade in a resealable plastic freezer bag. To use, thaw in refrigerator overnight. Drain chicken, discarding marinade. Grill as directed.

Per 1 chicken breast half: 231 cal., 9g fat (2g sat. fat), 94mg chol., 156mg sod., 1g carb. (0 sugars, 0 fiber), 34g pro.
Diabetic Exchanges: 5 lean meat, 1 fat.

FAST FIX ▶

CHICKEN & GARLIC WITH FRESH HERBS

The key to this savory chicken is the combo of garlic, rosemary and thyme.

—JAN VALDEZ LOMBARD, IL

START TO FINISH: 30 MIN.
MAKES: 6 SERVINGS

- 6 boneless skinless chicken thighs (about 1½ pounds)
- ½ teaspoon salt
- ¼ teaspoon pepper
- 1 tablespoon olive oil
- 10 garlic cloves, peeled and halved
- 2 tablespoons brandy or chicken stock
- 1 cup chicken stock
- 1 teaspoon minced fresh rosemary or ¼ teaspoon dried rosemary, crushed
- ½ teaspoon minced fresh thyme or ⅛ teaspoon dried thyme
- 1 tablespoon minced fresh chives

1. Sprinkle the chicken with salt and pepper. In a large skillet, heat oil over medium-high heat. Brown chicken on both sides. Remove from pan.
2. Remove skillet from heat; add garlic and brandy. Return to heat; cook and stir over medium heat 1-2 minutes or until liquid is almost evaporated.
3. Stir in stock, rosemary and thyme; return chicken to pan. Bring to a boil. Reduce heat; simmer, uncovered, 6-8 minutes or until a thermometer reads 170°. Sprinkle with chives.

Per 1 thigh with 2 tablespoons cooking juices: 203 cal., 11g fat (3g sat. fat), 76mg chol., 346mg sod., 2g carb. (0 sugars, 0 fiber), 22g pro.
Diabetic Exchanges: 3 lean meat, ½ fat.

ROASTED CHICKEN THIGHS WITH PEPPERS & POTATOES

Peppers and herbs transform chicken and potatoes in an easy-to-make dish.

—**PATRICIA PRESCOTT** MANCHESTER, NH

PREP: 20 MIN. • **BAKE:** 35 MIN.
MAKES: 8 SERVINGS

- 2 pounds red potatoes (about 6 medium)
- 2 large sweet red peppers
- 2 large green peppers
- 2 medium onions
- 2 tablespoons olive oil, divided
- 4 teaspoons minced fresh thyme or 1½ teaspoons dried thyme, divided
- 3 teaspoons minced fresh rosemary or 1 teaspoon dried rosemary, crushed, divided
- 8 boneless skinless chicken thighs (about 2 pounds)
- ½ teaspoon salt
- ¼ teaspoon pepper

1. Preheat oven to 450°. Cut potatoes, peppers and onions into 1-in. pieces. Place the vegetables in a roasting pan. Drizzle with 1 tablespoon oil; sprinkle with 2 teaspoons each of thyme and rosemary; toss to coat. Place chicken over vegetables. Brush chicken with remaining oil; sprinkle with remaining thyme and rosemary. Sprinkle the vegetables and chicken thighs with salt and pepper.
2. Roast 35-40 minutes or until a thermometer inserted in chicken reads 170° and vegetables are tender.

Per 1 thigh with 1 cup vegetables: 308 cal., 12g fat (3g sat. fat), 76mg chol., 221mg sod., 25g carb. (5g sugars, 4g fiber), 24g pro.
Diabetic Exchanges: 3 lean meat, 1 starch, 1 vegetable, ½ fat.

FAST FIX ▶

SPRING CHICKEN & PEA SALAD

Endive, radicchio and chicken salad with a surprising minty dressing is wonderful to serve for luncheon or a light dinner.

—**ROXANNE CHAN** ALBANY, CA

START TO FINISH: 20 MIN.
MAKES: 4 SERVINGS

- 1 cup fresh peas
- 2 cups torn curly or Belgian endive
- 2 cups torn radicchio
- 2 cups chopped rotisserie chicken
- ½ cup sliced radishes
- 2 tablespoons chopped red onion
- 2 tablespoons fresh mint leaves, torn

DRESSING
- 2 tablespoons olive oil
- ¼ teaspoon grated lemon peel
- 1 tablespoon lemon juice
- 1 tablespoon mint jelly
- 1 garlic clove, minced
- ¼ teaspoon salt
- ¼ teaspoon pepper
  Toasted pine nuts, optional

1. In a large saucepan, bring ½ in. of water to a boil. Add peas; cover and cook 5-8 minutes or until tender.
2. Drain the peas and place in a large bowl. Add endive, radicchio, chicken, radishes, onion and mint. In a small saucepan, combine oil, lemon peel, juice, jelly, garlic, salt and pepper; cook and stir over medium-low heat 4-6 minutes or until jelly is melted. Drizzle over the salad; toss to coat. If desired, sprinkle with pine nuts.

Per 1½ cups: 250 cal., 12g fat (2g sat. fat), 62mg chol., 225mg sod., 12g carb. (6g sugars, 3g fiber), 23g pro.
Diabetic Exchanges: 3 lean meat, 1½ fat, 1 vegetable, ½ starch.

FAST FIX ▶

THAI CHICKEN LINGUINE

When I'm feeding a crowd, I multiply this Thai-inspired favorite. Even kids love it!

—**TERI RUMBLE** JENSEN BEACH, FL

START TO FINISH: 30 MIN.
MAKES: 6 SERVINGS

- 8 ounces uncooked whole wheat linguine
- ⅓ cup reduced-sodium soy sauce
- ¼ cup lime juice
- 3 tablespoons brown sugar
- 2 tablespoons rice vinegar
- 1 tablespoon Thai chili sauce
- 2 tablespoons peanut oil, divided
- 1 pound boneless skinless chicken breasts, cubed
- 1 cup fresh snow peas
- 1 medium sweet red pepper, julienned
- 4 garlic cloves, minced
- 2 large eggs, beaten
- ⅓ cup chopped unsalted peanuts

1. Cook linguine according to package directions. Meanwhile, in a small bowl, mix soy sauce, lime juice, brown sugar, vinegar and chili sauce until blended.
2. In a large nonstick skillet, heat 1 tablespoon oil over medium-high heat. Add chicken; stir-fry until no longer pink. Remove from pan. Stir-fry peas and pepper in remaining oil until crisp-tender. Add garlic; cook 1 minute longer. Add eggs; cook and stir until set.
3. Drain linguine; add to vegetable mixture. Stir soy sauce mixture and add to pan. Bring to a boil. Add chicken; heat through. Sprinkle with peanuts.

Per 1⅓ cups: 377 cal., 13g fat (2g sat. fat), 104mg chol., 697mg sod., 44g carb. (12g sugars, 5g fiber), 25g pro.
Diabetic Exchanges: 3 starch, 3 lean meat, 2 fat.

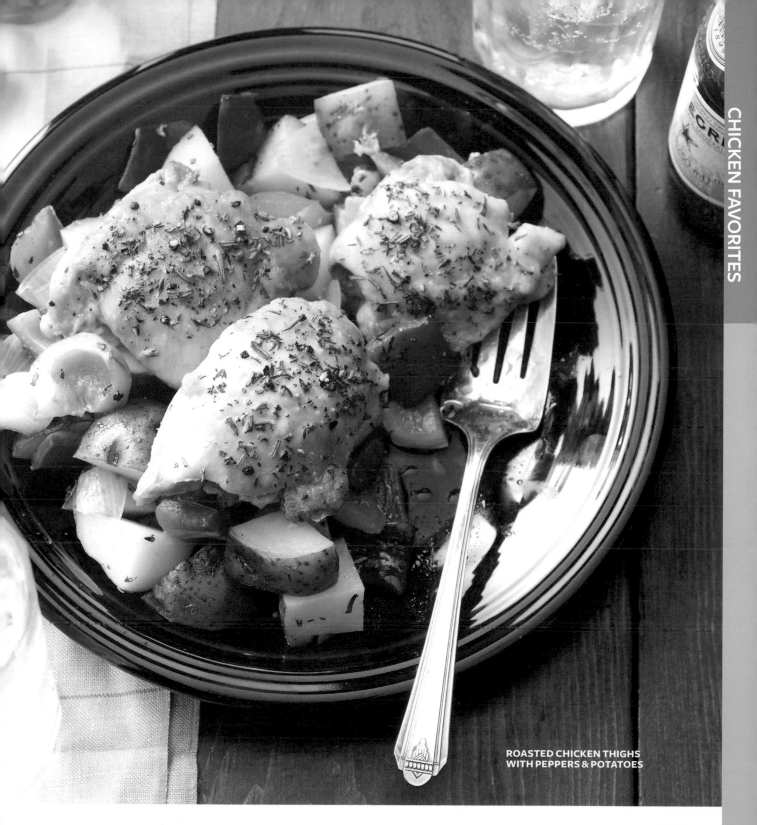

ROASTED CHICKEN THIGHS
WITH PEPPERS & POTATOES

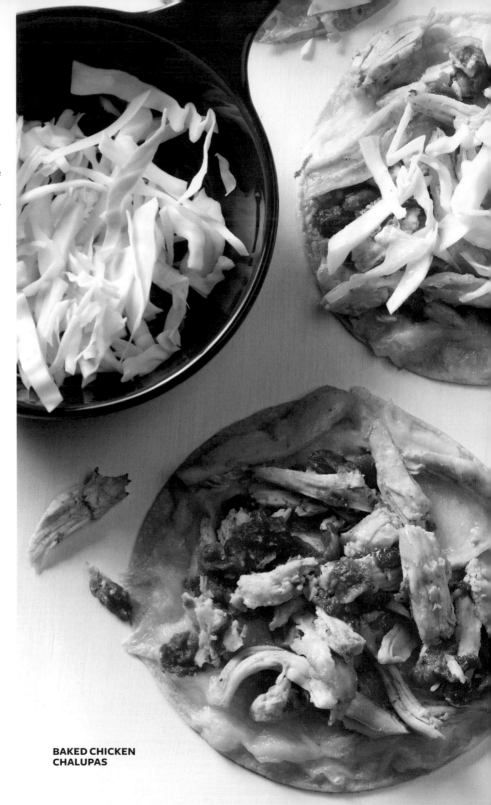

BAKED CHICKEN CHALUPAS

I wanted an easy alternative to deep-fried chalupas, so I bake them with the filling on top.

—**MAGDALENA FLORES** ABILENE, TX

PREP: 20 MIN. • **BAKE:** 15 MIN.
MAKES: 6 SERVINGS

- 6 corn tortillas (6 inches)
- 2 teaspoons olive oil
- ¾ cup shredded part-skim mozzarella cheese
- 2 cups chopped cooked chicken breast
- 1 can (14½ ounces) diced tomatoes with mild green chilies, undrained
- 1 teaspoon garlic powder
- 1 teaspoon onion powder
- 1 teaspoon ground cumin
- ¼ teaspoon salt
- ¼ teaspoon pepper
- ½ cup finely shredded cabbage

1. Preheat oven to 350°. Place the tortillas on an ungreased baking sheet. Brush each tortilla with oil; sprinkle with mozzarella cheese.

2. Place the chicken, tomatoes and seasonings in a large skillet; cook and stir over medium heat 6-8 minutes or until most of the liquid is evaporated. Spoon over tortillas. Bake 15-18 minutes or until tortillas are crisp and cheese is melted. Top with cabbage.

Per chalupa: 206 cal., 6g fat (2g sat. fat), 45mg chol., 400mg sod., 17g carb. (3g sugars, 3g fiber), 19g pro.
Diabetic Exchanges: 2 lean meat, 1 starch, ½ fat.

BAKED CHICKEN CHALUPAS

SPICY LEMON CHICKEN KABOBS

When I see Meyer lemons in the store, I know that spring has arrived. I like using them for these easy, smoky chicken kabobs, but regular grilled lemons can also get the job done.

—TERRI CRANDALL GARDNERVILLE, NV

PREP: 15 MIN. + MARINATING
GRILL: 10 MIN. • **MAKES:** 6 SERVINGS

- ¼ cup lemon juice
- 4 tablespoons olive oil, divided
- 3 tablespoons white wine
- 1½ teaspoons crushed red pepper flakes
- 1 teaspoon minced fresh rosemary or ¼ teaspoon dried rosemary, crushed
- 1½ pounds boneless skinless chicken breasts, cut into 1-inch cubes
- 2 medium lemons, halved
  Minced chives

1. In a large resealable plastic bag, combine lemon juice, 3 tablespoons oil, wine, pepper flakes and rosemary. Add chicken; seal the bag and turn to coat. Refrigerate up to 3 hours.
2. Drain chicken, discarding marinade. Thread the chicken onto six metal or soaked wooden skewers. Grill, covered, over medium heat 10-12 minutes or until no longer pink, turning once.
3. Place lemons on grill, cut side down. Grill for 8-10 minutes or until lightly browned. Squeeze lemon halves over chicken. Drizzle with remaining oil; sprinkle with chives.
Per kabob: 182 cal., 8g fat (2g sat. fat), 63mg chol., 55mg sod., 2g carb. (1g sugars, 1g fiber), 23g pro.
Diabetic Exchanges: 3 lean meat, 1 fat.

OVEN-FRIED CHICKEN DRUMSTICKS

This fabulous chicken recipe uses Greek yogurt to create an amazing marinade that makes the chicken incredibly moist. No one will guess that it's been lightened up and baked, not fried!

—KIMBERLY WALLACE DENNISON, OH

PREP: 20 MIN. + MARINATING
BAKE: 40 MIN. • **MAKES:** 4 SERVINGS

- 1 cup fat-free plain Greek yogurt
- 1 tablespoon Dijon mustard
- 2 garlic cloves, minced
- 8 chicken drumsticks (4 ounces each), skin removed
- ½ cup whole wheat flour
- 1½ teaspoons paprika
- 1 teaspoon baking powder
- 1 teaspoon salt
- 1 teaspoon pepper
  Olive oil-flavored cooking spray

1. In a large resealable plastic bag, combine yogurt, mustard and garlic. Add chicken; seal bag and turn to coat. Refrigerate 8 hours or overnight.
2. Preheat oven to 425°. In another plastic bag, mix flour, paprika, baking powder, salt and pepper. Remove the chicken from marinade and add, one piece at a time, to flour mixture; close bag and shake to coat. Place on a wire rack over a baking sheet; spritz with cooking spray. Bake 40-45 minutes or until a thermometer reads 180°.
Per 2 chicken drumsticks: 227 cal., 7g fat (1g sat. fat), 81mg chol., 498mg sod., 9g carb. (2g sugars, 1g fiber), 31g pro.
Diabetic Exchanges: 4 lean meat, ½ starch.

CHICKEN BURRITO SKILLET

This burrito-inspired dish is big at our house on Mexican nights!

—**KRISTA MARSHALL** FORT WAYNE, IN

PREP: 15 MIN. • **COOK:** 30 MIN.
MAKES: 6 SERVINGS

- 1 pound boneless skinless chicken breasts, cut into 1½-inch pieces
- ⅛ teaspoon salt
- ⅛ teaspoon pepper
- 2 tablespoons olive oil, divided
- 1 cup uncooked long grain rice
- 1 can (15 ounces) black beans, rinsed and drained
- 1 can (14½ ounces) diced tomatoes, drained
- 1 teaspoon ground cumin
- ½ teaspoon onion powder
- ½ teaspoon garlic powder
- ½ teaspoon chili powder
- 2½ cups reduced-sodium chicken broth
- 1 cup shredded Mexican cheese blend
- 1 medium tomato, chopped
- 3 green onions, chopped

1. Toss chicken with salt and pepper. In a skillet, heat 1 tablespoon oil over medium-high heat; saute until browned, about 2 minutes. Remove from pan.
2. In same pan, heat remaining oil over medium-high heat; saute the rice until lightly browned, 1-2 minutes. Stir in beans, canned tomatoes, seasonings and broth; bring to a boil. Place chicken on top (do not stir into rice). Simmer, covered, until rice is tender and chicken is no longer pink, 20-25 minutes.
3. Remove from heat; sprinkle with the cheese. Let stand, covered, until cheese is melted. Top with the chopped tomato and green onions.

Per 1⅓ cups: 403 cal., 13g fat (4g sat. fat), 58mg chol., 690mg sod., 43g carb. (4g sugars, 5g fiber), 27g pro.
Diabetic Exchanges: 3 starch, 3 lean meat, 1½ fat.

FAST FIX
TANDOORI CHICKEN THIGHS

I spent time in India, so I love reminders of this vibrant culture. Serving tandoori chicken truly makes me happy.

—**CLAIRE ELSTON** SPOKANE, WA

START TO FINISH: 30 MIN.
MAKES: 4 SERVINGS

- 1 cup (8 ounces) reduced-fat plain yogurt
- 1 tablespoon minced fresh gingerroot
- 1 teaspoon ground cumin
- 1 garlic clove, minced
- ¾ teaspoon kosher salt
- ½ teaspoon curry powder
- ½ teaspoon pepper
- ¼ teaspoon cayenne pepper
- 4 boneless skinless chicken thighs (about 1 pound)

1. In a small bowl, mix the first eight ingredients until blended. Add chicken to marinade; turn to coat. Let stand 10 minutes.
2. Place chicken on greased grill rack. Grill thighs, covered, over medium heat for 6-8 minutes on each side or until a thermometer reads 170°.

Per 1 thigh: 193 cal., 9g fat (3g sat. fat), 78mg chol., 333mg sod., 4g carb. (3g sugars, 0 fiber), 23g pro.
Diabetic Exchanges: 3 lean meat, ½ fat.

FAST FIX
COOL & CRUNCHY CHICKEN SALAD

When the weather sizzles, get your chill on with a cool chicken salad. Mine uses grapes, pecans and celery to give it that signature crunch.

—**SARAH SMILEY** BANGOR, ME

START TO FINISH: 25 MIN.
MAKES: 6 SERVINGS

- ½ cup reduced-fat mayonnaise
- 2 tablespoons minced fresh parsley
- 1 tablespoon lemon juice
- 1 tablespoon cider vinegar
- 1 teaspoon spicy brown mustard
- ½ teaspoon sugar
- ¼ teaspoon salt
- ¼ teaspoon pepper
- 3 cups cubed cooked chicken
- 1 cup seedless red grapes, halved
- 1 cup thinly sliced celery
- 1 cup pecan halves, toasted
  Lettuce leaves

In a large bowl, mix the first eight ingredients until blended. Add chicken, grapes, celery and pecans; toss to coat. Serve on lettuce.
Note: To toast nuts, bake in a shallow pan in a 350° oven for 5-10 minutes or cook in a skillet over low heat until lightly browned, stirring occasionally.
Per 1 cup: 340 cal., 24g fat (3g sat. fat), 69mg chol., 311mg sod., 10g carb. (7g sugars, 2g fiber), 22g pro.
Diabetic Exchanges: 3 lean meat, 3 fat, ½ starch.

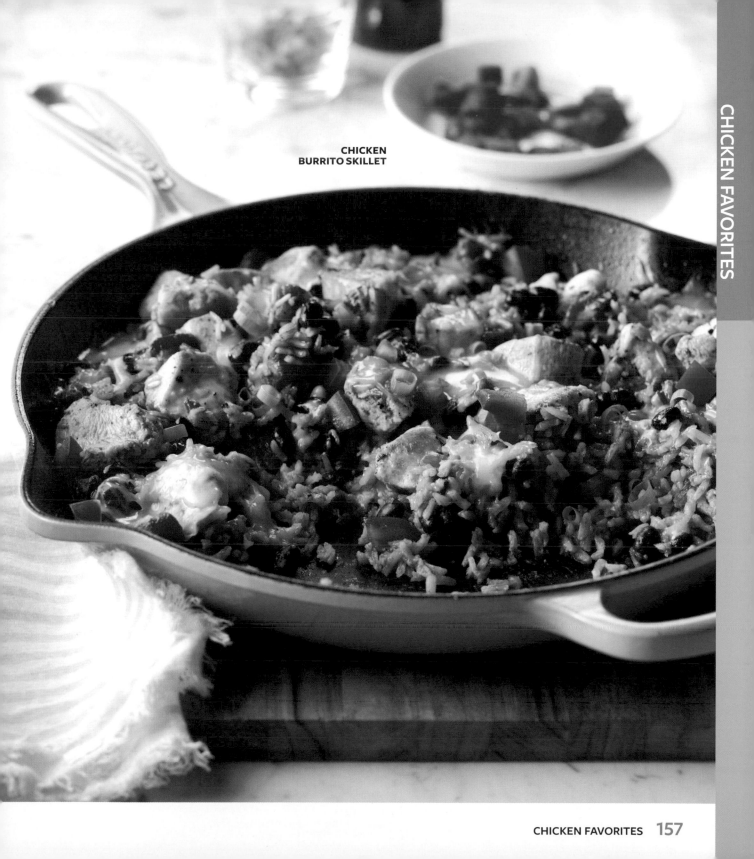

CHICKEN
BURRITO SKILLET

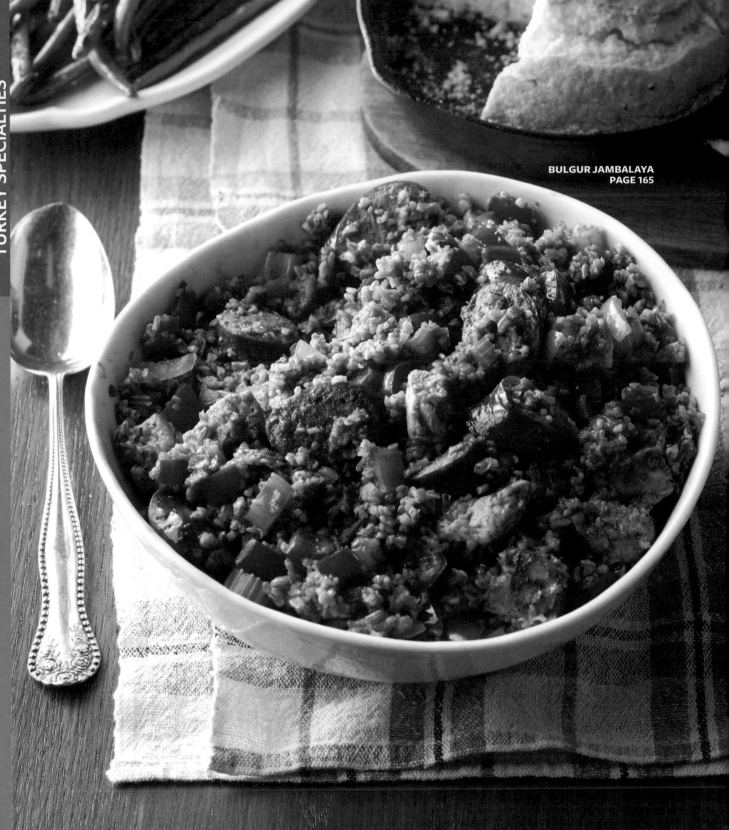

BULGUR JAMBALAYA
PAGE 165

Turkey Specialties

We're talking turkey! Lean and full of protein,
it works in an array of dishes, including stir-fries,
pizzas, casseroles and other mouthwatering meals
ideal for the entire family. Turn the page
and gobble up the goodness!

SAUSAGE-TOPPED WHITE PIZZA

FAST FIX

SAUSAGE-TOPPED WHITE PIZZA

Pizza is one of my favorite dishes to prepare, especially with ricotta cheese.

—**TRACY BROWN** RIVER EDGE, NJ

START TO FINISH: 30 MIN.
MAKES: 6 SERVINGS

- 2 hot Italian turkey sausage links, casings removed
- 1 cup reduced-fat ricotta cheese
- ¼ teaspoon garlic powder
- 1 prebaked 12-inch thin whole wheat pizza crust
- 1 medium sweet red pepper, julienned
- 1 small onion, halved and thinly sliced
- ½ teaspoon Italian seasoning
- ¼ teaspoon freshly ground pepper
- ¼ teaspoon crushed red pepper flakes, optional
- ½ cup shredded part-skim mozzarella cheese
- 2 cups arugula or baby spinach

1. Preheat oven to 450°. In a large skillet, cook and crumble sausage over medium-high heat until no longer pink, 4-6 minutes. Mix ricotta cheese and garlic powder.
2. Place crust on a baking sheet; spread with ricotta cheese mixture. Top with sausage, red pepper and onion; sprinkle with seasonings, then with the shredded mozzarella cheese.
3. Bake on a lower oven rack until edge is lightly browned and cheese is melted, 8-10 minutes. Top with arugula.
Per slice: 242 cal., 8g fat (4g sat. fat), 30mg chol., 504mg sod., 28g carb. (5g sugars, 4g fiber), 16g pro.
Diabetic Exchanges: 2 starch, 2 medium-fat meat.

FAST FIX

CURRY-ROASTED TURKEY & POTATOES

Honey mustard is the condiment around here, so I wanted a healthy recipe to serve it with. Roasted turkey with a dash of curry is perfect.

—**CAROL WIT** TINLEY PARK, IL

START TO FINISH: 30 MIN.
MAKES: 4 SERVINGS

- 1 pound Yukon Gold potatoes (about 3 medium), cut into ½-inch cubes
- 2 medium leeks (white portion only), thinly sliced
- 2 tablespoons canola oil, divided
- ½ teaspoon pepper, divided
- ¼ teaspoon salt, divided
- 3 tablespoons Dijon mustard
- 3 tablespoons honey
- ¾ teaspoon curry powder
- 1 package (17.6 ounces) turkey breast cutlets
  Minced fresh cilantro or thinly sliced green onions, optional

1. Preheat the oven to 450°. Place potatoes and leeks in a 15x10x1-in. baking pan coated with cooking spray. Drizzle with 1 tablespoon oil; sprinkle with ¼ teaspoon pepper and ⅛ teaspoon salt. Stir to coat. Roast for 15 minutes, stirring once.
2. Meanwhile, in a bowl, combine mustard, honey, curry powder and remaining oil. Sprinkle turkey with remaining salt and pepper.
3. Drizzle 2 tablespoons of mustard mixture over potatoes; stir to coat. Place turkey over the potato mixture; drizzle with remaining mustard mixture. Roast 6-8 minutes longer or until turkey is no longer pink and the potatoes are tender. If desired, sprinkle with cilantro.

Per 3 ounces cooked turkey with ¾ cup potato mixture: 393 cal., 9g fat (1g sat. fat), 71mg chol., 582mg sod., 44g carb. (16g sugars, 3g fiber), 33g pro.
Diabetic Exchanges: 4 lean meat, 3 starch, 1½ fat.

TURKEY MEAT LOAF

I first made this recipe when my husband and I started watching our diet. It's now a favorite that others request, too.

—**RUBY RATH** NEW HAVEN, IN

PREP: 15 MIN.
BAKE: 1 HOUR + STANDING
MAKES: 10 SERVINGS

- 1 cup quick-cooking oats
- 1 medium onion, chopped
- ½ cup shredded carrot
- ½ cup fat-free milk
- ¼ cup egg substitute
- 2 tablespoons ketchup
- 1 teaspoon garlic powder
- ¼ teaspoon pepper
- 2 pounds ground turkey breast
TOPPING
- ¼ cup ketchup
- ¼ cup quick-cooking oats

1. Preheat oven to 350°. Combine first eight ingredients. Add turkey; mix lightly but thoroughly.
2. Transfer to a 9x5-in. loaf pan coated with cooking spray. Mix the topping ingredients; spread over loaf. Bake until a thermometer reads 165°, 60-65 minutes. Let the loaf stand 10 minutes before slicing.
Per slice: 195 cal., 8g fat (2g sat. fat), 63mg chol., 188mg sod., 12g carb. (4g sugars, 1g fiber), 20g pro.
Diabetic Exchanges: 3 lean meat, 1 starch.

FAST FIX ▶
ASIAN LETTUCE WRAPS

This recipe replicates the lettuce wraps found in national restaurants, but it's healthier! You can make the filling ahead.

—**LINDA ROWLEY** RICHARDSON, TX

START TO FINISH: 25 MIN.
MAKES: 4 SERVINGS

- 1 tablespoon canola oil
- 1 pound lean ground turkey
- 1 jalapeno pepper, seeded and minced
- 2 green onions, thinly sliced
- 2 garlic cloves, minced
- 2 tablespoons minced fresh basil
- 2 tablespoons lime juice
- 2 tablespoons reduced-sodium soy sauce
- 1 to 2 tablespoons chili garlic sauce
- 1 tablespoon sugar or sugar substitute blend equivalent to 1 tablespoon sugar
- 12 Bibb or Boston lettuce leaves
- 1 medium cucumber, julienned
- 1 medium carrot, julienned
- 2 cups bean sprouts

1. In a skillet, heat oil over medium heat. Add turkey; cook 6-8 minutes or until no longer pink, breaking into crumbles. Add jalapeno, green onions and garlic; cook 2 minute longer. Stir in basil, lime juice, soy sauce, chili garlic sauce and sugar; heat through.

2. To serve, place turkey mixture in lettuce leaves; top with cucumber, carrot and bean sprouts. Fold lettuce over filling.

Per 3 lettuce wraps: 259 cal., 12g fat (3g sat. fat), 78mg chol., 503mg sod., 12g carb. (6g sugars, 3g fiber), 26g pro.
Diabetic Exchanges: 3 lean meat, 1 vegetable, ½ starch, ½ fat.

TURKEY PINTO BEAN SALAD WITH SOUTHERN MOLASSES DRESSING

This salad is a welcome alternative to the usual leftover turkey fare. Even better, it's loaded with good-for-you protein.

—**LILY JULOW** LAWRENCEVILLE, GA

PREP: 35 MIN. + CHILLING
MAKES: 6 SERVINGS

- ½ cup oil-packed sun-dried tomatoes
- 1 garlic clove, peeled and halved
- ½ cup molasses
- 3 tablespoons cider vinegar
- 1 teaspoon prepared mustard
- ½ teaspoon salt
- ¼ teaspoon coarsely ground pepper
- 3 cups cubed cooked turkey breast
- 2 cans (15 ounces each) pinto beans, rinsed and drained
- 1 medium green pepper, diced
- 2 celery ribs, diced
- 1 cup chopped sweet onion
- ¼ cup minced fresh parsley

1. Drain the tomatoes, reserving 2 tablespoons oil. Place the garlic and tomatoes in a food processor; cover and process until chopped. Add the molasses, vinegar, mustard, salt, pepper and reserved oil. Cover and process until smooth.

2. In a large bowl, combine the turkey, beans, green pepper, celery, onion and parsley. Add dressing and toss to coat. Cover mixture and refrigerate for at least 2 hours.

Per 1⅓ cups: 379 cal., 7g fat (1g sat. fat), 60mg chol., 483mg sod., 49g carb. (19g sugars, 7g fiber), 29g pro.
Diabetic Exchanges: 4 lean meat, 2½ starch, 1 vegetable, 1 fat.

FAST FIX ▶
GREEK SAUSAGE PITAS

I nicknamed my sandwich Thor's Pita because it's robust and lightning-quick. The ingredient amounts don't really matter. Use more or less depending on what you have.

—**TERESA ALEKSANDROV** YPSILANTI, MI

START TO FINISH: 20 MIN.
MAKES: 4 SERVINGS

- 4 whole wheat pita breads (6 inches)
- 1 cup plain yogurt
- 2 green onions, chopped
- 2 tablespoons minced fresh parsley
- 1 teaspoon lemon juice
- 1 garlic clove, minced
- ¾ pound Italian turkey sausage links or other sausage links of your choice, casings removed
- 1 medium cucumber, seeded and chopped
- 1 medium tomato, chopped
  Additional minced fresh parsley

1. Preheat oven to 325°. Wrap pita breads in foil; warm in oven while preparing toppings.

2. In a small bowl, mix yogurt, green onions, parsley, lemon juice and garlic. In a large skillet, cook sausage over medium heat 4-6 minutes or until no longer pink, breaking into crumbles.

3. To assemble, spoon sausage over pitas. Top with the cucumber, tomato and yogurt mixture; sprinkle with the additional parsley.

Per open-faced sandwich: 309 cal., 9g fat (3g sat. fat), 39mg chol., 667mg sod., 42g carb. (5g sugars, 6g fiber), 19g pro.
Diabetic Exchanges: 3 starch, 2 lean meat.

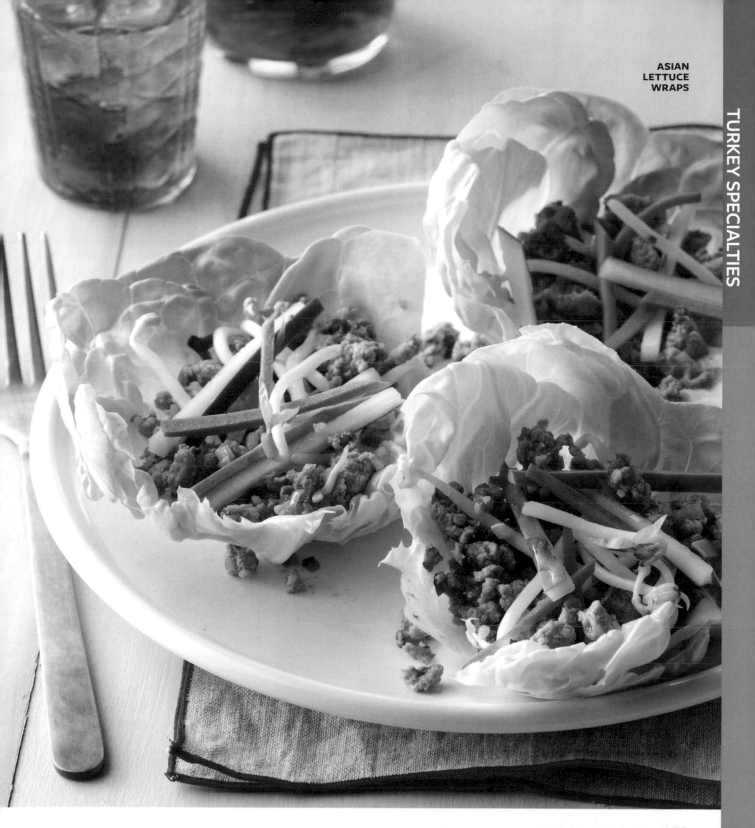

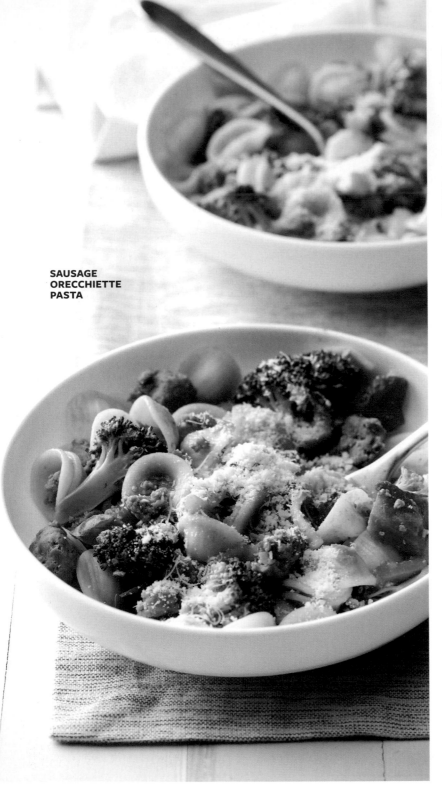

SAUSAGE
ORECCHIETTE
PASTA

FAST FIX

SAUSAGE ORECCHIETTE PASTA

I adapted this pasta to be like my favorite Italian restaurant version, only lighter— and tastier. I often use spicy sausage and broccoli rabe.

—MELANIE TRITTEN CHARLOTTE, NC

START TO FINISH: 25 MIN.
MAKES: 6 SERVINGS

- 4 cups uncooked orecchiette or small tube pasta
- 1 package (19½ ounces) Italian turkey sausage links, casings removed
- 3 garlic cloves, minced
- 1 cup white wine or chicken broth
- 4 cups small fresh broccoli florets
- 1 can (14½ ounces) diced tomatoes, drained
- ⅓ cup grated or shredded Parmesan cheese

1. Cook pasta according to package directions. Meanwhile, in a large skillet, cook the sausage over medium heat for 6-8 minutes or until no longer pink, breaking into crumbles. Add garlic; cook 1 minute longer. Add the wine, stirring to loosen browned bits from pan. Bring the mixture to a boil; cook 1-2 minutes or until liquid is reduced by half.

2. Stir in the broccoli and tomatoes. Reduce heat and simmer, covered, 4-6 minutes or until broccoli is crisp-tender. Drain pasta; add to skillet and toss to coat. Serve with cheese.

Per 1⅔ cups: 363 cal., 8g fat (2g sat. fat), 38mg chol., 571mg sod., 48g carb. (4g sugars, 5g fiber), 20g pro.
Diabetic Exchanges: 3 lean meat, 2½ starch, 1 vegetable.

FAST FIX

BULGUR JAMBALAYA

This dish lets me stay on track for losing weight while still eating foods I love.

—NICHOLAS MONFRE OAK RIDGE, NJ

START TO FINISH: 30 MIN.
MAKES: 4 SERVINGS

- 8 ounces boneless skinless chicken breasts, cut into ¾-inch pieces
- 1 teaspoon Cajun seasoning
- 2 teaspoons olive oil
- 6 ounces smoked turkey sausage, sliced
- 1 medium sweet red pepper, diced
- 2 celery ribs, diced
- 1 small onion, chopped
- ½ cup no-salt-added tomato sauce
- 1 cup bulgur
- 1 cup reduced-sodium chicken broth
- ¾ cup water
- ¼ teaspoon cayenne pepper, optional

1. Toss chicken with Cajun seasoning. In a large saucepan, heat the oil over medium heat; saute chicken until browned, 2-3 minutes. Remove from the pan.
2. In the same pan, saute sausage until browned, 1-2 minutes. Add the red pepper, celery and onion; cook and stir 2 minutes. Stir in tomato sauce; cook 30 seconds. Stir in bulgur, broth, water, chicken and, if desired, cayenne; bring to a boil. Reduce heat; simmer, covered, until the bulgur is tender and the liquid is almost absorbed, about 10 minutes, stirring occasionally.
Per 1 cup: 287 cal., 6g fat (2g sat. fat), 58mg chol., 751mg sod., 34g carb. (5g sugars, 6g fiber), 24g pro.
Diabetic Exchanges: 3 lean meat, 2 starch, ½ fat.

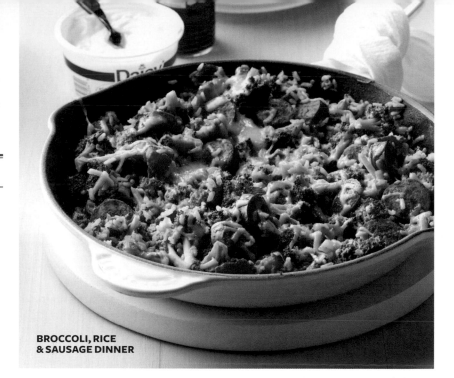

BROCCOLI, RICE & SAUSAGE DINNER

FAST FIX

BROCCOLI, RICE & SAUSAGE DINNER

The first recipe my kids wanted to take with them when they left home was broccoli with sausage and rice. If fresh zucchini or summer squash is available, add it to the mix.

—JOANN PARMENTIER BRANCH, MI

START TO FINISH: 25 MIN.
MAKES: 6 SERVINGS

- 1 tablespoon canola oil
- 1 package (13 ounces) smoked turkey sausage, sliced
- 4 cups small fresh broccoli florets
- 2 cups water
- 1 can (14½ ounces) diced tomatoes, drained
- ¼ teaspoon seasoned salt
- ¼ teaspoon garlic powder
- ¼ teaspoon dried oregano
- 2 cups uncooked instant brown rice
- ½ cup shredded sharp cheddar cheese

Reduced-fat sour cream and Louisiana-style hot sauce, optional

1. In a large skillet, heat the oil over medium-high heat. Add sausage; cook and stir 2-3 minutes or until browned. Stir in the broccoli; cook and stir 2 minutes longer.
2. Add water, tomatoes and seasonings; bring to a boil. Stir in rice. Reduce heat; simmer, covered, 5 minutes.
3. Remove from heat; stir rice mixture and sprinkle with cheese. Let stand, covered, 5 minutes or until liquid is almost absorbed and cheese is melted. If desired, serve with sour cream and hot sauce.
Per 1 cup without sour cream and hot sauce: 276 cal., 10g fat (3g sat. fat), 48mg chol., 853mg sod., 30g carb. (3g sugars, 4g fiber), 17g pro.
Diabetic Exchanges: 2 lean meat, 1½ starch, 1 vegetable, ½ fat.

FAST FIX

ASPARAGUS TURKEY STIR-FRY

When people try this dish, they ask for the recipe, just as I did when I first tasted it at my friend's house. With its delicious lemon sauce, the skillet dinner is sure to satisfy, and it's such a great dinner for the busiest of nights.

—MAY EVANS CORINTH, KY

START TO FINISH: 20 MIN.
MAKES: 4 SERVINGS

- 2 teaspoons cornstarch
- ¼ cup chicken broth
- 1 tablespoon lemon juice
- 1 teaspoon soy sauce
- 1 pound turkey breast tenderloins, cut into ½-inch strips
- 1 garlic clove, minced
- 2 tablespoons canola oil, divided
- 1 pound fresh asparagus, trimmed and cut into 1½-inch pieces
- 1 jar (2 ounces) sliced pimientos, drained

1. In a bowl, combine the cornstarch, broth, lemon juice and soy sauce until smooth; set aside. In a large skillet or wok, stir-fry the turkey and garlic in 1 tablespoon oil until meat is no longer pink; remove and keep warm.

2. Stir-fry asparagus in remaining oil until crisp-tender. Add pimientos. Stir broth mixture and add to the pan; cook and stir for 1 minute or until thickened. Return turkey to the pan; heat through.

Per 1¼ cups: 205 cal., 9g fat (1g sat. fat), 56mg chol., 204mg sod., 5g carb. (1g sugars, 1g fiber), 28g pro.

Diabetic Exchanges: 3 lean meat, 1½ fat, 1 vegetable.

⑤ INGREDIENTS   FAST FIX

SAUSAGE & FETA STUFFED TOMATOES

As a professional weight loss coach, I'm all about healthy eating. Clients and friends love these tomatoes so much that I had to put them in my cookbook, Getting Fit with Food, and share them here as well.

—SHANA CONRADT GREENVILLE, WI

START TO FINISH: 25 MIN.
MAKES: 4 SERVINGS

- 3 Italian turkey sausage links (4 ounces each), casings removed
- 1 cup (4 ounces) crumbled feta cheese, divided
- 8 plum tomatoes
- ¼ teaspoon salt
- ¼ teaspoon pepper
- 3 tablespoons balsamic vinegar
  Minced fresh parsley

1. Preheat oven to 350°. In a large skillet, cook sausage over medium heat 4-6 minutes or until no longer pink, breaking into crumbles. Transfer to a small bowl; stir in ½ cup cheese.

2. Cut tomatoes in half lengthwise. Scoop out pulp, leaving a ½-in. shell; discard pulp. Sprinkle the tomatoes with salt and pepper; transfer to an ungreased 13x9-in. baking dish. Spoon sausage mixture into tomato shells; drizzle with vinegar. Sprinkle with remaining cheese.

3. Bake, uncovered, for 10-12 minutes or until heated through. Sprinkle with the parsley.

Per 4 stuffed tomato halves: 200 cal., 10g fat (4g sat. fat), 46mg chol., 777mg sod., 12g carb. (8g sugars, 3g fiber), 16g pro.

Diabetic Exchanges: 2 medium-fat meat, 1 vegetable, ½ starch.

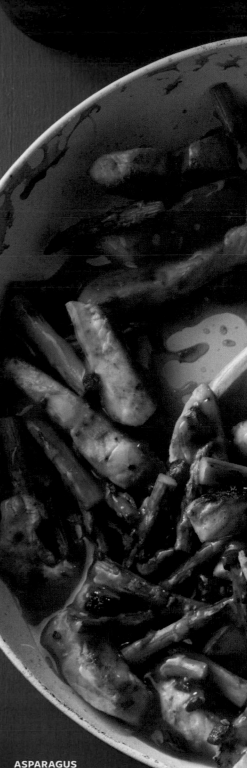

**ASPARAGUS
TURKEY STIR-FRY**

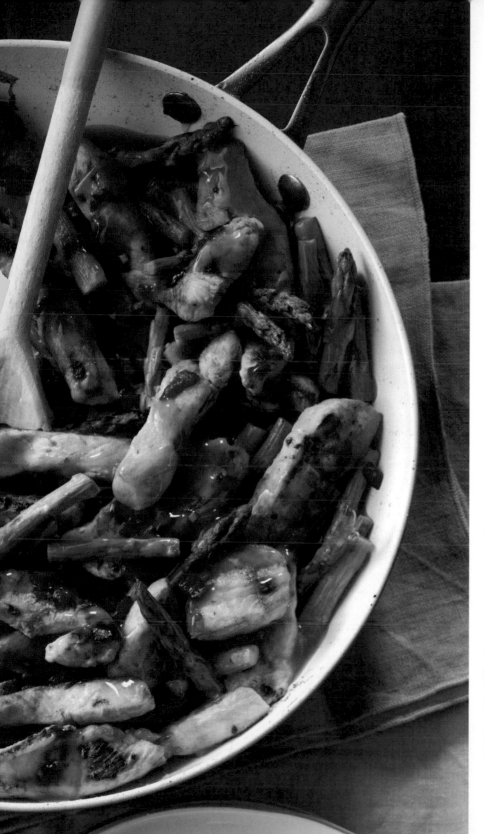

FAST FIX

WALDORF TURKEY SALAD

Crisp apples, celery and walnuts teamed with lean poultry turn any meal into a picnic. The combination of tastes and textures makes this Waldorf Turkey Salad a cool classic.

—**MITZI SENTIFF** ANNAPOLIS, MD

START TO FINISH: 25 MIN.
MAKES: 4 SERVINGS

- 1 cup (8 ounces) plain yogurt
- 2 tablespoons honey
- ⅛ to ¼ teaspoon ground ginger
- ¼ teaspoon salt
- 2 cups cubed cooked turkey breast
- 1 cup cubed apple
- 1 cup seedless red grapes, halved
- ½ cup thinly sliced celery
- ½ cup raisins
- 4 lettuce leaves
- 2 tablespoons chopped walnuts

1. In a small bowl, whisk the yogurt, honey, ginger and salt. In a large bowl, combine the turkey, apple, grapes, celery and raisins; add yogurt mixture and toss to coat.

2. Serve on lettuce leaves; sprinkle with chopped walnuts.

Per 1¼ cup: 294 cal., 5g fat (2g sat. fat), 68mg chol., 233mg sod., 39g carb. (33g sugars, 2g fiber), 25g pro.

Diabetic Exchanges: 3 lean meat, 1½ fruit, 1 starch, ½ fat.

✱

DID YOU KNOW?

Created by famed dining room manager Oscar Tschirky at the Waldorf Astoria New York in the 1890s, the original Waldorf salad included apples and mayonnaise atop a bed of lettuce. Chopped walnuts were added later.

ZUCCHINI-CRUSTED PIZZA

Great flavor, easy, nutritious and fun to make with the kids. What's not to like?

—RUTH HARTUNIAN-ALUMBAUGH
WILLIMANTIC, CT

PREP: 20 MIN. • **BAKE:** 25 MIN.
MAKES: 6 SERVINGS

- 2 large eggs, lightly beaten
- 2 cups shredded zucchini (about 1½ medium), squeezed dry
- ½ cup shredded part-skim mozzarella cheese
- ½ cup grated Parmesan cheese
- ¼ cup all-purpose flour
- 1 tablespoon olive oil
- 1 tablespoon minced fresh basil
- 1 teaspoon minced fresh thyme

TOPPINGS

- 1 jar (12 ounces) roasted sweet red peppers, julienned
- 1 cup (4 ounces) shredded part-skim mozzarella cheese
- ½ cup sliced turkey pepperoni

1. Preheat oven to 450°. Mix first eight ingredients; transfer to a 12-in. pizza pan coated generously with cooking spray. Spread mixture to an 11-in. circle.
2. Bake until light golden brown, 13-16 minutes. Reduce oven setting to 400°. Add toppings. Bake until the cheese is melted, 10-12 minutes.

Per slice: 219 cal., 12g fat (5g sat. fat), 95mg chol., 680mg sod., 10g carb. (4g sugars, 1g fiber), 14g pro.
Diabetic Exchanges: 2 medium-fat meat, ½ starch, ½ fat.

FAST FIX

CHILLED TURKEY PASTA SALAD

A Waldorf salad inspired my pasta dish. I use smoked turkey, apples, strawberries and orecchiette. Rotisserie chicken and other fruits would also taste great.

—SONYA LABBE WEST HOLLYWOOD, CA

START TO FINISH: 30 MIN.
MAKES: 4 SERVINGS

- 2 cups uncooked orecchiette or small tube pasta (about 6 ounces)
- ¼ cup reduced-fat plain yogurt
- 2 tablespoons mayonnaise
- 2 tablespoons 2% milk
- 4 teaspoons Dijon mustard
- ½ teaspoon dried thyme, optional
- 1 medium apple, chopped
- 1 tablespoon lemon juice
- ½ pound thick-sliced deli smoked turkey, cut into bite-size pieces
- 1 cup quartered fresh strawberries
- 1 celery rib, sliced
- ¼ cup toasted chopped walnuts, optional

1. Cook pasta according to package directions. Drain; rinse with cold water and drain well.
2. Meanwhile, in a small bowl, mix the yogurt, mayonnaise, milk, mustard and, if desired, thyme until blended. Toss apple with lemon juice.
3. In a large bowl, combine pasta, apple, turkey, strawberries and celery. Add dressing; toss gently to coat. If desired, sprinkle with the walnuts. Refrigerate until serving.

Per 1½ cups without walnuts: 313 cal., 8g fat (1g sat. fat), 24mg chol., 606mg sod., 42g carb. (8g sugars, 3g fiber), 19g pro.
Diabetic Exchanges: 2 starch, 2 lean meat, 1 fat, ½ fruit.

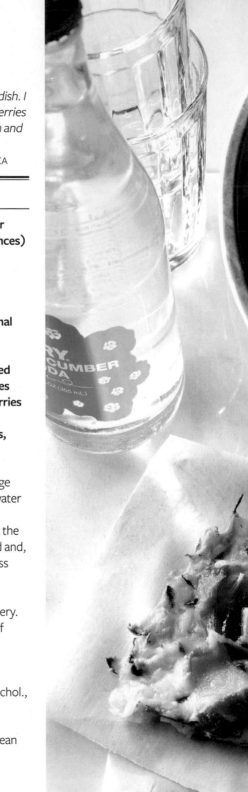

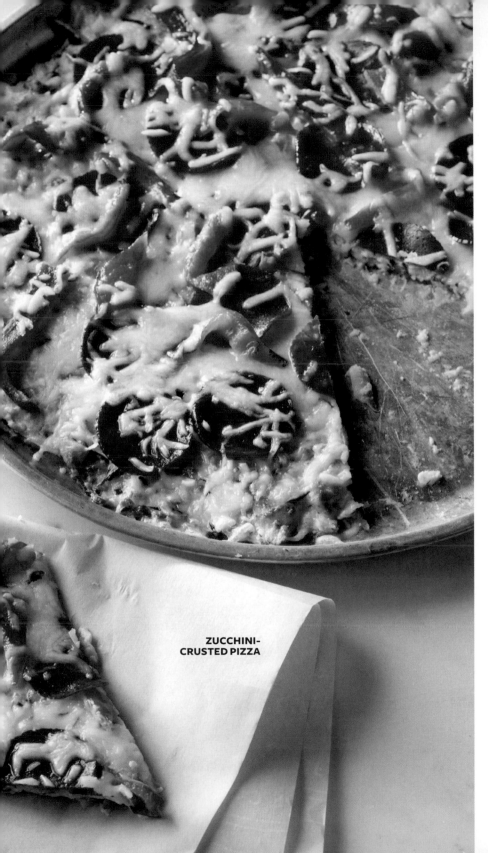

ZUCCHINI-CRUSTED PIZZA

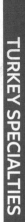

TURKEY SAUSAGE ZUCCHINI BOATS

My library co-workers were my taste testers when I worked there. They approved this spin on stuffed zucchini.
—**STEPHANIE COTTERMAN** ALEXANDRIA, OH

PREP: 30 MIN. • **BAKE:** 35 MIN.
MAKES: 6 SERVINGS

- 6 medium zucchini
- 1 pound lean ground turkey
- 1 small onion, chopped
- 1 celery rib, chopped
- 1 garlic clove, minced
- 1½ teaspoons Italian seasoning
- ¾ teaspoon salt
- ¼ teaspoon cayenne pepper
- ¼ teaspoon paprika
- 1 cup salad croutons, coarsely crushed
- 1 cup shredded part-skim mozzarella cheese, divided

1. Preheat oven to 350°. Cut each zucchini lengthwise in half. Scoop out pulp, leaving a ¼-in. shell; chop pulp.
2. In a large skillet, cook turkey, onion, celery, garlic and seasonings over medium heat 6-8 minutes or until turkey is no longer pink, breaking up turkey into crumbles. Stir in croutons, ½ cup cheese and zucchini pulp. Spoon into zucchini shells.
3. Transfer to two ungreased 13x9-in. baking dishes; add ¼ in. water. Bake, covered, 30-35 minutes or until zucchini is tender. Sprinkle with the remaining cheese. Bake, uncovered, for about 5 minutes or until cheese is melted.

Per 2 stuffed zucchini halves: 240 cal., 11g fat (4g sat. fat), 63mg chol., 556mg sod., 13g carb. (5g sugars, 2g fiber), 23g pro.
Diabetic Exchanges: 3 lean meat, 1 vegetable, ½ starch.

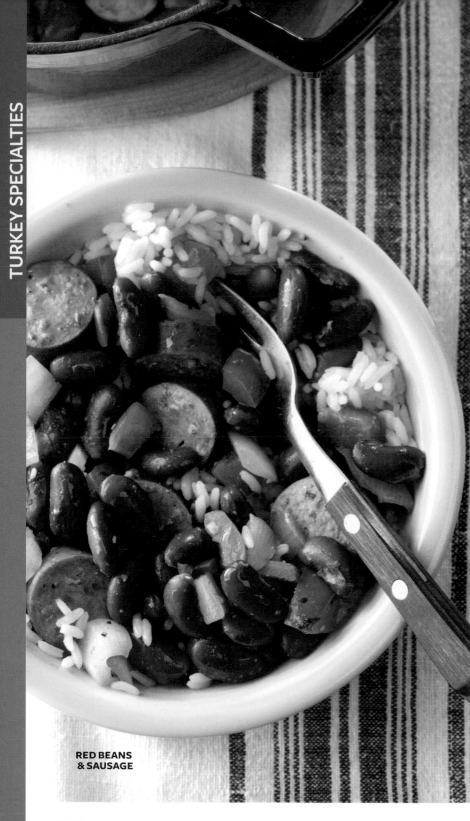

RED BEANS & SAUSAGE

RED BEANS & SAUSAGE

Turkey sausage can make a traditional dish appeal to more health-conscious cooks and eaters, while a zesty blend of seasonings keeps its sensational spark.
—CATHY WEBSTER MORRIS, IL

START TO FINISH: 25 MIN.
MAKES: 6 SERVINGS

- 1 tablespoon canola oil
- 1 medium green pepper, diced
- 1 medium onion, chopped
- 2 garlic cloves, minced
- 2 cans (16 ounces each) kidney beans, rinsed and drained
- ½ pound smoked turkey sausage, sliced
- 1 teaspoon Cajun seasoning
- ⅛ teaspoon hot pepper sauce
- ¾ cup water
  Hot cooked rice, optional

1. In a large saucepan, heat oil over medium heat; saute pepper and onion until tender. Add garlic; cook and stir 1 minute.

2. Stir in the beans, sausage, Cajun seasoning, pepper sauce and water; bring to a boil. Reduce heat; simmer, uncovered, until heated through, 5-7 minutes. If desired, serve with rice.

Per ⅔ cup without rice: 212 cal., 4g fat (1g sat. fat), 24mg chol., 706mg sod., 27g carb. (4g sugars, 8g fiber), 16g pro.
Diabetic Exchanges: 2 lean meat, 1½ starch, ½ fat.

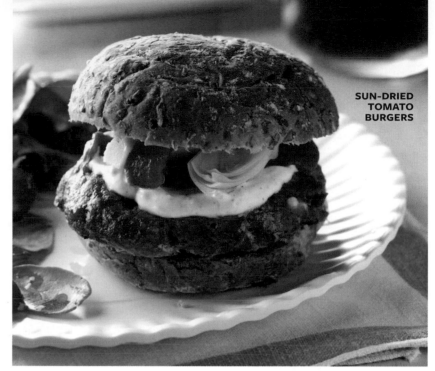

SUN-DRIED TOMATO BURGERS

TURKEY & FRUIT SALAD

We have our own turkeys, so I am always on the lookout for good recipes that are a little different. Salad with fruit and nuts is a great change of pace for leftovers.

—HARRIET STICHTER MILFORD, IN

START TO FINISH: 25 MIN.
MAKES: 5 SERVINGS

- ¼ cup fat-free plain yogurt
- ¼ cup reduced-fat mayonnaise
- 1 tablespoon honey
- 1 tablespoon spicy brown mustard
- ½ teaspoon dried marjoram
- ⅛ teaspoon ground ginger
- 3 cups cubed cooked turkey breast
- 1 large red apple, finely chopped
- 2 celery ribs, thinly sliced
- ½ cup dried cranberries
- ¼ cup chopped walnuts, toasted

Mix first six ingredients. In a large bowl, combine remaining ingredients. Stir in yogurt mixture. Refrigerate, covered, until serving.

Per 1 cup: 278 cal., 9g fat (1g sat. fat), 77mg chol., 208mg sod., 23g carb. (17g sugars, 2g fiber), 28g pro.
Diabetic Exchanges: 3 lean meat, 1 starch, 1 fat.

✳

TEST KITCHEN TIP
Turkey & Fruit Salad is perfect for a potluck. Serve it as is or bring along a box of wheat crackers for guests to top. Just make sure you keep the dish on ice, and don't leave it out for more than 2 hours—less if it's hot outside.

SUN-DRIED TOMATO BURGERS

I made a meat loaf similar to this once but changed it into grilled burgers for an outdoor option when the weather gets warm. My fiance and I really love the hearty flavor.

—MELISSA OBERNESSER UTICA, NY

PREP: 30 MIN. • **GRILL:** 10 MIN.
MAKES: 4 SERVINGS

- ½ cup reduced-fat sour cream
- 2 teaspoons lemon juice
- 1 garlic clove, minced
- ¼ teaspoon dried oregano
- ¼ teaspoon pepper

BURGERS
- ¼ cup oil-packed sun-dried tomatoes, chopped
- ¼ cup sun-dried tomato pesto
- 1 tablespoon salt-free Greek seasoning
- 1 pound lean ground turkey
- ¼ cup crumbled feta cheese
- 4 whole wheat hamburger buns, split
- ¼ cup chopped water-packed artichoke hearts
- ¼ cup julienned roasted sweet red peppers

1. In a small bowl, mix the first five ingredients. Refrigerate until serving.
2. In a large bowl, combine tomatoes, pesto and Greek seasoning. Add turkey and cheese; mix lightly but thoroughly. Shape into four ½-in.-thick patties.
3. On a greased grill rack, grill burgers, covered, over medium heat, or broil 4 in. from heat, 4-6 minutes on each side or until a thermometer reads 165°. Serve on buns with sour cream mixture, artichoke hearts and peppers.

Per burger: 391 cal., 17g fat (5g sat. fat), 92mg chol., 640mg sod., 30g carb. (8g sugars, 5g fiber), 31g pro.
Diabetic Exchanges: 3 lean meat, 2 starch, 2 fat.

TURKEY BREAST WITH CRANBERRY BROWN RICE

Here's a perfect meal for anyone who is cooking for a small household but wants a bit leftover for sandwiches!

—**NANCY HEISHMAN** LAS VEGAS, NV

PREP: 20 MIN.
BAKE: 45 MIN. + STANDING
MAKES: 6 SERVINGS

- 2 tablespoons jellied cranberry sauce
- 2 tablespoons chopped celery
- 2 tablespoons minced red onion
- 1 tablespoon olive oil
- 1½ teaspoons minced fresh parsley
- ½ teaspoon grated orange peel
- ⅛ teaspoon garlic powder
- ½ teaspoon poultry seasoning, divided
- 1 boneless skinless turkey breast half (2 pounds)
- ½ teaspoon kosher salt
- ¼ teaspoon pepper
- ¼ cup orange juice

RICE

- 1⅓ cups uncooked long grain brown rice
- 2⅔ cups water
- ¼ cup chopped celery
- 3 tablespoons minced red onion
- ¾ teaspoon salt
- ¼ teaspoon pepper
- ⅔ cup dried cranberries
- ⅔ cup sliced almonds, toasted
- 1 tablespoon minced fresh parsley
- ½ teaspoon grated orange peel

1. Preheat oven to 350°. Mix the first seven ingredients and ¼ teaspoon of poultry seasoning.

2. Place turkey in a greased foil-lined 13x9-in. baking pan; rub with salt, pepper and the remaining poultry seasoning. Spread with cranberry mixture. Roast until a thermometer reads 165°, 45-55 minutes, drizzling with orange juice halfway.

3. Meanwhile, in a saucepan, combine first six rice ingredients; bring to a boil. Reduce heat; simmer, covered, until rice is tender and liquid is absorbed, 40-45 minutes. Stir in remaining ingredients.

4. Remove turkey from oven; tent with foil. Let stand 10 minutes before slicing. Serve with rice.

Note: To toast nuts, bake in a shallow pan in a 350° oven for 5-10 minutes or cook in a skillet over low heat until lightly browned, stirring occasionally.

Per 5 ounces cooked turkey with ⅔ cup rice: 465 cal., 11g fat (1g sat fat), 86mg chol., 642mg sod., 50g carb. (13g sugars, 5g fiber), 42g pro.
Diabetic Exchanges: 5 lean meat, 3 starch, 1½ fat.

FAST FIX
MIGHTY HERO SANDWICH

The first time my friend served this sub sandwich, I had to ask her the secret to its change-of-pace flavor. It's the zesty marinated veggies!

—**KELLEY BOYCE** TULSA, OK

START TO FINISH: 30 MIN.
MAKES: 8 SERVINGS

- ¼ cup balsamic vinegar
- 1 tablespoon minced fresh parsley
- 1 tablespoon olive oil
- 2 garlic cloves, minced
- ¼ teaspoon dried oregano
- ¼ teaspoon pepper
- 1 large tomato, halved and sliced
- 1 cup sliced fresh mushrooms
- 2 thin slices red onion, separated into rings
- 1 round loaf (1 pound) sourdough bread
- 1 small zucchini, shredded
- ½ pound sliced deli turkey
- 6 slices part-skim mozzarella cheese

1. In a large bowl, whisk the first six ingredients until blended. Add tomato, mushrooms and onion; toss gently to coat. Let stand 15 minutes.

2. Meanwhile, cut loaf horizontally in half. Hollow out both parts, leaving a ½-in.-thick shell (save removed bread for another use).

3. Drain the marinated vegetables, reserving marinade. Brush marinade over inside of bread halves. Top bottom half with zucchini. Layer with half of the marinated vegetables, ¼ pound turkey and three slices cheese; repeat layers. Replace top of loaf. Cut into wedges.
Per piece: 233 cal., 7g fat (3g sat. fat), 24mg chol., 636mg sod., 26g carb. (6g sugars, 1g fiber), 16g pro.
Diabetic Exchanges: 2 starch, 2 lean meat, ½ fat.

★ ★ ★ ★ ★ **READER REVIEW**

"The marinated veggies add great flavor, and it was easy to assemble. This would be fantastic for a party."

DELICIOUSLYRESOURCEFUL_GINA
TASTEOFHOME.COM

TURKEY BREAST WITH
CRANBERRY BROWN RICE

SOUTHWEST-STYLE SHEPHERD'S PIE

I combined a few different flavors into this hearty shepherd's pie.
—LYNN PRICE MILLVILLE, MA

PREP: 20 MIN. • **BAKE:** 25 MIN.
MAKES: 6 SERVINGS

- 1¼ pounds lean ground turkey
- 1 small onion, chopped
- 2 garlic cloves, minced
- ½ teaspoon salt, divided
- 1 can (14¾ ounces) cream-style corn
- 1 can (4 ounces) chopped green chilies
- 1 to 2 tablespoons chipotle hot pepper sauce, optional
- 2⅔ cups water
- 2 tablespoons butter
- 2 tablespoons half-and-half cream
- ½ teaspoon pepper
- 2 cups mashed potato flakes

1. Preheat oven to 425°. In a large skillet, cook turkey, onion, garlic and ¼ teaspoon salt over medium heat 8-10 minutes or until turkey is no longer pink and onion is tender, breaking up turkey into crumbles. Stir in corn, green chilies and, if desired, pepper sauce. Transfer to a greased 8-in. square baking dish.

2. Meanwhile, in a saucepan, bring the water, butter, cream, pepper and remaining salt to a boil. Remove from heat. Stir in potato flakes. Spoon over turkey mixture, spreading to cover. Bake for 25-30 minutes or until bubbly and potatoes are light brown.

Per 1 cup: 312 cal., 12g fat (5g sat. fat), 78mg chol., 583mg sod., 31g carb. (4g sugars, 3g fiber), 22g pro.
Diabetic Exchanges: 3 lean meat, 2 starch, 1 fat.

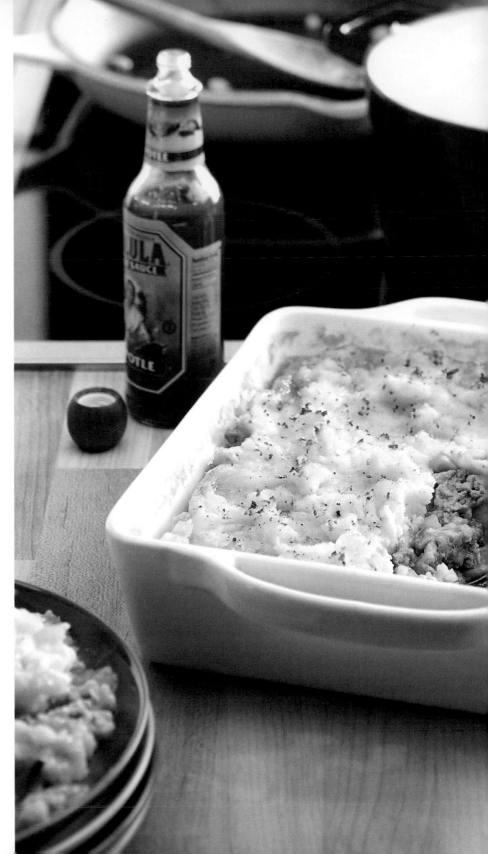

QUICK & EASY TURKEY SLOPPY JOES

When we were first married, I found a simple recipe and adjusted it to suit our tastes. The fresh bell pepper and red onion give sloppy joes wonderful flavor.

—KALLEE TWINER MARYVILLE, TN

START TO FINISH: 30 MIN.
MAKES: 8 SERVINGS

- 1 pound lean ground turkey
- 1 large red onion, chopped
- 1 large green pepper, chopped
- 1 can (8 ounces) tomato sauce
- ½ cup barbecue sauce
- 1 teaspoon dried oregano
- 1 teaspoon ground cumin
- 1 teaspoon chili powder
- ¼ teaspoon salt
- 8 hamburger buns, split

1. In a large skillet, cook turkey, onion and pepper over medium heat for 6-8 minutes or until turkey is no longer pink and vegetables are tender, breaking up turkey into crumbles.

2. Stir in tomato sauce, barbecue sauce and seasonings. Bring to a boil. Reduce heat; simmer, uncovered, for 10 minutes to allow the flavors to blend, stirring occasionally. Serve on buns.

Per sandwich: 251 cal., 6g fat (2g sat. fat), 39mg chol., 629mg sod., 32g carb. (10g sugars, 2g fiber), 16g pro.
Diabetic Exchanges: 2 lean meat, 1½ starch, 1 vegetable.

✱

DID YOU KNOW?
Sloppy joes go by different names around the country, like "dynamites" in Rhode Island or "slushburgers" in parts of the Midwest. With turkey, some call them "sloppy toms."

TURKEY LO MEIN

I love Chinese dishes but not the required veggie chopping. Using presliced mushrooms and ready-made sauce, I came up with a quick, easy and versatile meal. I sometimes add peanuts or cashews for extra crunch and flavor.

—CHRISTI PAULTON PHELPS, WI

START TO FINISH: 30 MIN.
MAKES: 8 SERVINGS

- 8 ounces uncooked linguine
- 2 pounds turkey breast tenderloins, cut into ¼-inch strips
- 2 tablespoons canola oil, divided
- 1⅔ cups julienned sweet red, yellow and/or green peppers
- ⅓ cup chopped onion
- ½ pound sliced fresh mushrooms
- ⅔ cup stir-fry sauce

1. Cook linguine according to package directions. Meanwhile, in a large skillet or wok, stir-fry the turkey in batches in 1 tablespoon hot oil for 5-6 minutes or until no longer pink. Remove turkey and keep warm.

2. In the same pan, stir-fry the peppers and onion in the remaining oil for 4-5 minutes or until crisp-tender. Add the mushrooms; stir-fry for 3-4 minutes or until vegetables are tender. Add turkey and stir-fry sauce; cook and stir for 2-3 minutes or until heated through. Drain linguine; add to turkey mixture and toss to coat.

Per 1 cup: 287 cal., 6g fat (1g sat. fat), 56mg chol., 771mg sod., 28g carb. (4g sugars, 2g fiber), 33g pro.
Diabetic Exchanges: 3 lean meat, 2 starch.

SOUTHWEST-STYLE
SHEPHERD'S PIE

TURKEY-THYME STUFFED PEPPERS

Chloe, my toddler, is a big fan of these healthy peppers, which have a great thyme flavor. She likes to help mix the ingredients and make meals with me.

—JENNIFER KENT PHILADELPHIA, PA

PREP: 30 MIN. • **COOK:** 10 MIN.
MAKES: 4 SERVINGS

- 1 pound lean ground turkey
- 1 medium onion, finely chopped
- 3 garlic cloves, minced
- ½ teaspoon dried thyme
- ¼ teaspoon salt
- ¼ teaspoon dried rosemary, crushed
- ⅛ teaspoon pepper
- 1 can (14½ ounces) diced tomatoes, undrained
- 1 package (8.8 ounces) ready-to-serve brown rice
- ½ cup seasoned bread crumbs
- 4 medium sweet yellow or orange peppers
- ¼ cup shredded part-skim mozzarella cheese

1. In a large skillet, cook turkey and onion over medium heat 8-10 minutes or until the turkey is no longer pink and onion is tender, breaking up turkey into crumbles. Add garlic and seasonings; cook 1 minute longer. Stir in tomatoes, rice and bread crumbs.

2. Cut sweet peppers lengthwise in half; remove seeds. Arrange pepper halves in a 13x9-in. microwave-safe dish; fill with turkey mixture. Sprinkle with cheese. Microwave, covered, on high for 7-9 minutes or until peppers are crisp-tender.

Note: This recipe was tested in a full-size 1,100-watt microwave. If your microwave does not accommodate a 13x9-in. dish, microwave stuffed peppers, half at a time, in an 8-in.-square dish for 6-8 minutes or until peppers are crisp-tender.

Per 2 stuffed pepper halves: 423 cal., 13g fat (3g sat. fat), 82mg chol., 670mg sod., 43g carb. (10g sugars, 6g fiber), 31g pro.

Diabetic Exchanges: 3 medium-fat meat, 2 starch, 2 vegetable.

FAST FIX

TURKEY CHOP SUEY

I use leftover turkey for my fast-to-fix dinner. Water chestnuts and bean sprouts add a nice crunch to the mix.

—RUTH PETERSON JENISON, MI

START TO FINISH: 20 MIN.
MAKES: 4 SERVINGS

- 1 small onion, sliced
- 2 celery ribs, sliced
- 1 tablespoon butter
- 2 cups cubed cooked turkey breast
- 1 can (8 ounces) sliced water chestnuts, drained
- 1¼ cups reduced-sodium chicken broth
- 2 tablespoons cornstarch
- ¼ cup cold water
- 3 tablespoons reduced-sodium soy sauce
- 1 can (14 ounces) bean sprouts, drained
  Hot cooked rice

1. In a large skillet, saute onion and celery in butter until tender. Add the turkey, water chestnuts and broth; bring to a boil. Reduce heat.

2. In a small bowl, combine the cornstarch, water and soy sauce until smooth; add to turkey mixture. Bring to a boil; cook and stir for 2 minutes or until thickened. Add bean sprouts. Serve with rice.

Per 1¼ cup: 204 cal., 4g fat (2g sat. fat), 68mg chol., 762mg sod., 17g carb. (3g sugars, 3g fiber), 25g pro.

Diabetic Exchanges: 3 lean meat, 2 vegetable, ½ starch.

⑤INGREDIENTS FAST FIX

TURKEY & APRICOT WRAPS

For these wraps, I combined the Southern appetizer of jam and cream cheese on crackers with turkey sandwiches. I sneak fresh baby spinach into all sorts of recipes because it has such nice crunch, color and flavor.

—KIM BEAVERS NORTH AUGUSTA, SC

START TO FINISH: 15 MIN.
MAKES: 4 SERVINGS

- ½ cup reduced-fat cream cheese
- 3 tablespoons apricot preserves
- 4 whole wheat tortillas (8 inches), room temperature
- ½ pound sliced reduced-sodium deli turkey
- 2 cups fresh baby spinach or arugula

In a small bowl, mix cream cheese and preserves. Spread about 2 tablespoons over each tortilla to within ½ in. of edges. Layer with turkey and spinach. Roll up tightly. Serve immediately or wrap in plastic wrap and refrigerate until serving.

Per wrap: 312 cal., 10g fat (4g sat. fat), 41mg chol., 655mg sod., 33g carb. (8g sugars, 2g fiber), 20g pro.

Diabetic Exchanges: 2 starch, 2 lean meat, 1 fat.

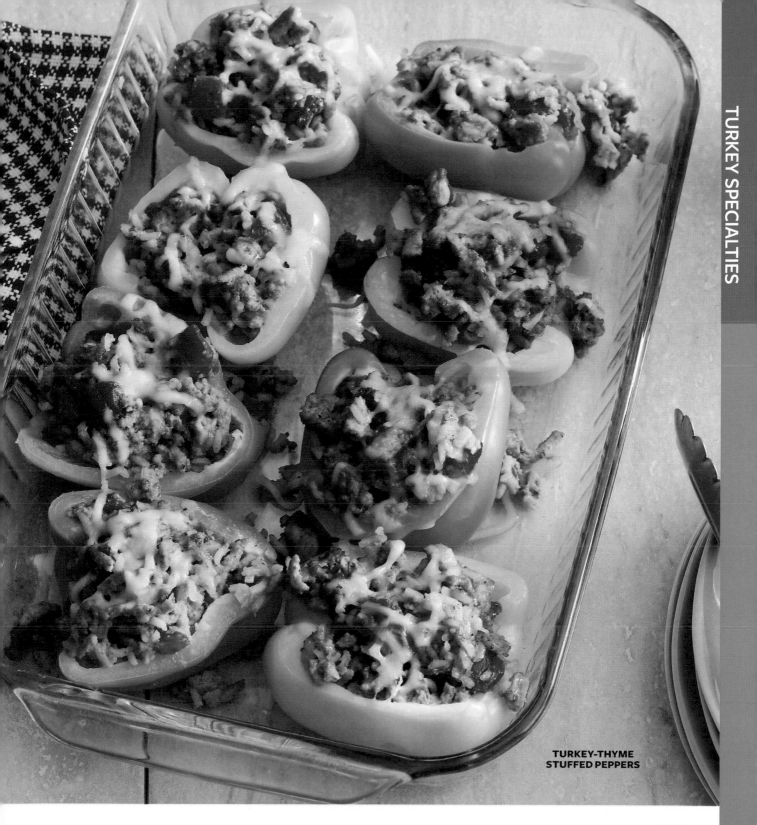

**TURKEY-THYME
STUFFED PEPPERS**

PIZZAIOLA CHOPS
PAGE 199

Pork, Ham & More

A welcome change from beef and chicken,
pork is a lean, tasty alternative. Roasted, stir-fried or
served in a salad, there are so many meaty possibilities
to sink your teeth into. Add some bacon
and even lamb—no ho-hum dinners here!

PORK TENDERLOIN WITH FENNEL & CRANBERRIES

This delicious entree is quick to prepare at home and easy to take to a potluck. Fresh rosemary, fennel and sweet-tart cranberries are a lovely combination.

—**JUDY ARMSTRONG** PRAIRIEVILLE, LA

PREP: 25 MIN. • **BAKE:** 20 MIN.
MAKES: 8 SERVINGS

- 1 teaspoon kosher salt
- 1 teaspoon fennel seeds, crushed
- 1 teaspoon paprika
- ¼ teaspoon cayenne pepper
- 2 pork tenderloins (1 pound each)
- 2 tablespoons olive oil, divided
- 2 medium fennel bulbs, halved and thinly sliced
- 2 shallots, thinly sliced
- 3 garlic cloves, minced
- 1½ cups dry white wine or chicken broth
- 1 cup dried cranberries
- 2 tablespoons minced fresh rosemary or 2 teaspoons dried rosemary, crushed
  Fennel fronds, optional

1. Preheat oven to 425°. In a small bowl, mix salt, fennel seeds, paprika and cayenne. Rub over pork.

2. In a large skillet, heat 1 tablespoon oil over medium-high heat. Brown the pork on all sides. Transfer to a rack in a shallow roasting pan. Roast for 20-25 minutes or until a thermometer reads 145°. Remove tenderloins from oven; tent with foil. Let stand for 5 minutes before slicing.

3. Meanwhile, in same skillet, heat remaining oil over medium-high heat. Add fennel and shallots; cook and stir 4-6 minutes or until tender. Add garlic; cook 1 minute longer.

4. Stir in the wine, cranberries and rosemary. Bring to a boil. Reduce heat; simmer, uncovered, 10 minutes.

5. To serve, spoon fennel mixture onto a serving platter. Using a slotted spoon, top with tenderloin slices and, if desired, fennel fronds.

Per 3 ounces cooked pork with ½ cup fennel mixture: 273 cal., 7g fat (2g sat. fat), 63mg chol., 374mg sod., 20g carb. (11g sugars, 3g fiber), 24g pro.
Diabetic Exchanges: 3 lean meat, 1 starch, 1 vegetable, 1 fat.

PORK ROAST WITH HERB RUB

Marinating pork loin with herbs like marjoram and sage gives it a mild but out-of-this-world flavor. People flock to the table for this tender roast.

—**CAROLYN POPE** MASON CITY, IA

PREP: 5 MIN. + CHILLING
BAKE: 1¼ HOURS + STANDING
MAKES: 12 SERVINGS

- 2 tablespoons sugar
- 2 teaspoons dried marjoram
- 2 teaspoons rubbed sage
- 1 teaspoon salt
- ½ teaspoon celery seed
- ½ teaspoon ground mustard
- ⅛ teaspoon pepper
- 1 boneless pork loin roast (4 pounds)

1. Mix first seven ingredients; rub over roast. Refrigerate at least 4 hours.

2. Preheat oven to 350°. Place roast on a rack in a roasting pan, fat side up. Roast until a thermometer reads 145°, 1¼ to 1¾ hours.

3. Remove roast from oven; tent with foil. Let stand 15 minutes before slicing.

Applesauce Pork Roast: Omit herb rub. Combine 1½ cups unsweetened applesauce with 1½ teaspoons each salt and rubbed sage; spread over the roast. Omit refrigeration time. Bake pork as directed, covering with foil for the first hour.

Old-World Pork Roast: Omit herb rub. Combine 1 teaspoon each salt, caraway seeds and rubbed sage with ¼ teaspoon pepper; rub over the roast. Omit the refrigeration time. Bake as directed. If desired, thicken pan drippings for gravy.

Tuscan Pork Roast: In a food processor, combine 5 to 8 peeled garlic cloves, 1 tablespoon dried rosemary, 1 tablespoon olive oil and ½ teaspoon salt; cover and process until mixture becomes a paste. Rub over roast; refrigerate as directed. Bake as directed.

Per 4 ounces cooked pork with herb rub: 198 cal., 7g fat (3g sat. fat), 75mg chol., 240mg sod., 2g carb. (2g sugars, 0 fiber), 29g pro.
Diabetic Exchanges: 4 lean meat.

✳

TEST KITCHEN TIP
Before cooking meat that's been marinated in the refrigerator, let it come to room temperature to take the chill off the meat's surface. This helps it more quickly reach the optimal temperature for browning when you place it into a hot oven.

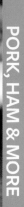

**PORK TENDERLOIN WITH
FENNEL & CRANBERRIES**

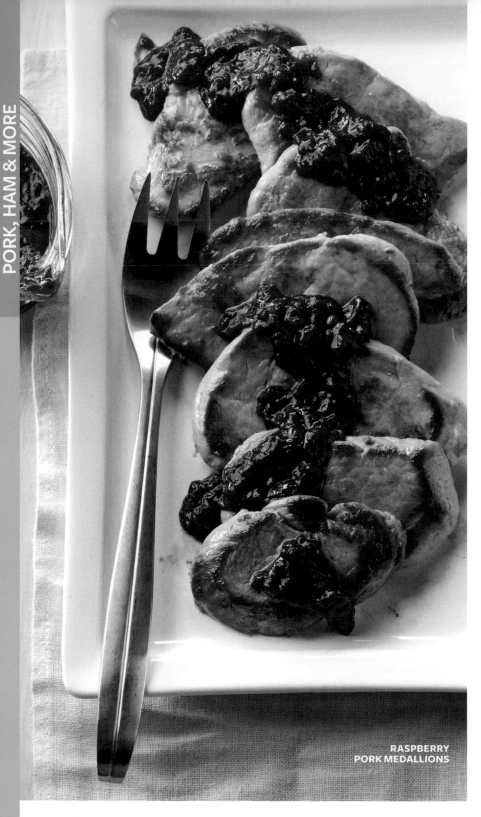

RASPBERRY PORK MEDALLIONS

With a ruby red berry sauce, these pork medallions are special enough for your guests. I like to round out the meal with sides of wild rice and steamed veggies.

—TRISHA KRUSE EAGLE, ID

START TO FINISH: 25 MIN.
MAKES: 4 SERVINGS

- 1 pork tenderloin (1 pound)
- 1 tablespoon canola oil
- 2 tablespoons reduced-sodium soy sauce
- 1 garlic clove, minced
- ½ teaspoon ground ginger
- 1 cup fresh raspberries
- 2 tablespoons seedless raspberry spreadable fruit
- 2 teaspoons minced fresh basil
- ½ teaspoon minced fresh mint, optional

1. Cut tenderloin crosswise into eight slices; pound each with a meat mallet to ½-in. thickness. In a large skillet, heat oil over medium-high heat. Add pork; cook for 3-4 minutes on each side or until a thermometer reads 145°. Remove the meat from pan; keep warm.

2. Reduce heat to medium-low; add soy sauce, garlic and ginger to the pan, stirring to loosen browned bits from pan. Add raspberries, spreadable fruit, basil and, if desired, mint; cook and stir 2-3 minutes or until slightly thickened. Serve with pork.

Per 3 ounces cooked pork with 3 tablespoons sauce: 206 cal., 8g fat (2g sat. fat), 64mg chol., 333mg sod., 10g carb. (5g sugars, 2g fiber), 24g pro. **Diabetic Exchanges:** 3 lean meat, ½ starch, ½ fat.

RASPBERRY PORK MEDALLIONS

ZESTY GRILLED CHOPS

Tasty sauce makes pork chops a quick company dish. Our family enjoys them grilled outside, as the summer weather in our part of the country is hot and muggy. In the wintertime, they're just as wonderful prepared under the broiler.
—BLANCHE BABINSKI MINOT, ND

PREP: 10 MIN. + MARINATING
GRILL: 10 MIN. • **MAKES:** 6 SERVINGS

- ¾ cup soy sauce
- ¼ cup lemon juice
- 1 tablespoon chili sauce
- 1 tablespoon brown sugar
- 1 garlic clove, minced
- 6 bone-in pork loin or rib chops (about 1½ inches thick)

1. In a large resealable plastic bag, combine first five ingredients; reserve ⅓ cup mixture for brushing over chops. Add pork chops to bag; seal bag and turn to coat. Refrigerate overnight.
2. Drain pork, discarding marinade. Grill chops, covered, over medium heat or broil 4 in. from heat until a thermometer reads 145°, 6-8 minutes per side. Brush occasionally with the reserved soy mixture during the last 5 minutes. Let stand about 5 minutes before serving.

Per 1 pork chop: 246 cal., 11g fat (4g sat. fat), 82mg chol., 598mg sod., 1g carb. (1g sugars, trace fiber), 34g pro.
Diabetic Exchanges: 5 lean meat.

❋

DID YOU KNOW?
Lemon juice in this zesty marinade is an acid, which breaks down the tough proteins in the pork and helps to tenderize it.

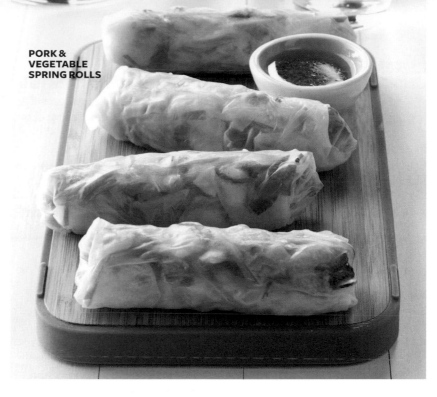
PORK & VEGETABLE SPRING ROLLS

FAST FIX
PORK & VEGETABLE SPRING ROLLS

I thought rice paper wrappers would be a quick, fun way to put salad ingredients into a hand-held snack or meal. Try your rolls with shrimp or add in cranberries.
—MARLA STRADER OZARK, MO

START TO FINISH: 30 MIN.
MAKES: 4 SERVINGS

- 2 cups thinly sliced romaine
- 1½ cups cubed cooked pork
- 1 cup thinly sliced fresh spinach
- ¾ cup julienned carrot
- ⅓ cup thinly sliced celery
- ⅓ cup dried cherries, coarsely chopped
- 1 tablespoon sesame oil
- 12 round rice paper wrappers (8 inches)
- ¼ cup sliced almonds
- ¼ cup wasabi-coated green peas
  Sesame ginger salad dressing

1. In a large bowl, combine the first six ingredients. Drizzle with the oil; toss to coat.
2. Fill a large shallow dish partway with warm water. Dip a rice paper wrapper into water just until pliable, about 45 seconds (do not soften completely); allow excess water to drip off.
3. Place the wrapper on a flat surface. Layer salad mixture, almonds and peas across bottom third of wrapper. Fold in both ends of wrapper; fold bottom side over filling, then roll up tightly. Place on a serving plate, seam side down. Repeat with remaining ingredients. Serve with the dressing.

Per 3 spring rolls without salad dressing: 255 cal., 12g fat (3g sat. fat), 48mg chol., 91mg sod., 19g carb. (10g sugars, 3g fiber), 18g pro.
Diabetic Exchanges: 3 lean meat, 1 starch, 1 vegetable, 1 fat.

FAST FIX ▶
CHARDONNAY PORK CHOPS

I began perfecting these juicy chops when I moved to another state and missed my stepdad's best pork recipe. His dish inspired my version, which includes a wine sauce.

—JOLEEN THOMPSON FARMINGTON, MN

START TO FINISH: 25 MIN.
MAKES: 4 SERVINGS

- 4 bone-in pork loin chops (6 ounces each)
- ½ teaspoon salt
- ¼ teaspoon pepper
- 1 cup seasoned bread crumbs
- 1 tablespoon olive oil
- 3 green onions, chopped
- 2 garlic cloves, minced
- 1 cup chardonnay or chicken broth
- 2 tablespoons lemon juice
- 1 teaspoon dried rosemary, crushed

1. Sprinkle pork chops with salt and pepper. Place bread crumbs in a shallow bowl. Dip pork chops in bread crumbs to coat both sides; shake off excess. In a large skillet, heat oil over medium heat; cook chops 4-5 minutes on each side or until golden and thermometer reads 145°. Remove from pan; keep warm.
2. In same pan, add green onions and garlic; cook and stir 1-2 minutes or until tender. Add chardonnay; stir to loosen browned bits from pan. Bring to a boil; cook for 1-2 minutes or until liquid is reduced by half. Stir in lemon juice and rosemary. Serve pork chops with sauce.

Per 1 pork chop with 3 tablespoons sauce: 270 cal., 11g fat (3g sat. fat), 74mg chol., 509mg sod., 9g carb. (1g sugars, 1g fiber), 28g pro.
Diabetic Exchanges: 4 lean meat, ½ starch, ½ fat.

FAST FIX ▶
QUICK TACOS AL PASTOR

We tried pork and pineapple tacos at a truck stand in Hawaii, and I decided to make my own version at home.

—LORI MCLAIN DENTON, TX

START TO FINISH: 25 MIN.
MAKES: 4 SERVINGS

- 1 package (15 ounces) refrigerated pork roast au jus
- 1 cup well-drained unsweetened pineapple chunks, divided
- 1 tablespoon canola oil
- ½ cup enchilada sauce
- 8 corn tortillas (6 inches), warmed
- ½ cup finely chopped onion
- ¼ cup chopped fresh cilantro
  Optional ingredients: crumbled queso fresco, salsa verde and lime wedges

1. Coarsely shred the pork, reserving juices. In a small bowl, crush half of the pineapple with a fork.
2. In a large nonstick skillet, heat oil over medium-high heat. Add whole pineapple chunks; cook 2-3 minutes or until lightly browned, turning pineapple occasionally. Remove from pan.
3. Add enchilada sauce and crushed pineapple to same skillet; stir in pork and reserved juices. Cook over medium-high heat 4-6 minutes or until liquid is evaporated, stirring occasionally.
4. Serve in tortillas with pineapple chunks, onion and cilantro. If desired, top with cheese and salsa and serve with lime wedges.

Per 2 tacos: 317 cal., 11g fat (3g sat. fat), 57mg chol., 573mg sod., 36g carb. (12g sugars, 5g fiber), 24g pro.
Diabetic Exchanges: 3 lean meat, 2 starch, 1 fat.

PORK PANCIT

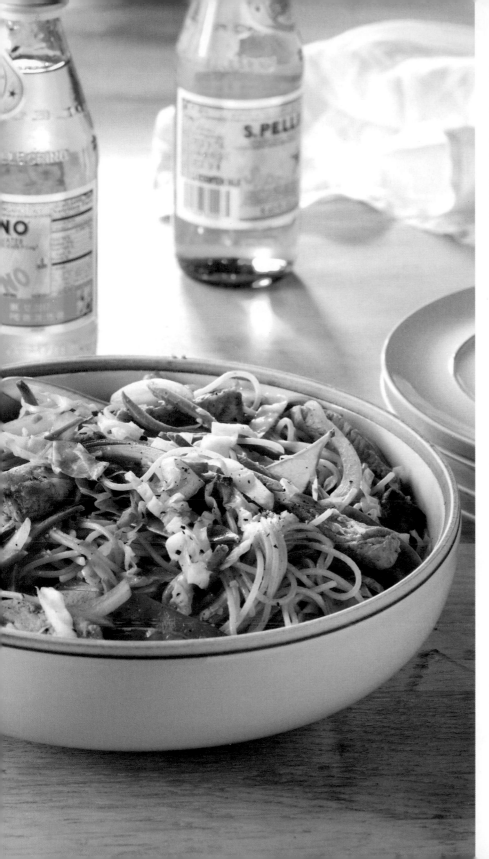

FAST FIX ▶
PORK PANCIT

My friend's noodle recipe is so tempting, we never have leftovers. It works with chicken too!

—PRISCILLA GILBERT
INDIAN HARBOUR BEACH, FL

START TO FINISH: 30 MIN.
MAKES: 6 SERVINGS

- 8 ounces uncooked vermicelli or angel hair pasta
- 1 pound boneless pork loin chops (½ inch thick), cut into thin strips
- 3 tablespoons canola oil, divided
- 4 garlic cloves, minced
- 1½ teaspoons salt, divided
- 1 medium onion, thinly sliced
- 2½ cups shredded cabbage
- 1 medium carrot, julienned
- 1 cup fresh snow peas
- ¼ teaspoon pepper

1. Break the vermicelli in half; cook according to package directions. Drain.
2. Meanwhile, in a bowl, toss pork with 2 tablespoons oil, garlic and ½ teaspoon salt. Place a large skillet over medium-high heat. Add half of the pork mixture; stir-fry 2-3 minutes or until browned. Remove pork from the pan. Repeat with remaining pork mixture.
3. In same skillet, heat remaining oil over medium-high heat. Add onion; stir-fry 1-2 minutes or until tender. Add remaining vegetables; stir-fry for 3-5 minutes or until crisp-tender. Stir in pepper and remaining salt. Return pork to pan. Add vermicelli; heat through, tossing to combine.

Per 1⅓ cups: 326 cal., 12g fat (2g sat. fat), 36mg chol., 627mg sod., 34g carb. (3g sugars, 3g fiber), 21g pro.
Diabetic Exchanges: 2 starch, 2 lean meat, 1 vegetable, 1 fat.

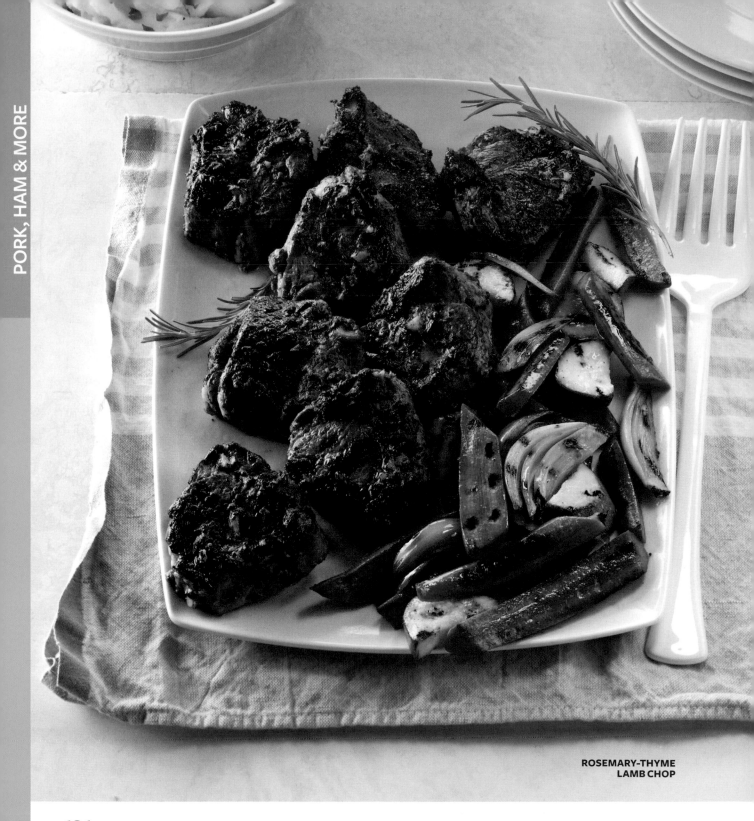

**ROSEMARY-THYME
LAMB CHOP**

⑤ INGREDIENTS FAST FIX
ROSEMARY-THYME LAMB CHOPS

My father loves lamb, so I make this dish whenever he visits. It's the perfect main course for holidays or get-togethers.
—**KRISTINA MITCHELL** CLEARWATER, FL

START TO FINISH: 30 MIN.
MAKES: 4 SERVINGS

- 8 lamb loin chops (3 ounces each)
- ½ teaspoon pepper
- ¼ teaspoon salt
- 3 tablespoons Dijon mustard
- 1 tablespoon minced fresh rosemary
- 1 tablespoon minced fresh thyme
- 3 garlic cloves, minced

1. Sprinkle lamb chops with pepper and salt. In a small bowl, mix mustard, rosemary, thyme and garlic.
2. Grill chops, covered, on an oiled rack over medium heat for 6 minutes. Turn; spread herb mixture over chops. Grill 6-8 minutes longer or until the meat reaches desired doneness (for medium-rare, a thermometer should read 135°; medium, 140°; medium-well, 145°;).

Per 2 lamb chops: 231 cal., 9g fat (4g sat. fat), 97mg chol., 493mg sod., 3g carb. (0 sugars, 0 fiber), 32g pro.
Diabetic Exchanges: 4 lean meat.

✳

DID YOU KNOW?
Loin chops sit between the rib and the leg of the lamb. A meaty cut, it's often easier to find at the grocery store—and more affordable than other types of chops.

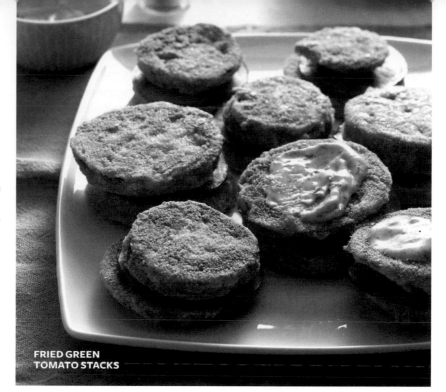
FRIED GREEN TOMATO STACKS

FRIED GREEN TOMATO STACKS

This recipe is for lovers of tomatoes, both red and green. When I ran across this recipe, I just had to try it, and the stacks proved to be delightful!
—**BARBARA MOHR** MILLINGTON, MI

PREP: 20 MIN. • **COOK:** 15 MIN.
MAKES: 4 SERVINGS

- ¼ cup fat-free mayonnaise
- ¼ teaspoon grated lime peel
- 2 tablespoons lime juice
- 1 teaspoon minced fresh thyme or ¼ teaspoon dried thyme
- ½ teaspoon pepper, divided
- ¼ cup all-purpose flour
- 2 large egg whites, lightly beaten
- ¾ cup cornmeal
- ¼ teaspoon salt
- 2 medium green tomatoes
- 2 medium red tomatoes
- 2 tablespoons canola oil
- 8 slices Canadian bacon

1. Mix the first four ingredients and ¼ teaspoon pepper; refrigerate until serving. Place flour in a shallow bowl; place egg whites in a separate shallow bowl. In a third bowl, mix cornmeal, salt and remaining pepper.
2. Cut each tomato crosswise into four slices. Lightly coat each slice in flour; shake off excess. Dip in the egg whites, then in cornmeal mixture.
3. In a large nonstick skillet, heat oil over medium heat. In batches, cook tomatoes until golden brown, about 4-5 minutes per side.
4. In same pan, lightly brown Canadian bacon on both sides. For each serving, stack one slice each green tomato, bacon and red tomato. Serve with the sauce.

Per 1 stack: 284 cal., 10g fat (1g sat. fat), 16mg chol., 679mg sod., 37g carb. (6g sugars, 3g fiber), 12g pro.
Diabetic Exchanges: 2 starch, 1½ fat, 1 lean meat, 1 vegetable.

SUNDAY PORK ROAST

Mom would prepare this delectable main dish for our family, friends and customers at the three restaurants she and Dad owned.

—**SANDI PICHON** MEMPHIS, TN

PREP: 20 MIN.
BAKE: 1 HOUR 10 MIN. + STANDING
MAKES: 12 SERVINGS

- 2 medium onions, chopped
- 2 medium carrots, chopped
- 1 celery rib, chopped
- 4 tablespoons all-purpose flour, divided
- 1 bay leaf, finely crushed
- ½ teaspoon dried thyme
- 1¼ teaspoons salt, divided
- 1¼ teaspoons pepper, divided
- 1 boneless pork loin roast (3 to 4 pounds)
- ⅓ cup packed brown sugar

1. Preheat oven to 350°. Place the vegetables on bottom of a shallow roasting pan. Mix 2 tablespoons flour, bay leaf, thyme and 1 teaspoon each salt and pepper; rub over roast. Place roast on top of vegetables, fat side up. Add 1 cup water to pan.

2. Roast 1 hour, basting once with pan juices if desired. Sprinkle brown sugar over roast. Roast 10-15 minutes longer or until a thermometer reads 140°. (Temperature of roast will continue to rise about 5-10° upon standing.)

3. Remove roast to a platter. Tent with foil; let stand 15 minutes before slicing.

4. Strain drippings from roasting pan into a measuring cup; skim off fat. Add enough water to drippings to measure 1½ cups.

5. In a small saucepan over medium heat, whisk remaining flour and ⅓ cup water until smooth. Gradually whisk in drippings mixture and remaining salt and pepper. Bring gravy to a boil over medium-high heat, stirring constantly; cook and stir for 2 minutes or until thickened. Serve roast with gravy.

To freeze: Freeze cooled sliced pork and gravy in freezer containers. To use, partially thaw in refrigerator overnight. Heat through in a covered saucepan, gently stirring and adding a little broth or water if necessary.

Per 3 ounces cooked pork with about 2 tablespoons gravy: 174 cal., 5g fat (2g sat. fat), 57mg chol., 280mg sod., 8g carb. (6g sugars, 0 fiber), 22g pro. **Diabetic Exchanges:** 3 lean meat, ½ starch.

★ ★ ★ ★ ★ **READER REVIEW**

"This is my new go-to for pork roast. Delightful in every way. My family loves the slightly sweet flavor of the roast and veggies."

DOT TASTEOFHOME.COM

SPICE-RUBBED LAMB CHOPS

One of my absolute favorite meals to eat anytime is lamb chops! My girls love watching me make the delicious chops, but they love eating them even more.

—**NAREMAN DIETZ** BEVERLY HILLS, MI

PREP: 15 MIN. + CHILLING • **BAKE:** 5 MIN.
MAKES: 2 SERVINGS

- 2 teaspoons lemon juice
- 2 teaspoons Worcestershire sauce
- 1½ teaspoons pepper
- 1¼ teaspoons ground cumin
- 1¼ teaspoons curry powder
- 1 garlic clove, minced
- ½ teaspoon sea salt
- ½ teaspoon onion powder
- ½ teaspoon crushed red pepper flakes
- 4 lamb rib chops
- 1 tablespoon olive oil

1. Mix first nine ingredients; spread over chops. Refrigerate, covered, overnight.

2. Preheat the oven to 450°. In an ovenproof skillet, heat the oil over medium-high heat; brown chops, about 2 minutes per side. Transfer chops to oven; roast until desired doneness (for medium-rare, a thermometer should read 145°; medium, 160°), 3-4 minutes.

Per 2 lamb chops: 290 cal., 17g fat (4g sat. fat), 90mg chol., 620mg sod., 5g carb. (1g sugars, 2g fiber), 29g pro. **Diabetic Exchanges:** 4 lean meat, 1½ fat.

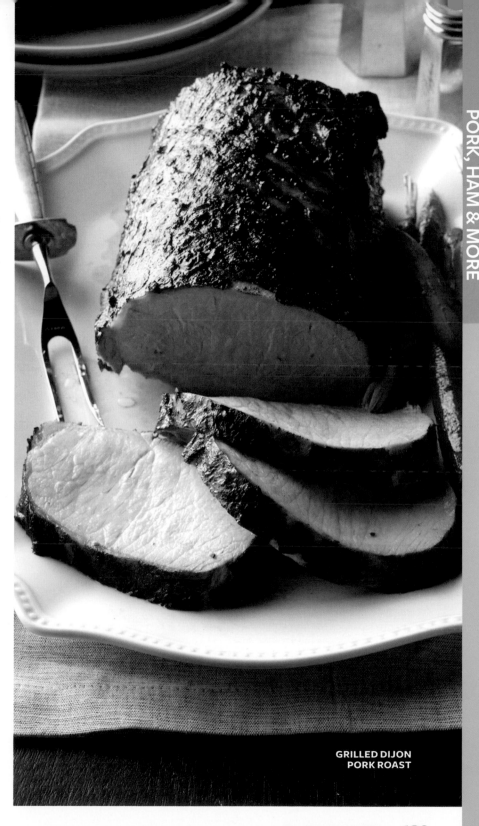

[5]INGREDIENTS

GRILLED DIJON PORK ROAST

I came up with this recipe one day after not having much in the house to eat. My husband loved it, and it has become the only way I make pork now.

—CYNDI LACY-ANDERSEN
WOODINVILLE, WA

PREP: 10 MIN. + MARINATING
GRILL: 1 HOUR + STANDING
MAKES: 12 SERVINGS

- ⅓ cup balsamic vinegar
- 3 tablespoons Dijon mustard
- 1 tablespoon honey
- 1 teaspoon salt
- 1 boneless pork loin roast (3 to 4 pounds)

1. In a large resealable plastic bag, whisk vinegar, mustard, honey and salt. Add pork; seal the bag and turn to coat. Refrigerate for at least 8 hours or overnight.

2. Prepare grill for indirect heat, using a drip pan.

3. Drain pork, discarding marinade. Place pork on a greased grill rack over drip pan and cook, covered, over indirect medium heat for 1 to 1½ hours or until a thermometer reads 145°, turning occasionally. Let stand for 10 minutes before slicing.

Per 3 ounces cooked pork: 149 cal., 5g fat (2g sat. fat), 56mg chol., 213mg sod., 2g carb. (1g sugars, 0 fiber), 22g pro.
Diabetic Exchanges: 3 lean meat.

GRILLED DIJON PORK ROAST

FAST FIX ▶

CHARD & BACON LINGUINE

I use Swiss chard every way I can, and that includes stirring it into this breezy linguine. When you're short on time, this dish keeps life simple.

—**DIANE NEMITZ** LUDINGTON, MI

START TO FINISH: 30 MIN.
MAKES: 4 SERVINGS

- 8 ounces uncooked whole wheat linguine
- 4 bacon strips, chopped
- 4 garlic cloves, minced
- ½ cup reduced-sodium chicken broth
- ½ cup dry white wine or additional chicken broth
- ¼ teaspoon salt
- 6 cups chopped Swiss chard (about 6 ounces)
- ⅓ cup shredded Parmesan cheese

1. Cook linguine according to package directions; drain. Meanwhile, in a large skillet, cook bacon over medium heat until crisp, stirring occasionally. Add garlic; cook 1 minute longer.
2. Add the broth, wine, salt and Swiss chard to skillet; bring to a boil. Cook and stir 4-5 minutes or until chard is tender.
3. Add linguine; heat through, tossing to combine. Sprinkle with cheese.
Per 1 cup: 353 cal., 14g fat (5g sat. fat), 23mg chol., 633mg sod., 47g carb. (2g sugars, 7g fiber), 14g pro.
Diabetic Exchanges: 3 starch, 1 medium-fat meat, 1 vegetable.

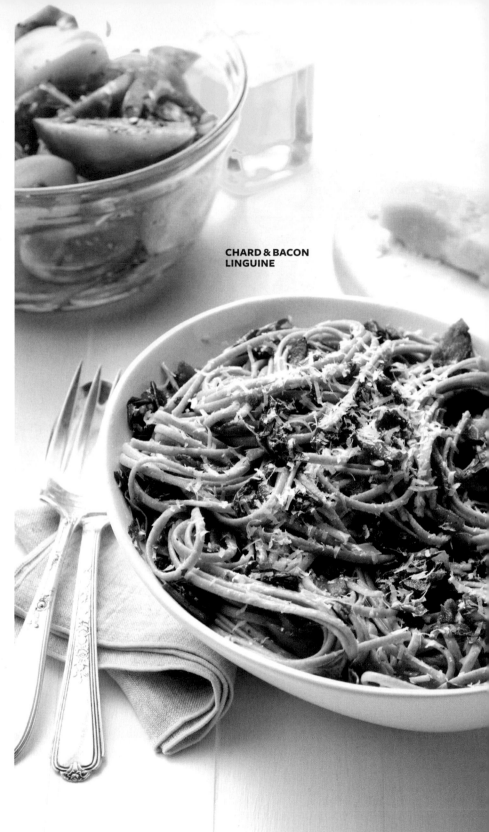

CHARD & BACON LINGUINE

EGG ROLL NOODLE BOWL

At our house, we love egg rolls. They can be challenging to make, so I simplified everything with this deconstructed version that is made on the stovetop in no time!

—**COURTNEY STULTZ** WEIR, KS

START TO FINISH: 30 MIN.
MAKES: 4 SERVINGS

- 1 tablespoon sesame oil
- ½ pound ground pork
- 1 tablespoon soy sauce
- 1 garlic clove, minced
- 1 teaspoon ground ginger
- ½ teaspoon salt
- ¼ teaspoon ground turmeric
- ¼ teaspoon pepper
- 6 cups shredded cabbage (about 1 small head)
- 2 large carrots, shredded (about 2 cups)
- 4 ounces rice noodles
- 3 green onions, thinly sliced
  Additional soy sauce, optional

1. In a large skillet, heat the oil over medium-high heat; cook and crumble pork until browned, 4-6 minutes. Stir in soy sauce, garlic and seasonings. Add cabbage and carrots; cook 4-6 minutes longer or until vegetables are tender, stirring occasionally.

2. Cook rice noodles according to the package directions; drain and add immediately to pork mixture, tossing to combine. Sprinkle with green onions. If desired, serve with additional soy sauce.

Per 1½ cups: 302 cal., 12g fat (4g sat. fat), 38mg chol., 652mg sod., 33g carb. (2g sugars, 4g fiber), 14g pro.

Diabetic Exchanges: 2 medium-fat meat, 2 vegetable, 1½ starch, ½ fat.

BRAISED PORK STEW

Pork tenderloin becomes an amazing treat in this hearty braised stew. It's a fantastic meal for a cold winter night.

—**NELLA PARKER** HERSEY, MI

START TO FINISH: 30 MIN.
MAKES: 4 SERVINGS

- 1 pound pork tenderloin, cut into 1-inch cubes
- ½ teaspoon salt
- ½ teaspoon pepper
- 5 tablespoons all-purpose flour, divided
- 1 tablespoon olive oil
- 1 package (16 ounces) frozen vegetables for stew
- 1½ cups reduced-sodium chicken broth
- 2 garlic cloves, minced
- 2 teaspoons stone-ground mustard
- 1 teaspoon dried thyme
- 2 tablespoons water

1. Sprinkle pork with salt and pepper; add 3 tablespoons flour and toss to coat. In a large skillet, heat oil over medium heat. Brown pork. Drain if necessary. Stir in vegetables, broth, garlic, mustard and thyme. Bring to a boil. Reduce heat; simmer, covered, for 10-15 minutes or until pork and vegetables are tender.

2. In a small bowl, mix remaining flour and water until smooth; stir into stew. Return to a boil, stirring constantly; cook and stir 1-2 minutes or until stew is thickened.

Per 1 cup: 275 cal., 8g fat (2g sat. fat), 63mg chol., 671mg sod., 24g carb. (2g sugars, 1g fiber), 26g pro.

Diabetic Exchanges: 3 lean meat, 1½ starch, ½ fat.

FAST FIX

PARMESAN PORK CHOPS WITH SPINACH SALAD

My pork chops needed a change, and I stumbled across this pan-fry method. With a few tiny changes and a yummy spinach salad, we transformed them.

—**LAUREL DALZELL** MANTECA, CA

START TO FINISH: 30 MIN.
MAKES: 4 SERVINGS

- 3 medium tomatoes, seeded and chopped
- 1 tablespoon olive oil
- 1 tablespoon lemon juice
- 1 small garlic clove, minced
- ½ teaspoon salt, divided
- ¼ teaspoon pepper, divided
- 2 large egg whites
- 1 tablespoon Dijon mustard
- ½ teaspoon dried oregano
- ½ cup dry bread crumbs
- 3 tablespoons grated Parmesan cheese
- 4 thin boneless pork loin chops (½ inch thick and 3 ounces each)
- 4 cups fresh baby spinach

1. In a large bowl, combine tomatoes, oil, lemon juice, garlic, ¼ teaspoon salt and ⅛ teaspoon pepper; toss gently to combine.

2. In a shallow bowl, whisk egg whites, mustard, oregano and remaining salt and pepper until blended. In another shallow bowl, mix bread crumbs with cheese. Dip pork chops in egg white mixture, then coat with the bread crumb mixture.

3. Place a large nonstick skillet coated with cooking spray over medium heat. Add pork chops; cook 2-3 minutes on each side or until golden brown and pork is tender.

4. Add spinach to tomato mixture; toss to combine. Serve with pork chops.

Per 1 pork chop with 1 cup salad: 223 cal., 10g fat (3g sat. fat), 43mg chol., 444mg sod., 12g carb. (3g sugars, 2g fiber), 22g pro.

Diabetic Exchanges: 3 lean meat, 2 vegetable, 1 fat.

FAST FIX

MELON ARUGULA SALAD WITH HAM

I love to think about all the healthy antioxidants in the melon salad I serve my summer dining guests! I save the melon rinds, cutting them into large wedges and using them as the serving dishes. It makes a lovely presentation, and cleanup is always a breeze.

—**SHAWN JACKSON** FISHERS, IN

START TO FINISH: 20 MIN.
MAKES: 8 SERVINGS

- ¼ cup olive oil
- 3 tablespoons white wine vinegar
- 3 tablespoons honey
- 3 cups cubed watermelon
- 2 cups cubed honeydew
- 2½ cups cubed fully cooked ham
- 1 small cucumber, coarsely chopped
- 8 cups fresh arugula
- ¾ cup crumbled feta cheese

1. In a large bowl, whisk together oil, vinegar and honey. Add both melons, ham and cucumber; toss to coat.

2. To serve, arrange the arugula on a platter. Top with the melon mixture; sprinkle with cheese.

Per 2 cups: 202 cal., 10g fat (3g sat. fat), 32mg chol., 646mg sod., 17g carb. (15g sugars, 2g fiber), 12g pro.

Diabetic Exchanges: 2 lean meat, 1½ fat, 1 vegetable, ½ fruit.

FAST FIX

PLUM-GLAZED PORK KABOBS

Get out there and fire up the grill for pork kabobs, a tasty change from beef and chicken. These sweet, gingery beauties make dinner a happy time!

—**TONYA BURKHARD** PALM COAST, FL

START TO FINISH: 30 MIN.
MAKES: 6 SERVINGS

- ⅓ cup plum jam
- 2 tablespoons reduced-sodium soy sauce
- 1 garlic clove, minced
- ½ teaspoon ground ginger
- 1 medium sweet red pepper
- 1 medium green pepper
- 1 small red onion
- 2 pork tenderloins (¾ pound each)

For glaze, in a small bowl, mix jam, soy sauce, garlic and ginger. Cut vegetables and pork into 1-in. pieces. On six metal or soaked wooden skewers, alternately thread pork and vegetables. On a lightly greased grill rack, grill kabobs, covered, over medium heat 12-15 minutes or until pork is tender, turning occasionally and brushing with ¼ cup glaze during the last 5 minutes. Brush with remaining glaze before serving.

Per 1 kabob: 196 cal., 4g fat (1g sat. fat), 64mg chol., 239mg sod., 15g carb. (12g sugars, 1g fiber), 24g pro.

Diabetic Exchanges: 3 lean meat, 1 starch.

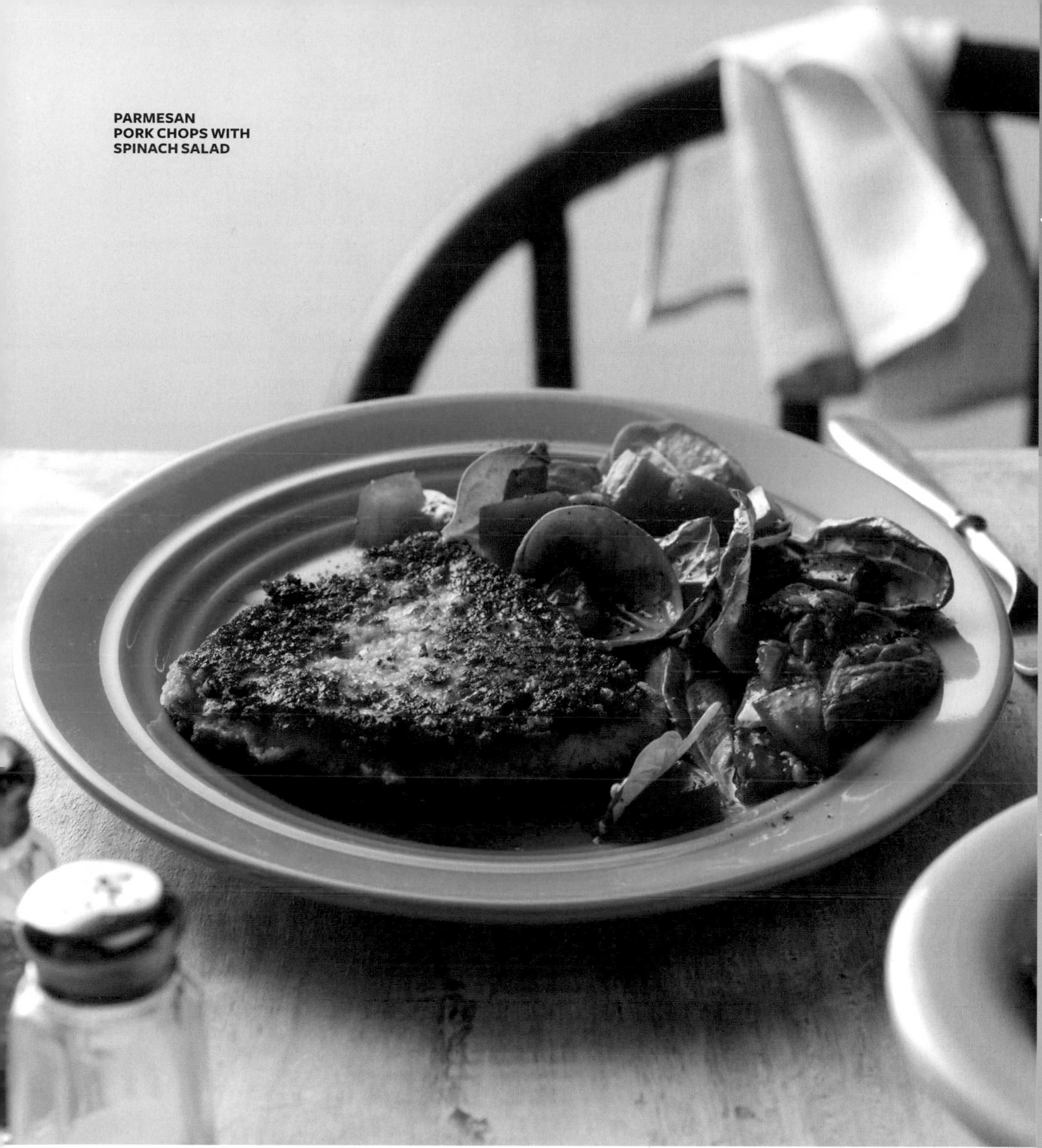

PARMESAN
PORK CHOPS WITH
SPINACH SALAD

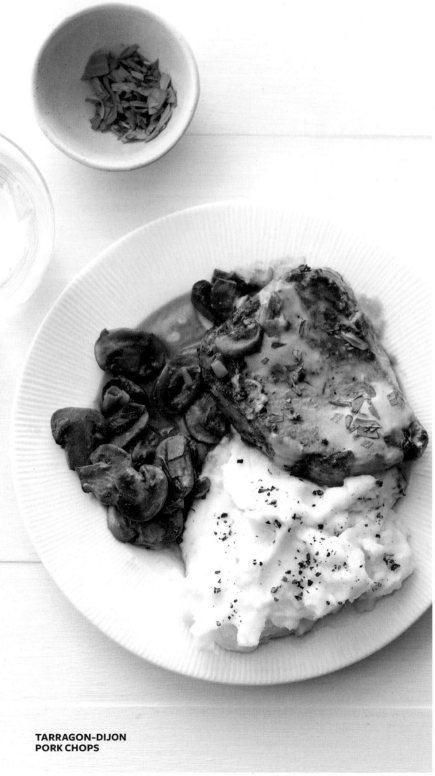

**TARRAGON-DIJON
PORK CHOPS**

TARRAGON-DIJON PORK CHOPS

For my smoky chops, I add tarragon to give a lovely hint of herbal flavor.

—JULIE DANLER BEL AIRE, KS

START TO FINISH: 30 MIN.
MAKES: 4 SERVINGS

- 4 boneless pork loin chops (¾ inch thick and 6 ounces each)
- ½ teaspoon garlic powder
- ¼ teaspoon pepper
- 2 tablespoons olive oil, divided
- 1 pound sliced fresh mushrooms
- 4 green onions, chopped
- ¼ cup Dijon mustard
- 1 to 1½ teaspoons chipotle or other hot pepper sauce
- 1 tablespoon red wine, optional
- 1 tablespoon minced fresh tarragon

1. Preheat oven to 400°. Sprinkle chops with garlic powder and pepper. In a large ovenproof skillet, heat 1 tablespoon oil over medium heat. Brown chops on both sides; remove from pan.

2. In same skillet, heat remaining oil over medium-high heat. Add the mushrooms and green onions; cook and stir 3 minutes. Place chops over mushroom mixture. Bake, uncovered, 8-10 minutes or until a thermometer inserted in pork reads 145°.

3. Meanwhile, mix mustard, pepper sauce and, if desired, wine; spread over chops. Bake about 2 minutes longer. Sprinkle with tarragon.

Per 1 pork chop with ⅓ cup mushroom mixture: 334 cal., 17g fat (5g sat. fat), 82mg chol., 417mg sod., 8g carb. (3g sugars, 2g fiber), 37g pro.
Diabetic Exchanges: 5 lean meat, 1½ fat, 1 vegetable.

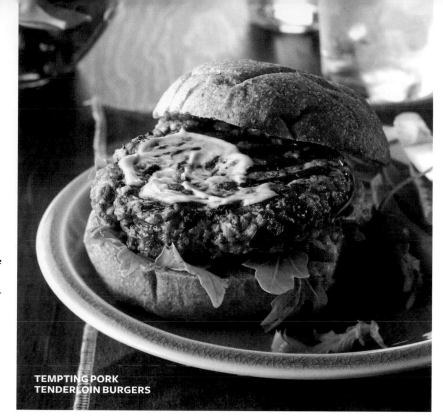

TEMPTING PORK TENDERLOIN BURGERS

FAST FIX ▶
TEMPTING PORK TENDERLOIN BURGERS

Pork tenderloin is a family favorite at my house. I'm always looking for new ways to cook it, so I came up with this burger recipe for a simple weeknight dinner. Chopped prunes, dried figs or dried blueberries can be substituted for the dried cranberries with great success!

—**DEBORAH BIGGS** OMAHA, NE

START TO FINISH: 30 MIN.
MAKES: 4 SERVINGS

- 1 large egg white, lightly beaten
- ⅓ cup panko (Japanese) bread crumbs
- 3 tablespoons dried cranberries, chopped
- ½ teaspoon poultry seasoning
- 1 pork tenderloin (1 pound), cubed
- 3 tablespoons Dijon mustard
- 3 tablespoons mayonnaise
- 1½ teaspoons maple syrup
- 4 whole wheat hamburger buns, split and lightly toasted
  Arugula or baby spinach

1. In a bowl, mix first four ingredients. In a food processor, pulse pork until finely chopped. Add to the egg white mixture; mix lightly but thoroughly. Shape into four ½-in.-thick patties. Mix mustard, mayonnaise and syrup.
2. Place patties on an oiled grill rack; grill, covered, over medium heat until a thermometer reads 160°, 4-6 minutes per side. Serve in buns with arugula and mustard mixture.
Per burger: 378 cal., 14g fat (3g sat. fat), 64mg chol., 620mg sod., 33g carb. (11g sugars, 4g fiber), 28g pro.
Diabetic Exchanges: 3 lean meat, 2 starch, 1 fat.

FAST FIX ▶
SPICY TOMATO PORK CHOPS

These have lots of flavor, but for even more pop, sprinkle garlic powder or Creole seasoning over the chops before you brown them.

—**HOLLY NEUHARTH** MESA, AZ

START TO FINISH: 30 MIN.
MAKES: 4 SERVINGS

- 1 tablespoon olive oil
- 4 boneless pork loin chops (5 ounces each)
- 1 large onion, chopped
- 1 can (8 ounces) tomato sauce
- ¼ cup water
- 2 teaspoons chili powder
- 1 teaspoon dried oregano
- 1 teaspoon Worcestershire sauce
- ½ teaspoon sugar
- ½ teaspoon crushed red pepper flakes

1. In a large skillet, heat oil over medium heat. Brown pork chops on both sides. Remove; keep warm. In same skillet, cook and stir onion until tender. Stir in remaining ingredients.
2. Return pork to skillet. Bring to a boil. Reduce heat; simmer, covered, 15-20 minutes or until tender. Let stand for 5 minutes before serving. Serve the pork chops with the sauce
Per 1 pork chop with ⅓ cup sauce: 257 cal., 12g fat (3g sat. fat), 68mg chol., 328mg sod., 8g carb. (3g sugars, 2g fiber), 29g pro.
Diabetic Exchanges: 4 lean meat, 1 vegetable, 1 fat.

PAN-ROASTED PORK CHOPS & POTATOES

A marinade gives these chops plenty of flavor, and the crumb coating packs on the crunch. For color, I like to tuck in a few handfuls of Brussels sprouts.

—**CHAR OUELLETTE** COLTON, OR

PREP: 20 MIN. + MARINATING
BAKE: 40 MIN.
MAKES: 4 SERVINGS

- 4   boneless pork loin chops (6 ounces each)
- ½   cup plus 2 tablespoons reduced-fat Italian salad dressing, divided
- 4   small potatoes (about 1½ pounds)
- ½   pound fresh Brussels sprouts, trimmed and halved
- ½   cup soft bread crumbs
- 1   tablespoon minced fresh parsley
- ¼   teaspoon salt
- ⅛   teaspoon pepper
- 2   teaspoons butter, melted

1. Place pork chops and ½ cup salad dressing in a large resealable plastic bag; seal bag and turn to coat. Refrigerate 8 hours or overnight. Refrigerate the remaining salad dressing.

2. Preheat oven to 400°. Cut each potato lengthwise into 12 wedges.

Arrange potatoes and Brussels sprouts in a 15x10x1-in. baking pan coated with cooking spray. Drizzle vegetables with remaining salad dressing; toss to coat. Roast 20 minutes.

3. Drain pork, discarding marinade. Pat pork dry with paper towels. Stir the vegetables; place pork chops over top. Roast 15-20 minutes longer or until a thermometer inserted in pork reads 145°. Preheat broiler.

4. In a small bowl, combine bread crumbs, parsley, salt and pepper; stir in butter. Top pork with crumb mixture. Broil 4-6 in. from heat 1-2 minutes or until bread crumbs are golden brown. Let stand 5 minutes.

Note: To make soft bread crumbs, tear bread into pieces and place in a food processor or blender. Cover and pulse until crumbs form. One slice of bread yields ½ to ¾ cup crumbs.

Per 1 pork chop with 1 cup vegetables: 451 cal., 16g fat (5g sat. fat), 87mg chol., 492mg sod., 38g carb. (3g sugars, 5g fiber), 38g pro.
Diabetic Exchanges: 5 lean meat, 2½ starch, 2 fat.

★ ★ ★ ★ ★   **READER REVIEW**

"This was an easy and delicious dinner! My husband said it was one of the best pork chops he's ever had. Our kids even ate the Brussels sprouts!"

MBDUMEE TASTEOFHOME.COM

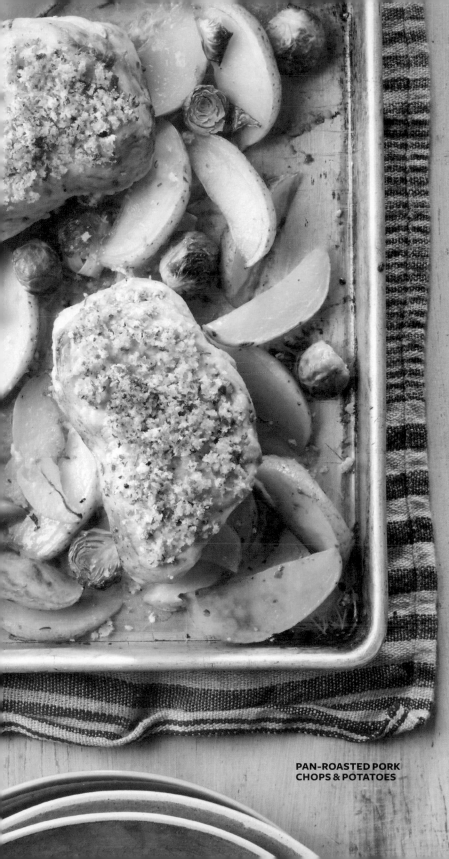

PAN-ROASTED PORK CHOPS & POTATOES

SPICE-BRINED PORK ROAST

This brined and barbecued pork roast is unbelievably tender. Adding seasonings to the coals produces an awesome aroma that draws guests to the grill!

—LORRAINE SCHROEDER ALBANY, OR

PREP: 15 MIN. + CHILLING
GRILL: 1½ HOURS • **MAKES:** 10 SERVINGS

- 2 **quarts water**
- 8 **orange peel strips (1 to 3 inches)**
- ½ **cup sugar**
- ¼ **cup salt**
- 3 **tablespoons fennel seed, crushed**
- 2 **tablespoons dried thyme**
- 2 **tablespoons whole peppercorns**
- 1 **boneless rolled pork loin roast (4 pounds)**

1. In a large saucepan, combine the first seven ingredients. Bring to a boil; cook and stir until salt and sugar are dissolved. Remove from the heat; cool to room temperature.

2. Place a large heavy-duty resealable plastic bag inside a second large resealable plastic bag; add the pork. Carefully pour cooled brine into bag. Squeeze out as much air as possible; seal bags and turn to coat. Refrigerate for 12-24 hours, turning several times. Strain brine; discard liquid and set aside seasonings. Lightly grease the grill rack. Prepare grill for indirect heat, using a drip pan. Add reserved seasonings to coals. Place pork over drip pan and grill, covered, over indirect medium heat for 1½-2 hours or until a thermometer reads 160°. Let stand for 5 minutes before slicing.

Per 6 ounces cooked pork: 225 cal., 8g fat (3g sat. fat), 90mg chol., 75mg sod., 0 carb. (0 sugars, 0 fiber), 35g pro.
Diabetic Exchanges: 6 lean meat.

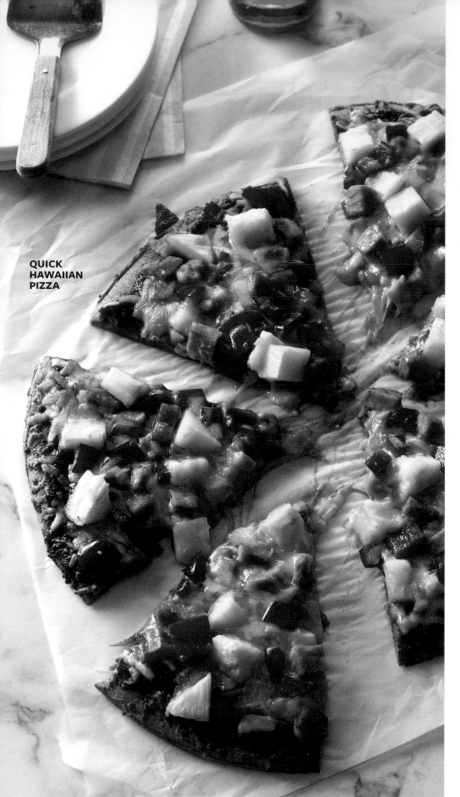

**QUICK
HAWAIIAN
PIZZA**

FAST FIX ▶

QUICK HAWAIIAN PIZZA

*Our family never quite liked the taste of
canned pizza sauce, so I tried mixing
BBQ sauce into spaghetti sauce to add
some sweetness. I've made my pizzas
with this easy special sauce ever since,
and my family loves it.*

—TONYA SCHIELER CARMEL, IN

START TO FINISH: 25 MIN.
MAKES: 6 SLICES

- 1 prebaked 12-inch thin whole
  wheat pizza crust
- ½ cup marinara sauce
- ¼ cup barbecue sauce
- 1 medium sweet yellow or red
  pepper, chopped
- 1 cup cubed fresh pineapple
- ½ cup chopped fully cooked ham
- 1 cup shredded part-skim
  mozzarella cheese
- ½ cup shredded cheddar cheese

1. Preheat oven to 425°. Place crust
on a baking sheet. Mix marinara and
barbecue sauces; spread over crust.
2. Top with remaining ingredients. Bake
until crust is browned and cheeses are
melted, 10-15 minutes.
Per slice: 290 cal., 10g fat (5g sat. fat),
29mg chol., 792mg sod., 36g carb.
(11g sugars, 5g fiber), 16g pro.
Diabetic Exchanges: 2 starch,
2 lean meat, ½ fat.

FAST FIX ▸
PIZZAIOLA CHOPS

My favorite cousin shared this recipe, and I tweaked it for our family. Try the Italian trick of sprinkling on a little extra oregano to give it more gusto.

—**LORRAINE CALAND** SHUNIAH, ON

START TO FINISH: 30 MIN.
MAKES: 4 SERVINGS

- 2 tablespoons olive oil, divided
- 4 boneless pork loin chops (6 ounces each)
- 1 teaspoon salt, divided
- ¼ teaspoon pepper, divided
- 1½ cups sliced baby portobello mushrooms
- 1 medium sweet yellow pepper, coarsely chopped
- 1 medium sweet red pepper, coarsely chopped
- 2 large tomatoes, chopped
- ½ cup white wine or chicken broth
- 1 tablespoon minced fresh oregano or ½ teaspoon dried oregano
- 2 garlic cloves, minced
  Hot cooked rice, optional

1. In a large skillet, heat 1 tablespoon oil over medium-high heat. Season pork chops with ½ teaspoon salt and ⅛ teaspoon pepper. Brown chops on both sides. Remove from pan.

2. In same pan, heat remaining oil over medium-high heat. Add mushrooms, yellow pepper and red pepper; cook and stir 3-4 minutes or until mushrooms are tender. Add the tomatoes, wine, oregano, garlic and the remaining salt and pepper. Bring to a boil. Reduce heat; simmer, uncovered, 2 minutes.

3. Return chops to pan. Cook, covered, 5-7 minutes or until a thermometer inserted in pork reads 145°. Let stand 5 minutes; if desired, serve with rice.

Per 1 pork chop and 1 cup vegetable mixture without rice: 351 cal., 17g fat (5g sat. fat), 82mg chol., 647mg sod., 10g carb. (4g sugars, 2g fiber), 35g pro.
Diabetic Exchanges: 5 lean meat, 1½ fat, 1 vegetable.

FARMERS MARKET PASTA

This recipe can be used almost any time of year, with almost any assortment of vegetables the season has to offer. By cooking without butter or oil, you can cut fat and calories.

—**WENDY G. BALL** BATTLE CREEK, MI

PREP: 20 MIN. • **COOK:** 20 MIN.
MAKES: 6 SERVINGS

- 9 ounces uncooked whole wheat linguine
- 1 pound fresh asparagus, trimmed and cut into 2-inch pieces
- 2 medium carrots, thinly sliced
- 1 small red onion, chopped
- 2 medium zucchini or yellow summer squash, thinly sliced
- ½ pound sliced fresh mushrooms
- 2 garlic cloves, minced
- 1 cup half-and-half cream
- ⅔ cup reduced-sodium chicken broth
- 1 cup frozen petite peas
- 2 cups cubed fully cooked ham
- 2 tablespoons julienned fresh basil
- ¼ teaspoon pepper
- ½ cup grated Parmesan cheese
  Additonal fresh basil and Parmesan cheese, optional

1. In a 6-qt. stockpot, cook linguine according to package directions, adding asparagus and carrots during the last 3-5 minutes of cooking. Drain; return to the pot.

2. Place a large skillet coated with cooking spray over medium heat. Add onion; cook and stir 3 minutes. Add squash, mushrooms, and garlic; cook and stir until crisp-tender, 4-5 minutes.

3. Add the cream and broth; bring to a boil, stirring to loosen browned bits from the pan. Reduce heat; simmer, uncovered, until the sauce is thickened slightly, for about 5 minutes. Stir in the peas, ham, basil and pepper; heat mixture through.

4. Add to linguine mixture; stir in ½ cup cheese. If desired, top with additional basil and cheese.

Per 2 cups without additional toppings: 338 cal., 9g fat (4g sat. fat), 53mg chol., 817mg sod., 46g carb. (8g sugars, 8g fiber), 23g pro.
Diabetic Exchanges: 2½ starch, 2 lean meat, 1 vegetable, ½ fat.

✱

TEST KITCHEN TIP
For the ultimate flavor, use fresh produce when it's in season. In spring, that means asparagus, peas, artichokes and fennel. In summer, eggplant, arugula, summer squash and tomatoes shine. Fall's finest? Butternut squash, Brussels sprouts and carrots, to name a few.

PORK CHOPS & MUSHROOMS

My mother-in-law gave me this recipe years ago, and I have used it ever since. Tarragon is such a special flavor—my family loves it.

—**HILARY RIGO** WICKENBURG, AZ

START TO FINISH: 25 MIN.
MAKES: 4 SERVINGS

- 4 boneless pork loin chops (6 ounces each)
- ¾ teaspoon salt, divided
- ⅛ teaspoon white pepper
- 3 teaspoons butter, divided
- ¾ pound sliced fresh mushrooms
- ½ cup dry white wine or reduced-sodium chicken broth
- ½ teaspoon dried tarragon

1. Sprinkle pork with ½ teaspoon salt and white pepper. In a large nonstick skillet coated with cooking spray, heat 2 teaspoons butter over medium heat. Add pork chops; cook 5-6 minutes on each side or until a thermometer reads 145°. Remove from pan.
2. In same skillet, heat remaining butter over medium-high heat. Add the mushrooms; cook and stir 6-8 minutes or until tender. Add wine, tarragon and remaining salt, stirring to loosen the browned bits from pan. Bring to a boil; cook until liquid is reduced by half. Return chops to pan; heat through.

Per 1 pork chop with ⅓ cup mushrooms: 299 cal., 13g fat (5g sat. fat), 89mg chol., 515mg sod., 4g carb. (1g sugars, 1g fiber), 35g pro.
Diabetic Exchanges: 5 lean meat, 1 vegetable, ½ fat.

ITALIAN PORK STEW

Don't skip the anchovy paste in this stew! It gives a savory, salty flavor, but it doesn't taste fishy at all. Add a salad and artisan bread for a wholesome meal.

—**LYNNE GERMAN** WOODLAND HILLS, CA

PREP: 30 MIN. • **COOK:** 2¼ HOURS
MAKES: 8 SERVINGS (2 QUARTS)

- ⅔ cup all-purpose flour
- 2 pounds boneless pork loin, cut into 1-inch pieces
- 4 tablespoons olive oil, divided
- 1 large onion, chopped
- 5 garlic cloves, crushed
- 1 can (28 ounces) diced tomatoes, undrained
- 1 cup dry red wine or beef broth
- 3 bay leaves
- 1 cinnamon stick (3 inches)
- 1 tablespoon tomato paste
- 1 tablespoon red wine vinegar
- 1 teaspoon anchovy paste
- 1 teaspoon each dried oregano, basil and sage leaves
- ½ teaspoon salt
- ½ teaspoon crushed red pepper flakes
- ¼ teaspoon pepper
- ¼ cup minced fresh parsley
  Hot cooked bow tie pasta
  Grated Parmesan cheese

1. Place flour in a large resealable plastic bag. Add pork, a few pieces at a time, and shake to coat. In a Dutch oven, brown pork in 3 tablespoons oil in batches. Remove and keep warm.
2. In the same pan, saute onion in remaining oil until crisp-tender. Add garlic; cook 1 minute longer. Stir in the tomatoes, wine, bay leaves, cinnamon, tomato paste, vinegar, anchovy paste, herbs, salt, pepper flakes, pepper and pork; bring to a boil.
3. Reduce heat; cover and simmer for 1½ hours, stirring occasionally. Stir in parsley. Cover and cook 30-40 minutes longer or until meat is tender. Skim fat; discard bay leaves and cinnamon.
4. Serve stew with the pasta; sprinkle with the cheese.

To freeze: Place individual portions of cooled stew in freezer containers and freeze. To use, partially thaw stew in refrigerator overnight. Heat through in a saucepan, stirring occasionally and adding a little water if necessary.

Per 1 cup: 256 cal., 12g fat (3g sat. fat), 59mg chol., 349mg sod., 12g carb. (4g sugars, 2g fiber), 24g pro.
Diabetic Exchanges: 3 lean meat, 1 vegetable, 1 fat.

✱

DID YOU KNOW?
Made from ground anchovies, salt and oil, anchovy paste adds a deep, savory flavor to food. Try a small amount—a little goes a long way—in pasta sauce or sauteed greens, stirred into garlic aioli or salad dressing, or mixed into various tapenades—or even a Bloody Mary.

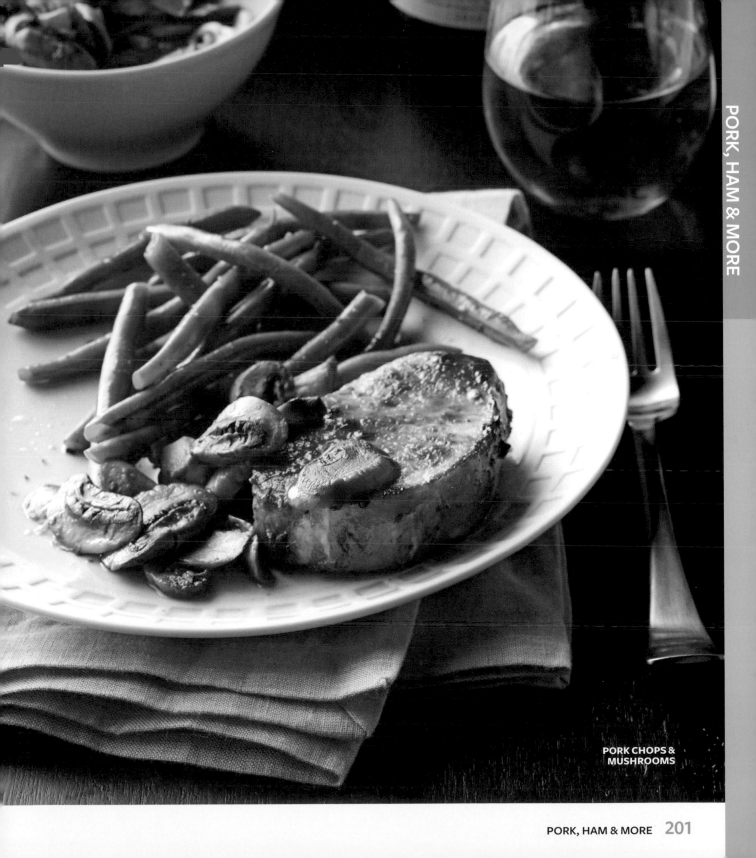

PORK, HAM & MORE

PORK CHOPS & MUSHROOMS

PORK, HAM & MORE   201

GARLIC-HERB SALMON
SLIDERS, PAGE 204

Fish & Seafood

These fresh fish dishes are sure to get along with your family just swimmingly. From succulent scallops to satisfying salmon, there's something for everyone— whether following a special diet or not! Make a splash at your table today!

GARLIC-HERB SALMON SLIDERS

I serve these as full-size burgers on kaiser rolls, too. I've found the fresh flavors of the salmon and herbs are unbeatable.

—MARGEE BERRY WHITE SALMON, WA

PREP: 25 MIN.
GRILL: 10 MIN.
MAKES: 4 SERVINGS

- ⅓ cup panko (Japanese) bread crumbs
- 4 teaspoons finely chopped shallot
- 2 teaspoons snipped fresh dill
- 1 tablespoon prepared horseradish
- 1 large egg, beaten
- ¼ teaspoon salt
- ⅛ teaspoon pepper
- 1 pound salmon fillet, skin removed, cut into 1-inch cubes
- 8 whole wheat dinner rolls, split and toasted
- ¼ cup reduced-fat garlic-herb spreadable cheese
- 8 small lettuce leaves

1. In a large bowl, combine the first seven ingredients. Place salmon in food processor; pulse until coarsely chopped and add to bread crumb mixture. Mix lightly but thoroughly. Shape into eight ½-in.-thick patties.

2. On a lightly greased grill rack, grill burgers, covered, over medium heat or broil 4 in. from heat 3-4 minutes on each side or until a thermometer reads 160°. Serve on rolls with spreadable cheese and lettuce.

Per 2 sliders: 442 cal., 17g fat (5g sat. fat), 119mg chol., 676mg sod., 42g carb. (7g sugars, 6g fiber), 30g pro.
Diabetic Exchanges: 3 starch, 3 lean meat, 1 fat.

FAST FIX
SHRIMP PICCATA

I typically serve this succulent pasta with French bread and asparagus. Cook it the next time you have company, and guests will beg for the recipe.

—HOLLY BAUER WEST BEND, WI

START TO FINISH: 25 MIN.
MAKES: 4 SERVINGS

- ½ pound uncooked angel hair pasta
- 2 shallots, finely chopped
- 2 garlic cloves, minced
- 2 tablespoons olive oil
- 1 pound uncooked large shrimp, peeled and deveined
- 1 teaspoon dried oregano
- ⅛ teaspoon salt
- 1 cup chicken broth
- 1 cup white wine or additional chicken broth
- 4 teaspoons cornstarch
- ⅓ cup lemon juice
- ¼ cup capers, drained
- 3 tablespoons minced fresh parsley

1. Cook angel hair pasta according to package directions.

2. Meanwhile, in a large skillet, saute shallots and garlic in oil for 1 minute. Add the shrimp, oregano and salt; cook and stir until shrimp turn pink. In small bowl, combine the broth, wine and cornstarch; gradually stir into pan. Bring to a boil; cook and stir for 2 minutes or until thickened. Remove from the heat.

3. Drain pasta. Add the pasta, lemon juice, capers and parsley to the skillet; toss to coat.

Per 1½ cups: 295 cal., 9g fat (1g sat. fat), 139mg chol., 715mg sod., 27g carb. (2g sugars, 2g fiber), 22g pro.
Diabetic Exchanges: 3 lean meat, 1½ starch, 1 fat.

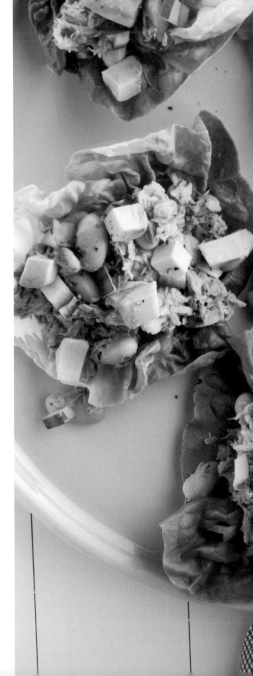

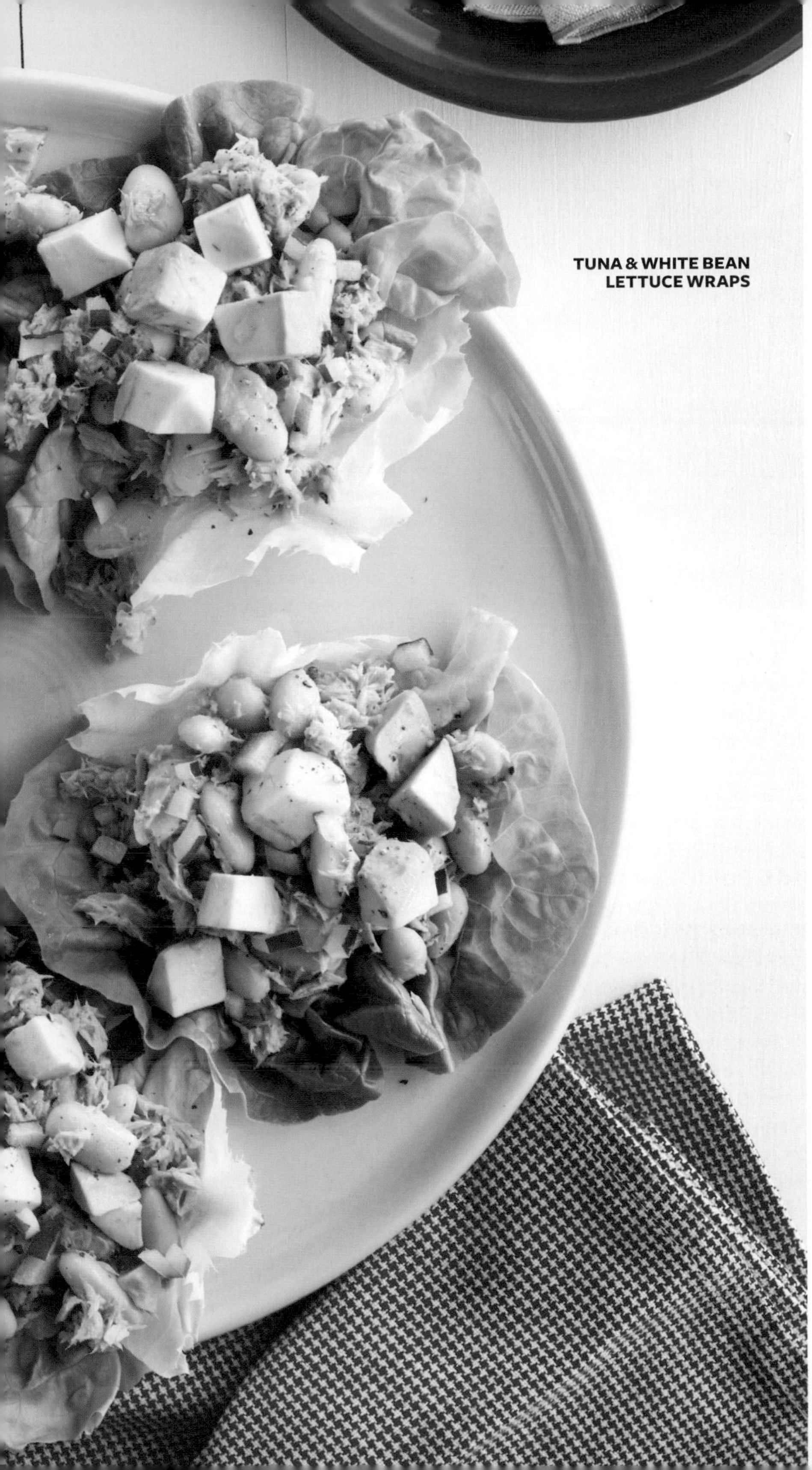

TUNA & WHITE BEAN LETTUCE WRAPS

FAST FIX ▸

TUNA & WHITE BEAN LETTUCE WRAPS

Here's a great way to dress up ordinary tuna salad. This quick recipe makes a quick dinner or lunch at the office, and it's good for you.

—HEATHER SENGER MADISON, WI

START TO FINISH: 20 MIN.
MAKES: 4 SERVINGS

- 1 can (12 ounces) light tuna in water, drained and flaked
- 1 can (15 ounces) cannellini beans, rinsed and drained
- ¼ cup chopped red onion
- 2 tablespoons olive oil
- 1 tablespoon minced fresh parsley
- ⅛ teaspoon salt
- ⅛ teaspoon pepper
- 12 Bibb or Boston lettuce leaves (about 1 medium head)
- 1 medium ripe avocado, peeled and cubed

In a small bowl, combine the first seven ingredients; toss lightly to combine. Serve tuna mixture in lettuce leaves; top with avocado.

Per 3 wraps: 279 cal., 13g fat (2g sat. fat), 31mg chol., 421mg sod., 19g carb. (1g sugars, 7g fiber), 22g pro.
Diabetic Exchanges: 3 lean meat, 2 fat, 1 starch.

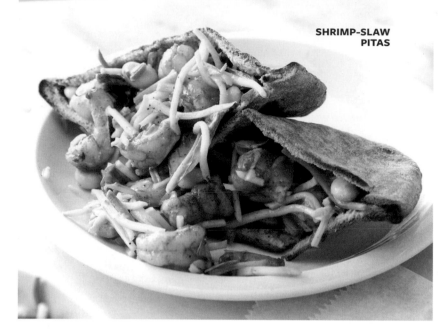

SHRIMP-SLAW PITAS

SHRIMP-SLAW PITAS

My mother brought me peach salsa from Georgia, inspiring this recipe for shrimp pitas. Edamame gives them awesome texture, or simply swap in some baby lima beans.

—ANGELA McCLURE CARY, NC

PREP: 30 MIN. • **BROIL:** 5 MIN.
MAKES: 6 SERVINGS

- 1½ pounds uncooked shrimp (31-40 per pound), peeled, deveined and coarsely chopped
- 1 tablespoon olive oil
- 1 teaspoon paprika

SLAW

- ⅓ cup reduced-fat plain Greek yogurt
- ⅓ cup peach salsa or salsa of your choice
- 1 tablespoon honey
- ½ teaspoon salt
- ½ teaspoon pepper
- 1 package (12 ounces) broccoli coleslaw mix
- 2 cups fresh baby spinach
- ¼ cup shredded carrots
- ¼ cup frozen shelled edamame, thawed
- 12 whole wheat pita pocket halves

1. Preheat broiler. In a small bowl, toss shrimp with oil and paprika. Transfer to a foil-lined 15x10x1-in. baking pan. Broil 4-5 in. from heat 3-4 minutes or until shrimp turn pink, stirring once.
2. In a small bowl, whisk yogurt, salsa, honey, salt and pepper. Add coleslaw mix, spinach, carrots, edamame and shrimp; toss to coat.
3. Place pita pockets on a baking sheet. Broil 4-5 in. from heat about 1-2 minutes on each side or until lightly toasted. Fill each pita half with ½ cup shrimp mixture.
Per 2 filled pita halves: 322 cal., 6g fat (1g sat. fat), 139mg chol., 641mg sod., 41g carb. (7g sugars, 7g fiber), 28g pro.
Diabetic Exchanges: 3 lean meat, 2 starch, 1 vegetable, ½ fat.

FAST FIX ▶
ASIAN SNAPPER WITH CAPERS

Here's a simple sauteed snapper with lots of flavor. It takes very little time and effort to prepare. Asian flavors really make this dish exciting.

—MARY ANN LEE CLIFTON PARK, NY

START TO FINISH: 20 MIN.
MAKES: 4 SERVINGS

- 4 red snapper fillets (6 ounces each)
- 4½ teaspoons Mongolian Fire oil or sesame oil
- ¼ cup apple jelly
- 3 tablespoons ketchup
- 2 tablespoons capers, drained
- 1 tablespoon lemon juice
- 1 tablespoon reduced-sodium soy sauce
- 1 teaspoon grated fresh gingerroot

1. In a large skillet, cook the fillets in oil over medium heat for 3-5 minutes on each side or until fish flakes easily with a fork; remove and keep warm.
2. Stir the jelly, ketchup, capers, lemon juice, soy sauce and ginger into skillet. Cook and stir for 2-3 minutes or until slightly thickened; serve alongside the red snapper.
Per 1 fillet with 2 tablespoons sauce: 275 cal., 7g fat (1g sat. fat), 60mg chol., 494mg sod., 17g carb. (15g sugars, 0 fiber), 34g pro.
Diabetic Exchanges: 4 lean meat, 1 starch, 1 fat.

✱

DID YOU KNOW?
When consuming fish and seafood on a regular basis, you should opt for low-mercury options, such as salmon, tilapia, shrimp and scallops. Avoid large predatory fish like shark, marlin and swordfish.

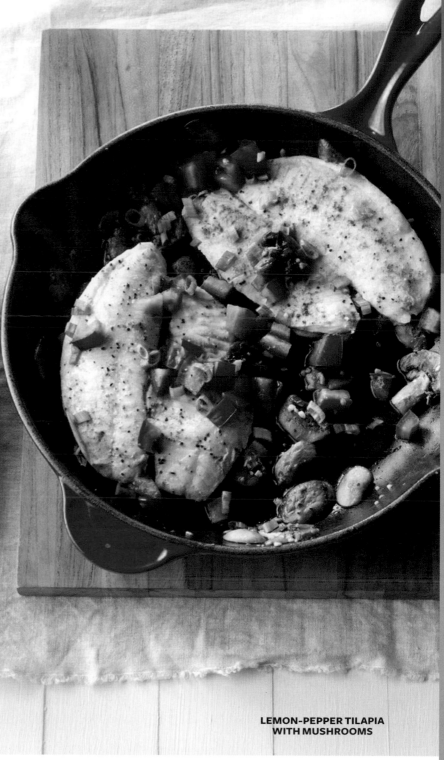

FAST FIX ▶

LEMON-PEPPER TILAPIA WITH MUSHROOMS

My husband and I are trying to add more fish and healthier entrees to our diet, and this one makes it easy. It comes together in less than 30 minutes, so it's perfect for hectic weeknights.

—DONNA MCDONALD LAKE ELSINORE, CA

START TO FINISH: 25 MIN.
MAKES: 4 SERVINGS

- 2 tablespoons butter
- ½ pound sliced fresh mushrooms
- ¾ teaspoon lemon-pepper seasoning, divided
- 3 garlic cloves, minced
- 4 tilapia fillets (6 ounces each)
- ¼ teaspoon paprika
- ⅛ teaspoon cayenne pepper
- 1 medium tomato, chopped
- 3 green onions, thinly sliced

1. In a 12-in. skillet, heat butter over medium heat. Add mushrooms and ¼ teaspoon lemon pepper; cook and stir 3-5 minutes or until tender. Add garlic; cook 30 seconds longer.

2. Place the fillets over mushrooms; sprinkle them with paprika, cayenne and remaining lemon pepper. Cook, covered, 5-7 minutes or until fish just begins to flake easily with a fork. Top with tomato and green onions.

Per serving: 216 cal., 8g fat (4g sat. fat), 98mg chol., 173mg sod., 5g carb. (2g sugars, 1g fiber), 34g pro.
Diabetic Exchanges: 4 lean meat, 1½ fat.

LEMON-PEPPER TILAPIA WITH MUSHROOMS

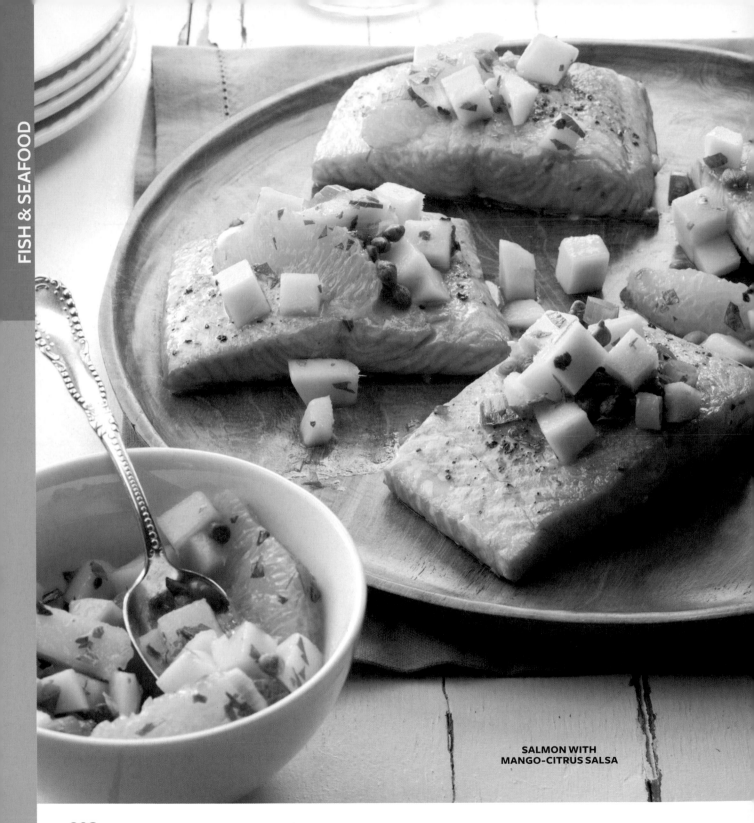

**SALMON WITH
MANGO-CITRUS SALSA**

<FAST FIX>

SALMON WITH MANGO-CITRUS SALSA

My mother would make this for us on weeknights in the summer—it was the only way we would eat fish. You can make the salsa a day ahead of time. Just keep it in the refrigerator covered with plastic wrap.

—NAJMUSSAHAR AHMED ANN ARBOR, MI

START TO FINISH: 30 MIN.
MAKES: 4 SERVINGS

- 1 large navel orange
- 1 medium lemon
- 2 tablespoons olive oil
- 1 tablespoon capers, drained and coarsely chopped
- 1½ teaspoons minced fresh mint
- 1½ teaspoons minced fresh parsley
- ¼ teaspoon crushed red pepper flakes
- ⅛ teaspoon plus ½ teaspoon salt, divided
- ⅛ teaspoon plus ¼ teaspoon pepper, divided
- 1 medium mango, peeled and chopped
- 1 green onion, thinly sliced
- 4 salmon fillets (6 ounces each)
- 1 tablespoon canola oil

1. For salsa, finely grate enough peel from orange to measure 2 teaspoons; finely grate enough peel from lemon to measure ½ teaspoon. Place citrus peels in a small bowl. Cut lemon crosswise in half; squeeze 2 tablespoons lemon juice and add to bowl.

2. Cut a thin slice from the top and bottom of orange; stand orange upright on a cutting board. With a knife, cut off the peel and outer membrane from the orange. Cut along the membrane of each segment to remove fruit.

3. Add olive oil, capers, mint, parsley, pepper flakes and ⅛ teaspoon each salt and pepper to lemon juice mixture. Gently stir in mango, green onion and orange sections.

4. Sprinkle salmon with the remaining salt and pepper. In a large skillet, heat canola oil over medium heat. Add the salmon; cook 5-6 minutes on each side or until fish just begins to flake easily with a fork. Serve with salsa.

Per 1 fillet with ½ cup salsa: 433 cal., 26g fat (4g sat. fat), 85mg chol., 516mg sod., 19g carb. (16g sugars, 3g fiber), 30g pro.
Diabetic Exchanges: 5 lean meat, 1½ fat, 1 fruit.

SPICY COCONUT SHRIMP WITH QUINOA

Help yourself to a big plate full because generous servings are still low in calories and big on protein. If you have company, you can add a salad and call it a day.

—KERI WHITNEY CASTRO VALLEY, CA

PREP: 20 MIN. • **COOK:** 20 MIN.
MAKES: 4 SERVINGS

- 1 cup quinoa, rinsed
- 2 cups water
- ¼ teaspoon salt

SHRIMP

- 1 teaspoon olive oil
- 1 medium onion, chopped
- 1 tablespoon minced fresh gingerroot
- ½ teaspoon curry powder
- ½ teaspoon ground cumin
- ¼ teaspoon salt
- ¼ teaspoon cayenne pepper
- 1 pound uncooked shrimp (26-30 per pound), peeled and deveined
- 2 cups fresh snow peas (about 7 ounces), trimmed
- 3 tablespoons light coconut milk
- 1 tablespoon orange juice
- ¼ cup flaked coconut, toasted
- ¼ cup minced fresh cilantro

1. In a large saucepan, combine quinoa, water and salt; bring to a boil. Reduce heat; simmer, covered, 12-15 minutes or until liquid is absorbed. Remove from heat; fluff with a fork.

2. Meanwhile, in a nonstick skillet, heat oil over medium heat. Add onion; cook and stir 4-6 minutes or until tender. Stir in ginger, curry powder, cumin, salt and cayenne; cook 1 minute longer.

3. Add shrimp and snow peas to skillet; cook and stir for 3-4 minutes or until shrimp turn pink and snow peas are crisp-tender. Stir in coconut milk and orange juice; heat through. Serve with quinoa; top each serving with coconut and cilantro.

Note: To toast the coconut, bake in a shallow pan in a 350° oven for 5-10 minutes or cook in a skillet over low heat until golden brown, stirring occasionally.

Per 1 cup shrimp mixture with ¾ cup quinoa: 330 cal., 8g fat (3g sat. fat), 138mg chol., 451mg sod., 37g carb. (6g sugars, 5g fiber), 26g pro.
Diabetic Exchanges: 3 lean meat, 2 starch, 1 vegetable, ½ fat.

★ ★ ★ ★ ★ **READER REVIEW**

"The coconut milk and toasted garnish give you the taste of fried shrimp without all the calories."

CURLYLIS85 TASTEOFHOME.COM

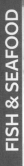
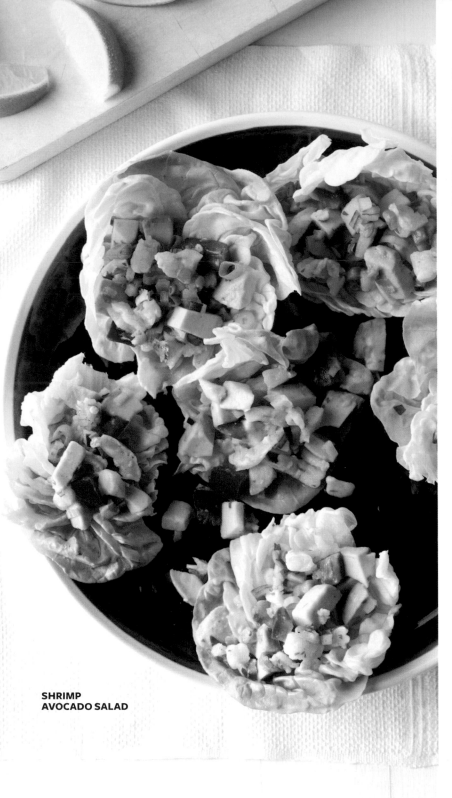

**SHRIMP
AVOCADO SALAD**

SHRIMP AVOCADO SALAD

This salad can be served as a cool and satisfying dinner or lunch. The delicious taste of avocados mixed with crisp shrimp salad is heavenly.

—**TERI RASEY** CADILLAC, MI

PREP: 25 MIN. + CHILLING
MAKES: 6 SERVINGS

- 1 pound peeled and deveined cooked shrimp, coarsely chopped
- 2 plum tomatoes, seeded and chopped
- 2 green onions, chopped
- ¼ cup finely chopped red onion
- 1 jalapeno pepper, seeded and minced
- 1 serrano pepper, seeded and minced
- 2 tablespoons minced fresh cilantro
- 2 tablespoons lime juice
- 2 tablespoons seasoned rice vinegar
- 2 tablespoons olive oil
- 1 teaspoon adobo seasoning
- 3 medium ripe avocados, peeled and cubed
  Bibb lettuce leaves
  Lime wedges

1. Place first seven ingredients in a large bowl. Mix lime juice, vinegar, oil and adobo seasoning; stir into shrimp mixture. Refrigerate, covered, to allow flavors to blend, about 1 hour.

2. To serve, stir in avocados. Serve over lettuce. Serve with lime wedges.

Note: Wear disposable gloves when cutting hot peppers; the oils can burn skin. Avoid touching your face.

Per ¾ cup avocado mixture: 252 cal., 16g fat (2g sat. fat), 115mg chol., 523mg sod., 11g carb. (3g sugars, 5g fiber), 17g pro.

Diabetic Exchanges: 3 fat, 2 lean meat, ½ starch.

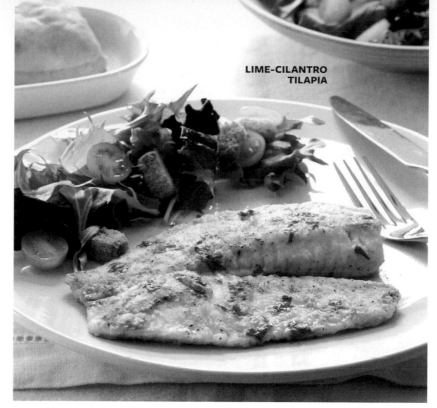

LIME-CILANTRO TILAPIA

FAST FIX

CRISPY FISH & CHIPS

A classic British pub favorite turns crown jewel when you add horseradish, panko and Worcestershire. Try it with any white fish, such as cod or haddock.

—**LINDA SCHEND** KENOSHA, WI

START TO FINISH: 30 MIN.
MAKES: 4 SERVINGS

- 4 cups frozen steak fries
- 4 salmon fillets (6 ounces each)
- 1 to 2 tablespoons prepared horseradish
- 1 tablespoon grated Parmesan cheese
- 1 tablespoon Worcestershire sauce
- 1 teaspoon Dijon mustard
- ¼ teaspoon salt
- ½ cup panko (Japanese) bread crumbs
  Cooking spray

1. Preheat oven to 450°. Arrange steak fries in a single layer on a baking sheet. Bake on lowest oven rack 18-20 minutes or until light golden brown.
2. Meanwhile, place salmon on a foil-lined baking sheet coated with cooking spray. In a small bowl, mix horseradish, cheese, Worcestershire sauce, mustard and salt; stir in panko. Press mixture onto fillets. Spritz tops with cooking spray.
3. Bake salmon on middle oven rack 8-10 minutes or until fish just begins to flake easily with a fork. Serve with fries.
Per 1 fillet with ¾ cup fries: 419 cal., 20g fat (4g sat. fat), 86mg chol., 695mg sod., 26g carb. (2g sugars, 2g fiber), 32g pro.
Diabetic Exchanges: 5 lean meat, 1½ starch.

FAST FIX

LIME-CILANTRO TILAPIA

I have so much fun serving this Mexican-inspired tilapia at summer parties. Finish it off with a side of rice and a crisp green salad that's loaded with sliced avocados and tomatoes.

—**NADINE MESCH** MOUNT HEALTHY, OH

START TO FINISH: 25 MIN.
MAKES: 4 SERVINGS

- ⅓ cup all-purpose flour
- ¾ teaspoon salt
- ½ teaspoon pepper
- ½ teaspoon ground cumin, divided
- 4 tilapia fillets (6 ounces each)
- 1 tablespoon olive oil
- ½ cup reduced-sodium chicken broth
- 2 tablespoons minced fresh cilantro
- 1 teaspoon grated lime peel
- 2 tablespoons lime juice

1. In a shallow bowl, mix flour, salt, pepper and ¼ teaspoon cumin. Dip fillets in flour mixture to coat both sides; shake off excess.
2. In a large nonstick skillet, heat oil over medium heat. Add fillets; cook, uncovered, 3-4 minutes on each side or until the fish flakes easily with a fork. Remove and keep warm.
3. To the same pan, add broth, cilantro, lime peel, lime juice and the remaining cumin; bring to a boil. Reduce the heat; simmer, uncovered, 2-3 minutes or until slightly thickened. Serve with tilapia.
Per 1 fillet with 2 tablespoons sauce: 198 cal., 5g fat (1g sat. fat), 83mg chol., 398 mg sod., 6g carb. (1g sugars, 0 fiber), 33g pro.
Diabetic Exchanges: 4 lean meat, ½ starch, ½ fat.

FANTASTIC FISH TACOS

Searching for a lighter substitute to traditional fried fish tacos, I came up with this entree. It's been a hit with friends and family. These fillets are so mild that even those who don't like fish are pleasantly surprised.

—JENNIFER PALMER
RANCHO CUCAMONGA, CA

START TO FINISH: 30 MIN.
MAKES: 4 SERVINGS

- ½ cup fat-free mayonnaise
- 1 tablespoon lime juice
- 2 teaspoons fat-free milk
- 1 large egg
- 1 teaspoon water
- ⅓ cup dry bread crumbs
- 2 tablespoons salt-free lemon-pepper seasoning
- 1 pound mahi mahi or cod fillets, cut into 1-inch strips
- 4 corn tortillas (6 inches), warmed

TOPPINGS

- 1 cup coleslaw mix
- 2 medium tomatoes, chopped
- 1 cup shredded reduced-fat Mexican cheese blend
- 1 tablespoon minced fresh cilantro

1. For the sauce, in a small bowl, mix the mayonnaise, lime juice and milk; refrigerate until serving.
2. In a shallow bowl, whisk together egg and water. In another bowl, toss bread crumbs with lemon pepper. Dip fish in egg mixture, then in crumb mixture, patting to help coating adhere.
3. Place a large nonstick skillet coated with cooking spray over medium-high heat. Add fish; cook 2-4 minutes per side or until golden brown and fish just begins to flake easily with a fork. Serve in tortillas with toppings and sauce.

Per taco: 321 cal., 10g fat (5g sat. fat), 148mg chol., 632mg sod., 29g carb. (5g sugars, 4g fiber), 34g pro.
Diabetic Exchanges: 4 lean meat, 2 starch.

SHRIMP & VEGETABLE BOIL

When my children were small, they liked picking out the ingredients for making this supper.

—JOYCE GUTH MOHNTON, PA

PREP: 20 MIN. • **COOK:** 30 MIN.
MAKES: 6 SERVINGS

- 4 cups water
- 4 cups chicken broth
- 2 teaspoons salt
- 2 teaspoons ground nutmeg
- ½ teaspoon sugar
- 2 pounds red potatoes (about 8 medium), cut into wedges
- 1 medium head cauliflower, broken into florets
- 2 large onions, quartered
- 3 medium carrots, sliced
- 1 pound fresh peas, shelled (about 1 cup)
- 2 pounds uncooked shell-on shrimp (26-30 per pound), deveined
- 6 ounces fresh baby spinach (about 8 cups)
- 1 tablespoon minced fresh parsley
  Salt and pepper to taste

1. In a stockpot, combine the first five ingredients; add potatoes, cauliflower, onions, carrots and peas. Bring to a boil. Reduce heat; simmer, uncovered, 12-15 minutes or until vegetables are tender.
2. Stir in shrimp and spinach; cook 3-5 minutes longer or until shrimp turn pink. Drain; transfer to a large serving bowl. Sprinkle with parsley; season with salt and pepper.

Per 2⅔ cups: 367 cal., 3g fat (1g sat. fat), 185mg chol., 721mg sod., 50g carb. (12g sugars, 11g fiber), 35g pro.
Diabetic Exchanges: 4 lean meat, 3 starch.

CRUNCHY TUNA WRAPS

We stuff our tortilla wraps with tuna and crunchies like celery, red pepper and water chestnuts for a bit of zip that shakes up standard tuna salad.

—EDIE FARM FARMINGTON, NM

START TO FINISH: 10 MIN.
MAKES: 2 SERVINGS

- 1 pouch (6.4 ounces) light tuna in water
- ¼ cup finely chopped celery
- ¼ cup chopped green onions
- ¼ cup sliced water chestnuts, chopped
- 3 tablespoons chopped sweet red pepper
- 2 tablespoons reduced-fat mayonnaise
- 2 teaspoons prepared mustard
- 2 spinach tortillas (8 inches), room temperature
- 1 cup shredded lettuce

In a small bowl, mix the first seven ingredients until blended. Spread over tortillas; sprinkle with lettuce. Roll up tightly jelly-roll style.

Per wrap: 312 cal., 10g fat (2g sat. fat), 38mg chol., 628mg sod., 34g carb. (2g sugars, 3g fiber), 23g pro.
Diabetic Exchanges: 3 lean meat, 2 starch, ½ fat.

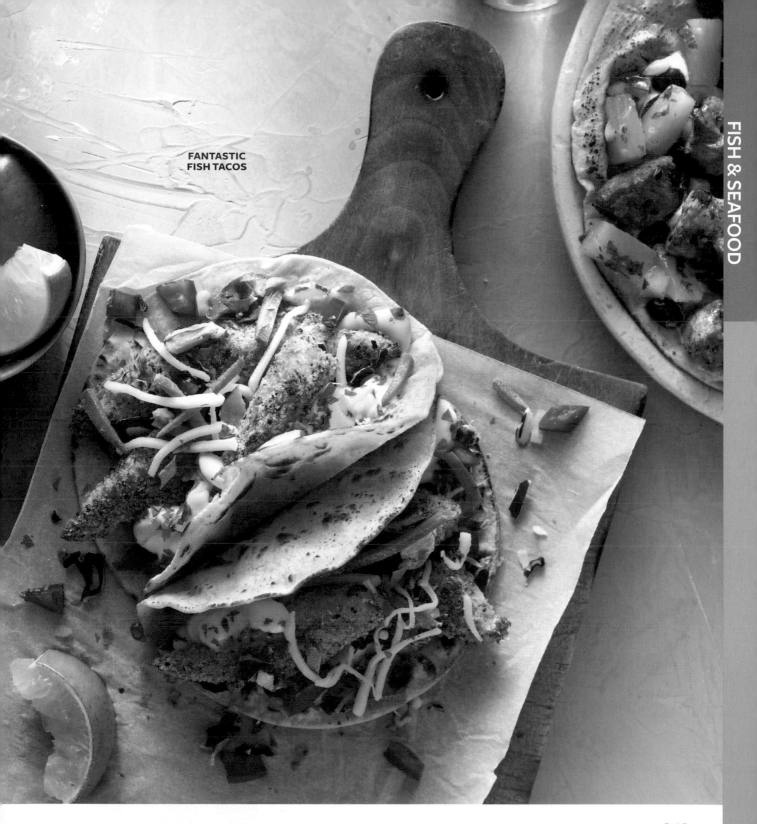

FANTASTIC
FISH TACOS

CILANTRO SHRIMP & RICE

I created this one-dish wonder for my son, who has the pickiest palate. The aroma of fresh herbs is so appetizing—even my son can't resist!
—NIBEDITA DAS FORT WORTH, TX

START TO FINISH: 30 MIN.
MAKES: 8 SERVINGS

- 2 packages (8½ ounces each) ready-to-serve basmati rice
- 2 tablespoons olive oil
- 2 cups frozen corn, thawed
- 2 medium zucchini, quartered and sliced
- 1 large sweet red pepper, chopped
- ½ teaspoon crushed red pepper flakes
- 3 garlic cloves, minced
- 1 pound peeled and deveined cooked large shrimp, tails removed
- ½ cup chopped fresh cilantro
- 1 tablespoon grated lime peel
- 2 tablespoons lime juice
- ¾ teaspoon salt
  Lime wedges, optional

1. Prepare the rice according to the package directions.
2. Meanwhile, in a large skillet, heat oil over medium-high heat. Add the corn, zucchini, red pepper and pepper flakes; cook and stir 3-5 minutes or until the zucchini is crisp-tender. Add garlic; cook 1 minute longer. Add shrimp; cook and stir 3-5 minutes or until heated through.
3. Stir in the rice, cilantro, lime peel, lime juice and salt. If desired, serve with lime wedges.

Per 1½ cups: 243 cal., 6g fat (1g sat. fat), 86mg chol., 324mg sod., 28g carb. (3g sugars, 3g fiber), 16g pro.
Diabetic Exchanges: 2 lean meat, 1½ starch, ½ fat.

COD WITH BACON & BALSAMIC TOMATOES

Everything is better with bacon. I fry it up, add cod fillets to the pan, and finish with a big, tomato-y pop.
—MAUREEN MCCLANAHAN ST. LOUIS, MO

START TO FINISH: 30 MIN.
MAKES: 4 SERVINGS

- 4 center-cut bacon strips, chopped
- 4 cod fillets (5 ounces each)
- ½ teaspoon salt
- ¼ teaspoon pepper
- 2 cups grape tomatoes, halved
- 2 tablespoons balsamic vinegar

1. In a large skillet, cook the bacon over medium heat until crisp, stirring occasionally. Remove with a slotted spoon; drain on paper towels.
2. Sprinkle fillets with salt and pepper. Add fillets to the bacon drippings; cook over medium-high heat 4-6 minutes on each side or until fish just begins to flake easily with a fork. Remove from pan and keep warm.
3. Add tomatoes to skillet; cook and stir 2-4 minutes or until tomatoes are softened. Stir in vinegar; reduce heat to medium-low. Cook 1-2 minutes longer or until sauce is thickened. Serve cod with tomato mixture and bacon.

Per 1 fillet with ¼ cup tomato mixture and 1 tablespoon bacon: 178 cal., 6g fat (2g sat. fat), 64mg chol., 485mg sod., 5g carb. (4g sugars, 1g fiber), 26g pro.
Diabetic Exchanges: 4 lean meat, 1 vegetable.

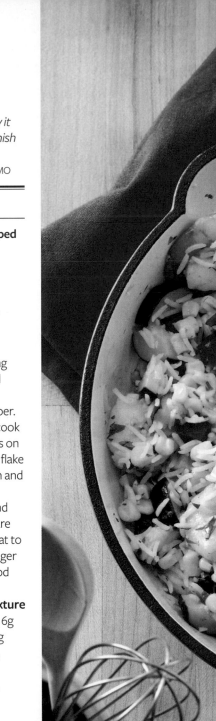

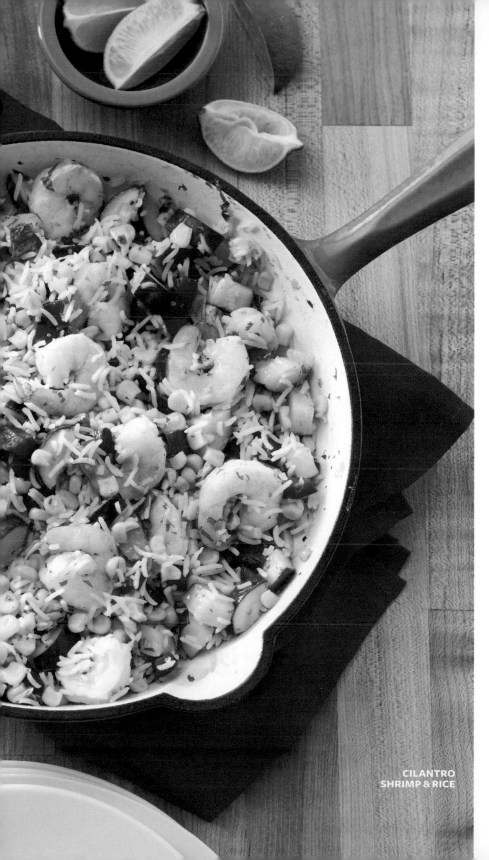

CILANTRO SHRIMP & RICE

FAST FIX

CRUNCHY OVEN-BAKED TILAPIA

This baked tilapia is perfectly crunchy. Dip it in the fresh lime mayo to send it over the top.

—LESLIE PALMER SWAMPSCOTT, MA

START TO FINISH: 25 MIN.
MAKES: 4 SERVINGS

- 4 tilapia fillets (6 ounces each)
- 1 tablespoon reduced-fat mayonnaise
- 1 tablespoon lime juice
- ¼ teaspoon grated lime peel
- ½ teaspoon salt
- ¼ teaspoon onion powder
- ¼ teaspoon pepper
- ½ cup panko (Japanese) bread crumbs
  Cooking spray
- 2 tablespoons minced fresh cilantro or parsley

1. Preheat oven to 425°. Place fillets on a baking sheet coated with cooking spray. In a small bowl, mix mayonnaise, lime juice and peel, salt, onion powder and pepper. Spread the mayonnaise mixture over fish. Sprinkle with bread crumbs; spritz with cooking spray.
2. Bake 15-20 minutes or until the fish just begins to flake easily with a fork. Sprinkle with cilantro.
Per fillet: 186 cal., 3g fat (1g sat. fat), 84mg chol., 401mg sod., 6g carb. (0 sugars, 0 fiber), 33g pro.
Diabetic Exchanges: 5 lean meat, ½ starch.

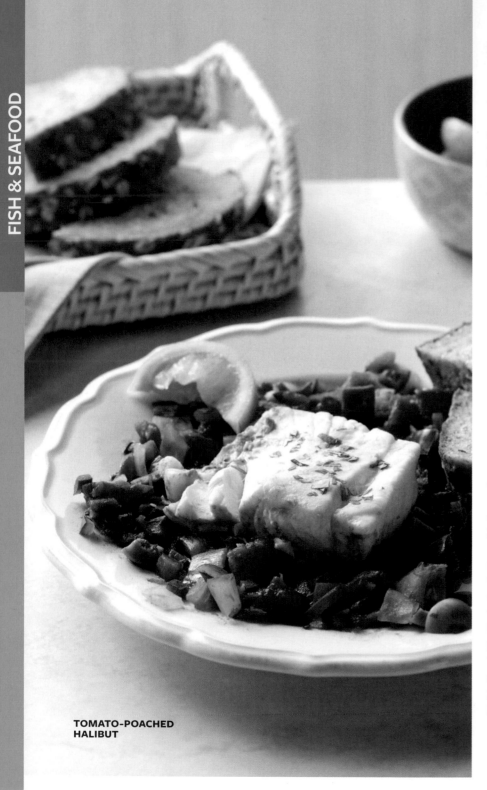

FAST FIX

TOMATO-POACHED HALIBUT

My simple halibut with a burst of lemon comes together in one pan. Try it with polenta or angel hair pasta.

—DANNA ROGERS WESTPORT, CT

START TO FINISH: 30 MIN.
MAKES: 4 SERVINGS

- 1 tablespoon olive oil
- 2 poblano peppers, finely chopped
- 1 small onion, finely chopped
- 1 can (14½ ounces) fire-roasted diced tomatoes, undrained
- 1 can (14½ ounces) no-salt-added diced tomatoes, undrained
- ¼ cup chopped pitted green olives
- 3 garlic cloves, minced
- ¼ teaspoon pepper
- ⅛ teaspoon salt
- 4 halibut fillets (4 ounces each)
- ⅓ cup chopped fresh cilantro
- 4 lemon wedges
  Crusty whole grain bread, optional

1. In a large nonstick skillet, heat oil over medium-high heat. Add poblano peppers and onion; cook and stir about 4-6 minutes or until tender.

2. Stir in tomatoes, olives, garlic, pepper and salt. Bring to a boil. Adjust heat to maintain a gentle simmer. Add fillets. Cook, covered, 8-10 minutes or until fish just begins to flake easily with a fork. Sprinkle with cilantro. Serve with lemon wedges and, if desired, bread.

Per 1 fillet with 1 cup sauce: 224 cal., 7g fat (1g sat. fat), 56mg chol., 651mg sod., 17g carb. (8g sugars, 4g fiber), 24g pro.

Diabetic Exchanges: 3 lean meat, 1 starch, ½ fat.

TOMATO-POACHED HALIBUT

⑤ INGREDIENTS
CEDAR PLANK SCALLOPS

I got this idea from the fishmonger at our local farmers market and a kitchen store that had cedar cooking planks on sale. All of my friends who tried these scallops have gone out and bought cedar planks for cooking.

—**ROBERT HALPERT** NEWBURYPORT, MA

PREP: 10 MIN. + SOAKING
GRILL: 15 MIN.
MAKES: 4 SERVINGS

- 2 cedar grilling planks
- ¼ cup dry white wine
- 2 tablespoons olive oil
- 2 teaspoons minced fresh basil
- 1 teaspoon minced fresh thyme
- 1 teaspoon lime juice
- 12 sea scallops (about 1½ pounds)

1. Soak planks in water at least 1 hour. In a large bowl, whisk wine, oil, basil, thyme and lime juice. Add the scallops and gently toss to coat. Let stand at least 15 minutes.

2. Place planks on grill rack over direct medium heat. Cover and heat 4-5 minutes or until light to medium smoke comes from the plank and the wood begins to crackle. (This indicates the plank is ready.) Turn plank over and place on indirect heat. Drain scallops, discarding marinade. Place scallops on plank. Grill, covered, over indirect medium heat 10-12 minutes or until firm and opaque.

Per 3 scallops: 142 cal., 3g fat (1g sat. fat), 41mg chol., 667mg sod., 6g carb. (0 sugars, 0 fiber), 21g pro.
Diabetic Exchanges: 3 lean meat, ½ starch, ½ fat.

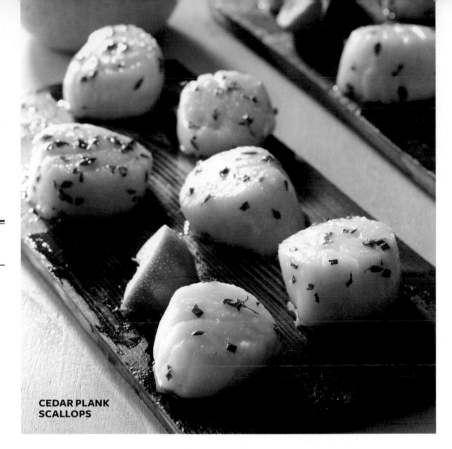

CEDAR PLANK SCALLOPS

GRILLED SHRIMP SCAMPI

When I was in second grade, my class put together a cookbook. This recipe was from one of my friends, and it quickly became a favorite in our house.

—**PEGGY ROOS** MINNEAPOLIS, MN

PREP: 15 MIN. + MARINATING
GRILL: 10 MIN.
MAKES: 6 SERVINGS

- 2 tablespoons olive oil
- 2 tablespoons lemon juice
- 3 garlic cloves, minced
- ¼ teaspoon salt
- ¼ teaspoon pepper
- 1½ pounds uncooked jumbo shrimp, peeled and deveined
  Hot cooked jasmine rice
  Minced fresh parsley

1. In a large bowl, whisk the first five ingredients. Add shrimp; toss to coat. Refrigerate, covered, 30 minutes.

2. Thread shrimp onto six metal or soaked wooden skewers. Grill, covered, over medium heat or broil 4 in. from heat 6-8 minutes or until shrimp turn pink, turning once. Serve with rice; sprinkle with parsley.

Per 1 skewer without rice: 118 cal., 4g fat (1g sat. fat), 138mg chol., 184mg sod., 1g carb. (0 sugars, 0 fiber), 18g pro.
Diabetic Exchanges: 2 meat, ½ fat.

**POACHED SALMON
WITH DILL & TURMERIC**

POACHED SALMON WITH DILL & TURMERIC

This meal-in-one dish is among my husband's favorites because the fish is always tender, juicy and delicious. It's a quick, simple way to prepare salmon, and the robust turmeric doesn't overpower at all.

—EVELYN BANKER ELMHURST, NY

START TO FINISH: 30 MIN.
MAKES: 4 SERVINGS

- 1 tablespoon canola oil
- ¼ teaspoon cumin seeds
- 1 pound Yukon Gold potatoes (about 2 medium), finely chopped
- 1¼ teaspoons salt, divided
- ⅛ teaspoon plus ¼ teaspoon ground turmeric, divided
- 2 tablespoons chopped fresh dill, divided
- 4 salmon fillets (1 inch thick and 4 ounces each)
- 8 fresh dill sprigs
- 2 teaspoons grated lemon peel
- 2 tablespoons lemon juice
- 1 cup (8 ounces) reduced-fat plain yogurt
- ¼ teaspoon pepper

1. In a large skillet, heat oil and cumin over medium heat 1-2 minutes or until seeds are toasted, stirring occasionally. Stir in potatoes, ½ teaspoon salt and ⅛ teaspoon turmeric. Cook, covered, on medium-low 10-12 minutes or until tender. Stir in 1 tablespoon chopped dill; cook, uncovered, 1 minute. Remove from heat.
2. Meanwhile, place salmon, skin side down, in a large skillet with high sides. Add dill sprigs, lemon peel, lemon juice, ½ teaspoon salt, remaining turmeric and enough water to cover salmon.

Bring just to a boil. Adjust the heat to maintain a gentle simmer. Cook it, uncovered, 7-9 minutes or until fish just begins to flake easily with a fork.
3. In a small bowl, mix yogurt, pepper and remaining 1 tablespoon chopped dill and ¼ teaspoon salt. Serve with salmon and potatoes.

Per 3 ounces cooked salmon with ½ cup potatoes and ¼ cup sauce: 350 cal., 15g fat (3g sat. fat), 61mg chol., 704mg sod., 27g carb. (6g sugars, 2g fiber), 25g pro.
Diabetic Exchanges: 3 lean meat, 2 starch, 1 fat.

TUNA VEGGIE KABOBS

This is such a quick and easy meal! My children love to help cut up the veggies and assemble the skewers. I serve it over brown rice cooked in low-salt chicken broth and garnish with parsley and lemon wedges.

—LYNN CARUSO SAN JOSE, CA

PREP: 30 MIN. + MARINATING
GRILL: 10 MIN. • **MAKES:** 8 KABOBS

- 2 pounds tuna steaks, cut into 1½-inch cubes
- 16 large fresh mushrooms
- 3 medium green peppers, seeded and cut into 2-inch pieces
- 3 medium ears sweet corn, cut into 2-inch pieces
- 3 medium zucchini, cut into 1-inch slices
- ¼ cup olive oil
- 2 tablespoons lemon juice
- 2 tablespoons finely chopped shallot
- 1 tablespoon rice vinegar
- 1 tablespoon minced garlic
- 1 teaspoon salt
- 1 teaspoon dried rosemary, crushed
- 1 teaspoon dried thyme
- ½ teaspoon pepper

1. Place the tuna in a large resealable plastic bag; place the vegetables in another large resealable plastic bag. In a small bowl, combine the remaining ingredients. Place half of the marinade in each bag. Seal bags and turn to coat; refrigerate for 1 hour.
2. Drain both bags and discard the marinade. On eight metal or soaked wooden skewers, alternately thread the tuna and vegetables. Using long-handled tongs, moisten a paper towel with cooking oil and lightly coat the grill rack.
3. Grill the tuna, covered, over medium heat or broil it 4 in. from the heat for 10-12 minutes for medium-rare or until the fish is slightly pink in the center and the vegetables are crisp-tender, turning occasionally.

Per kabob: 253 cal., 9g fat (1g sat. fat), 51mg chol., 348mg sod., 15g carb. (5g sugars, 3g fiber), 30g pro.
Diabetic Exchanges: 4 lean meat, 1 vegetable, 1 fat, ½ starch.

❋

TEST KITCHEN TIP
If fresh tuna steaks aren't available at your local grocery store, you can try these easy kabobs with another firm-flesh fish like sea bass, halibut, red snapper or salmon. A delicious result is a sure thing!

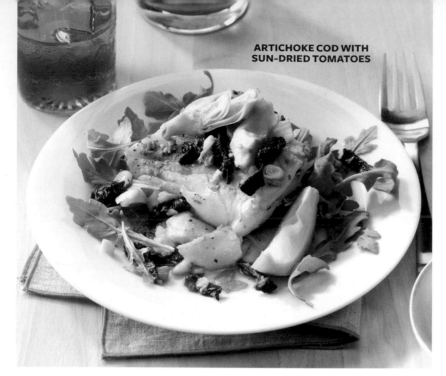

ARTICHOKE COD WITH SUN-DRIED TOMATOES

BASIL CRAB CAKES

I love crabmeat any way it's served, but especially in these crab cakes. If you don't have time to dash to the store, substitute 2 teaspoons of dried basil for the fresh.

—**PRISCILLA GILBERT**
INDIAN HARBOUR BEACH, FL

PREP: 15 MIN. + CHILLING
COOK: 10 MIN. • **MAKES:** 4 SERVINGS

- 1 large egg white
- ¼ cup mayonnaise
- 2 tablespoons minced fresh basil
- 2 teaspoons Dijon mustard
- 2 teaspoons Worcestershire sauce
- ¼ teaspoon salt
- ¼ teaspoon pepper
- 2 drops hot pepper sauce
- ½ pound lump crabmeat, drained
- 6 saltines, finely crushed
- 1 tablespoon canola oil
  Seafood cocktail sauce, optional

1. In a small bowl, combine the first eight ingredients. Stir in the crab and cracker crumbs. Refrigerate for at least 30 minutes.

2. Shape the mixture into four patties. In a large skillet, cook crab cakes in oil for 3-4 minutes on each side or until golden brown. Serve with cocktail sauce if desired.

Per 1 crab cake without cocktail sauce: 214 cal., 16g fat (2g sat. fat), 55mg chol., 568mg sod., 4g carb. (0 sugars, 0 fiber), 13g pro.
Diabetic Exchanges: 2½ fat, 2 lean meat.

FAST FIX
ARTICHOKE COD WITH SUN-DRIED TOMATOES

Cod offers a great break from really rich dishes around the holidays. I like to serve it over a bed of greens, pasta or quinoa. A squeeze of lemon gives it another layer of freshness.

—**HIROKO MILES** EL DORADO HILLS, CA

START TO FINISH: 30 MIN.
MAKES: 6 SERVINGS

- 1 can (14 ounces) quartered water-packed artichoke hearts, drained
- ½ cup julienned soft sun-dried tomatoes (not packed in oil)
- 2 green onions, chopped
- 3 tablespoons olive oil
- 1 garlic clove, minced
- 6 cod fillets (6 ounces each)
- 1 teaspoon salt
- ½ teaspoon pepper
  Salad greens and lemon wedges, optional

1. Preheat oven to 400°. In a small bowl, combine the first five ingredients; toss to combine.

2. Sprinkle both sides of cod with salt and pepper; place in a 13x9-in. baking dish coated with cooking spray. Top with artichoke mixture.

3. Bake, uncovered, 15-20 minutes or until fish just begins to flake easily with a fork. If desired, serve over greens with lemon wedges.

Note: This recipe was tested with sun-dried tomatoes that can be used without soaking. When using other sun-dried tomatoes that are not oil-packed, cover with boiling water and let stand until soft. Drain before using.

Per 1 fillet with ⅓ cup artichoke mixture: 231 cal., 8g fat (1g sat. fat), 65mg chol., 665mg sod., 9g carb. (3g sugars, 2g fiber), 29g pro.
Diabetic Exchanges: 4 lean meat, 1½ fat, 1 vegetable.

⑤INGREDIENTS | FAST FIX ▶

TERIYAKI SALMON

For this delectable glaze, I blend maple syrup with teriyaki sauce. It makes the salmon sweet, tender and delicious.

—LENITA SCHAFER ORMOND BEACH, FL

START TO FINISH: 30 MIN.
MAKES: 4 SERVINGS

- ¾ cup reduced-sodium teriyaki sauce
- ½ cup maple syrup
- 4 salmon fillets (6 ounces each)
  Mixed salad greens, optional

1. In a small bowl, whisk teriyaki sauce and syrup. Pour 1 cup marinade into a large resealable plastic bag. Add salmon; seal bag and turn to coat. Refrigerate 15 minutes. Cover and refrigerate any of the remaining marinade.

2. Drain the salmon, discarding the marinade in bag. Moisten a paper towel with cooking oil; using long-handled tongs, rub on grill rack to coat lightly.

3. Place salmon on grill rack, skin side down. Grill, covered, over medium heat or broil 4 in. from heat 8-12 minutes or until fish just begins to flake easily with a fork, basting frequently with reserved marinade. If desired, serve over mixed salad greens.

Per fillet: 362 cal., 18g fat (4g sat. fat), 100mg chol., 422mg sod., 12g carb. (12g sugars, 0 fiber), 35g pro.

Diabetic Exchanges: 5 lean meat, 1 starch.

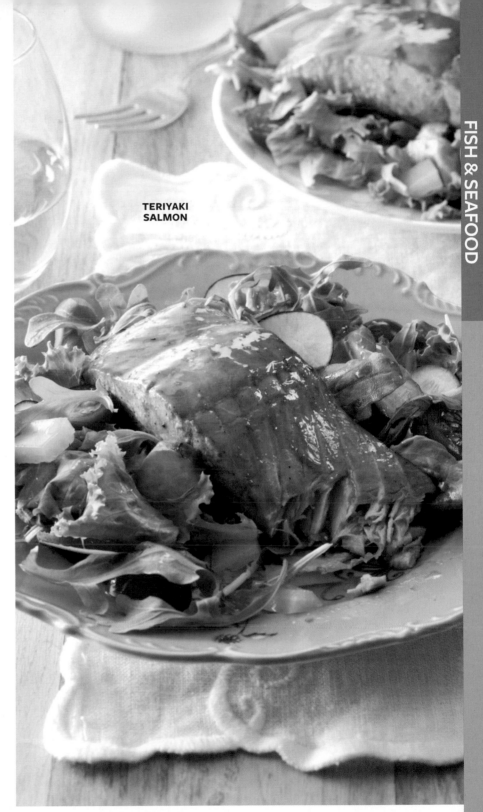

TERIYAKI SALMON

FAST FIX ▶
LEMON-PARSLEY BAKED COD

This is the first fish recipe that got two thumbs up from the picky meat-only eaters at my table. The tangy lemon gives the cod some oomph.
—TRISHA KRUSE EAGLE, ID

START TO FINISH: 30 MIN.
MAKES: 4 SERVINGS

- 3 tablespoons lemon juice
- 3 tablespoons butter, melted
- ¼ cup all-purpose flour
- ½ teaspoon salt
- ¼ teaspoon paprika
- ¼ teaspoon lemon-pepper seasoning
- 4 cod fillets (6 ounces each)
- 2 tablespoons minced fresh parsley
- 2 teaspoons grated lemon peel

1. Preheat oven to 400°. In a shallow bowl, mix lemon juice and butter. In a separate shallow bowl, mix flour and seasonings. Dip fillets in lemon juice mixture, then in flour mixture to coat both sides; shake off excess.
2. Place in a 13x9-in. baking dish coated with cooking spray. Drizzle with the remaining lemon juice mixture. Bake 12-15 minutes or until fish just begins to flake easily with a fork. Mix parsley and lemon peel; sprinkle over fish.
Per fillet: 232 cal., 10g fat (6g sat. fat), 87mg chol., 477mg sod., 7g carb. (0 sugars, 0 fiber), 28g pro.
Diabetic Exchanges: 4 lean meat, 2 fat, ½ starch.

FAST FIX ▶
GARLIC TILAPIA WITH SPICY KALE

When making this main dish and side together, adjust the amount of red pepper flakes to your liking.
—TARA CRUZ KERSEY, CO

START TO FINISH: 30 MIN.
MAKES: 4 SERVINGS

- 3 tablespoons olive oil, divided
- 2 garlic cloves, minced
- 1 teaspoon fennel seed
- ½ teaspoon crushed red pepper flakes
- 1 bunch kale, trimmed and coarsely chopped (about 16 cups)
- ⅔ cup water
- 4 tilapia fillets (6 ounces each)
- ¾ teaspoon pepper, divided
- ½ teaspoon garlic salt
- 1 can (15 ounces) cannellini beans, rinsed and drained
- ½ teaspoon salt

1. In 6-qt. stockpot, heat 1 tablespoon oil over medium heat. Add garlic, fennel and pepper flakes; cook and stir for 1 minute. Add kale and water; bring to a boil. Reduce heat; simmer, covered, 10-12 minutes or until the kale is tender.
2. Meanwhile, sprinkle tilapia with ½ teaspoon pepper and garlic salt. In large skillet, heat remaining oil over medium heat. Add tilapia; cook 3-4 minutes per side or until fish flakes easily with fork.
3. Add beans, salt and the remaining pepper to kale; heat through, stirring occasionally. Serve with tilapia.
Per 1 fillet with 1 cup kale mixture: 359 cal., 13g fat (2g sat. fat), 83mg chol., 645mg sod., 24g carb. (0 sugars, 6g fiber), 39g pro.
Diabetic Exchanges: 5 lean meat, 2 fat, 1½ starch.

FAST FIX ▶
CAJUN BAKED CATFISH

This well-seasoned fish earns praise from family and friends whenever I serve it. It's moist and flaky, and the coating is crispy, crunchy and flecked with paprika.
—JIM GALES MILWAUKEE, WI

START TO FINISH: 25 MIN.
MAKES: 2 SERVINGS

- 2 tablespoons yellow cornmeal
- 2 teaspoons Cajun or blackened seasoning
- ½ teaspoon dried thyme
- ½ teaspoon dried basil
- ¼ teaspoon garlic powder
- ¼ teaspoon lemon-pepper seasoning
- 2 catfish or tilapia fillets (6 ounces each)
- ¼ teaspoon paprika

1. Preheat oven to 400°. In a shallow bowl, mix the first six ingredients.
2. Dip the fillets in cornmeal mixture to evenly coat both sides. Place them on a baking sheet coated with cooking spray. Sprinkle with paprika.
3. Bake 20-25 minutes or until fish just begins to flake easily with a fork.
Per fillet: 242 cal., 10g fat (2g sat. fat), 94mg chol., 748mg sod., 8g carb. (0 sugars, 1g fiber), 27g pro.
Diabetic Exchanges: 4 lean meat, ½ starch.

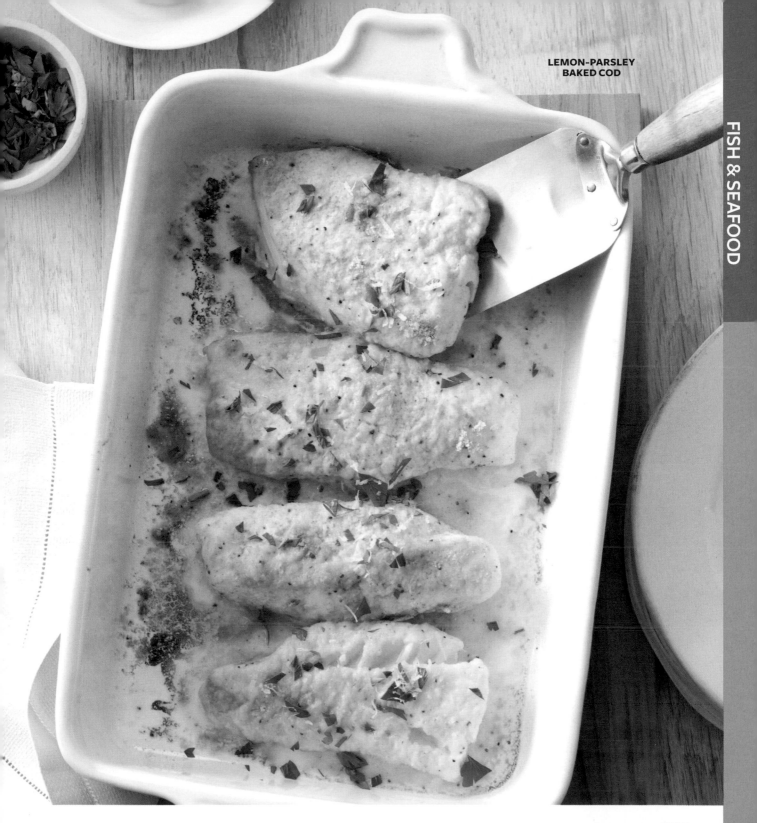

LEMON-PARSLEY BAKED COD

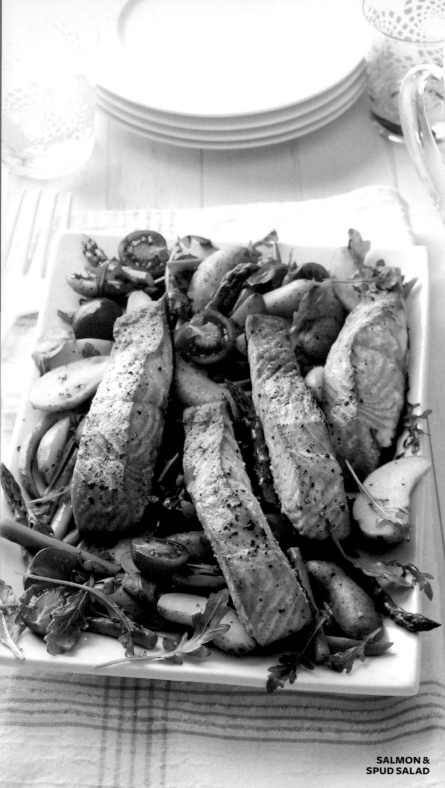

SALMON & SPUD SALAD

FAST FIX

SALMON & SPUD SALAD

Here's a meal that proves that smart choices can be simple and satisfying.
—MATTHEW TEIXEIRA MILTON, ON

START TO FINISH: 30 MIN.
MAKES: 4 SERVINGS

- 1 pound fingerling potatoes
- ½ pound fresh green beans
- ½ pound fresh asparagus
- 4 salmon fillets (6 ounces each)
- 1 tablespoon plus ⅓ cup red wine vinaigrette, divided
- ¼ teaspoon salt
- ¼ teaspoon pepper
- 4 cups fresh arugula or baby spinach
- 2 cups cherry tomatoes, halved
- 1 tablespoon minced fresh chives

1. Cut potatoes lengthwise in half. Trim and cut green beans and asparagus into 2-in. pieces. Place potatoes in a 6-qt. stockpot; add water to cover. Bring to a boil. Reduce heat; cook, uncovered, 10-15 minutes or until tender, adding green beans and asparagus during the last 4 minutes of cooking. Drain.

2. Meanwhile, brush salmon with 1 tablespoon vinaigrette; sprinkle with salt and pepper. Place fish on oiled grill rack, skin side down. Grill it, covered, over medium-high heat or broil 4 in. from heat 6-8 minutes or until fish just begins to flake easily with a fork.

3. In a large bowl, combine potato mixture, arugula, tomatoes and chives. Drizzle with remaining vinaigrette; toss to coat. Serve with salmon.

Per 1 salmon fillet with 2 cups salad: 480 cal., 23g fat (4g sat. fat), 85mg chol., 642mg sod., 33g carb. (8g sugars, 6g fiber), 34g pro.
Diabetic Exchanges: 5 lean meat, 2 vegetable, 1½ starch, 1½ fat.

FAST FIX ▶
SOLE FILLETS IN LEMON BUTTER

This provides such a speedy, no-fuss and delicious way to prepare fish! My son started requesting this fish with crackers as a little boy, and he still asks for it as an adult today.

—BARB SHARON PLYMOUTH, WI

START TO FINISH: 20 MIN.
MAKES: 4 SERVINGS

- 4 sole fillets (4 ounces each)
- ¼ teaspoon salt
- ⅛ teaspoon pepper
- 3 tablespoons butter, melted
- ½ cup minced fresh parsley
- 1 tablespoon lemon juice
- ¼ cup crushed butter-flavored crackers
- ½ teaspoon paprika

1. Place the sole in an ungreased microwave-safe 11x7-in. dish; sprinkle with salt and pepper. Cover and microwave on high for 3-4 minutes.
2. In a small bowl, combine the butter, parsley and lemon juice; pour mixture over fillets. Then sprinkle with cracker crumbs. Microwave, uncovered, for 3-4 minutes or until fish flakes easily with a fork. Sprinkle with paprika.
Note: This recipe was tested in a 1,100-watt microwave.
Per fillet: 213 cal., 11g fat (6g sat. fat), 77mg chol., 377mg sod., 5g carb. (1g sugars, 0 fiber), 22g pro.
Diabetic Exchanges: 3 lean meat, 2 fat.

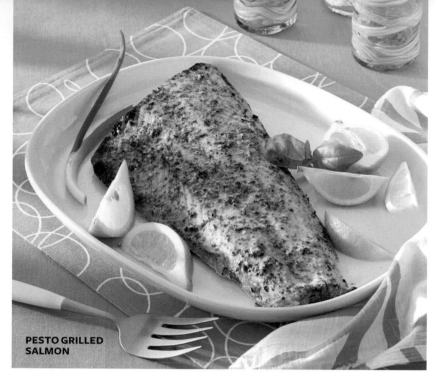
PESTO GRILLED SALMON

⑤ INGREDIENTS   FAST FIX ▶
PESTO GRILLED SALMON

Using just a few ingredients, this fresh and easy summertime dish is sure to become a family favorite.

—SONYA LABBE WEST HOLLYWOOD, CA

START TO FINISH: 30 MIN.
MAKES: 12 SERVINGS

- 1 salmon fillet (3 pounds)
- ½ cup prepared pesto
- 2 green onions, finely chopped
- ¼ cup lemon juice
- 2 garlic cloves, minced

1. Moisten a paper towel with cooking oil; using long-handled tongs, lightly coat the grill rack. Place salmon skin side down on grill rack. Grill, covered, over medium heat or broil 4 in. from the heat for 5 minutes.
2. In a small bowl, combine the pesto, onions, lemon juice and garlic. Carefully spoon some of the pesto mixture over salmon. Grill for about 15-20 minutes longer or until the fish flakes easily with a fork, basting occasionally with the remaining pesto mixture.
Per 3 ounces cooked salmon: 262 cal., 17g fat (4g sat. fat), 70mg chol., 147mg sod., 1g carb. (0 sugars, 0 fiber), 25g pro.
Diabetic Exchanges: 3 lean meat, 3 fat.

★ ★ ★ ★ ★ **READER REVIEW**

"Just delicious! I've made it with salmon and other types of fish."

ANNAMARIATU TASTEOFHOME.COM

RICOTTA-STUFFED
PORTOBELLO
MUSHROOMS, PAGE 232

Meatless Mains

No matter what kind of diet you follow,
vegetables are the cornerstone for healthy eating.
Pizzas, pastas and more keep blood sugars level,
vitamins high and everyone happy. Add a colorful side
dish or salad for a satisfying meal everyone will love.

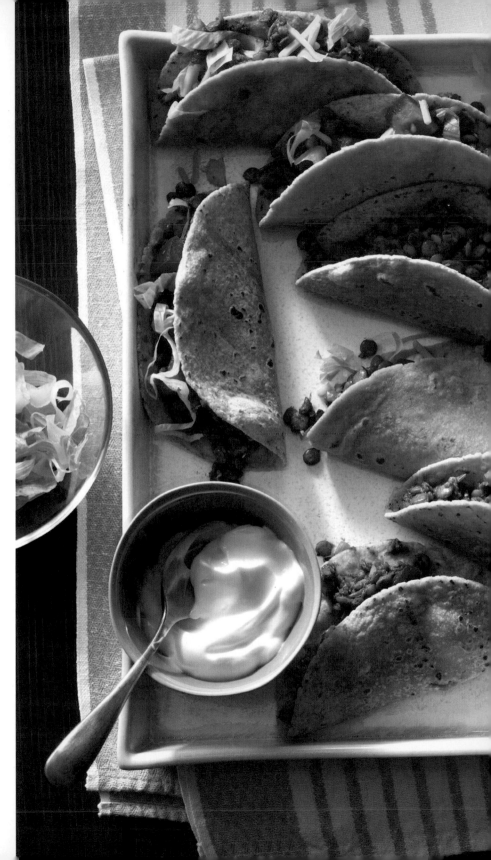

TASTY LENTIL TACOS

My husband watches his cholesterol, and I found a dish that's healthy for him and yummy for our kids.

—MICHELLE THOMAS BANGOR, ME

PREP: 15 MIN. • **COOK:** 40 MIN.
MAKES: 6 SERVINGS

- 1 teaspoon canola oil
- 1 medium onion, finely chopped
- 1 garlic clove, minced
- 1 cup dried lentils, rinsed
- 1 tablespoon chili powder
- 2 teaspoons ground cumin
- 1 teaspoon dried oregano
- 2½ cups vegetable or reduced-sodium chicken broth
- 1 cup salsa
- 12 taco shells
- 1½ cups shredded lettuce
- 1 cup chopped fresh tomatoes
- 1½ cups shredded reduced-fat cheddar cheese
- 6 tablespoons fat-free sour cream

1. In a large nonstick skillet, heat oil over medium heat; saute onion and garlic until tender. Add the lentils and seasonings; cook and stir 1 minute. Stir in broth; bring to a boil. Reduce heat; simmer, covered, until lentils are tender, 25-30 minutes.

2. Cook, uncovered, until mixture is thickened, for 6-8 minutes, stirring occasionally. Mash lentils slightly; stir in salsa and heat through. Serve in taco shells. Top with remaining ingredients.

Per 2 tacos: 365 cal., 12g fat (5g sat. fat), 21mg chol., 777mg sod., 44g carb. (5g sugars, 6g fiber), 19g pro.
Diabetic Exchanges: 2½ starch, 2 lean meat, 1 vegetable, 1 fat.

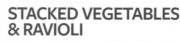

TASTY LENTIL TACOS

STACKED VEGETABLES & RAVIOLI

Yellow squash, zucchini and basil meet ricotta and ravioli in this crowd-pleasing entree with delicious summer flavors. One bite and you'll know—this is what summer fresh tastes like.

—**TASTE OF HOME** TEST KITCHEN

PREP: 20 MIN.
BAKE: 30 MIN. + STANDING
MAKES: 6 SERVINGS

- 2 yellow summer squash
- 2 medium zucchini
- 1 package (9 ounces) refrigerated cheese ravioli
- 1 cup ricotta cheese
- 1 large egg
- ½ teaspoon garlic salt
- 1 jar (24 ounces) marinara or spaghetti sauce
- 10 fresh basil leaves, divided
- ¾ cup shredded Parmesan cheese

1. Preheat oven to 350°. Using a vegetable peeler, cut the squash and zucchini into very thin lengthwise strips. In a Dutch oven, cook ravioli according to package directions, adding vegetable strips during last 3 minutes of cooking.
2. Meanwhile, in a small bowl, combine the ricotta cheese, egg and garlic salt; set aside. Drain ravioli and vegetables.
3. Spread ½ cup marinara sauce into a greased 11x7-in. baking dish. Layer with half of the ravioli and vegetables, half of ricotta mixture, seven basil leaves and 1 cup marinara sauce. Layer with the remaining ravioli, vegetables and marinara sauce. Dollop the remaining ricotta mixture over top; sprinkle with Parmesan cheese.
4. Cover and bake 25 minutes. Uncover and bake 5-10 minutes longer or until cheese is melted. Let stand 10 minutes

before cutting. Thinly slice remaining basil; sprinkle over top.
Per serving: 323 cal., 11g fat (6g sat. fat), 76mg chol., 779mg sod., 39g carb. (15g sugars, 4g fiber), 19g pro.
Diabetic Exchanges: 2 starch, 2 medium-fat meat, 1 vegetable.

FAST FIX
ZESTY VEGGIE PITAS

Cilantro adds oomph wherever it goes. That's why I use it with ingredients from the fridge to make a zesty, refreshing sandwich combo.

—**KRISTA FRANK** RHODODENDRON, OR

START TO FINISH: 20 MIN.
MAKES: 4 SERVINGS

- ½ cup hummus
- 4 whole pocketless pita breads or flatbreads, warmed
- 4 slices pepper jack cheese
- 1 cup thinly sliced cucumber
- 1 large tomato, cut into wedges
- ¼ cup sliced pepperoncini
- ¼ cup sliced ripe olives
- ¼ cup fresh cilantro leaves

Spread hummus over pita breads. Top with the remaining ingredients; fold the pitas to serve.
Per sandwich: 323 cal., 11g fat (4g sat. fat), 23mg chol., 758mg sod., 42g carb. (2g sugars, 4g fiber), 14g pro.
Diabetic Exchanges: 3 starch, 1 medium-fat meat.

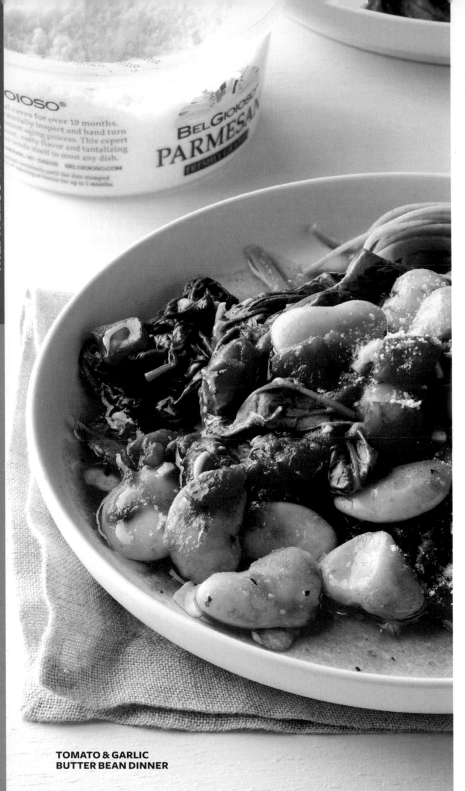

**TOMATO & GARLIC
BUTTER BEAN DINNER**

(5)INGREDIENTS | FAST FIX >

TOMATO & GARLIC BUTTER BEAN DINNER

*For days when I get home late and just
want a warm meal, I stir up tomatoes,
garlic and butter beans. Ladle it over
noodles on the days you think you can
afford the carbs.*

—JESSICA MEYERS AUSTIN, TX

START TO FINISH: 15 MIN.
MAKES: 4 SERVINGS

- 1 tablespoon olive oil
- 2 garlic cloves, minced
- 2 cans (14½ ounces) no-salt-added petite diced tomatoes, undrained
- 1 can (16 ounces) butter beans, rinsed and drained
- 6 cups fresh baby spinach (about 6 ounces)
- ½ teaspoon Italian seasoning
- ¼ teaspoon pepper
  Hot cooked pasta and grated
      Parmesan cheese, optional

In a large skillet, heat oil over medium-high heat. Add garlic; cook and stir 30-45 seconds or until tender. Add tomatoes, beans, spinach, Italian seasoning and pepper; cook until spinach wilts, stirring occasionally. If desired, serve with pasta and cheese.

To freeze: Freeze cooled bean mixture in freezer containers. To use, partially thaw in refrigerator overnight. Heat through in a saucepan, stirring occasionally and adding a little water if necessary.

Per 1¼ cups without pasta and cheese: 147 cal., 4g fat (1g sat. fat), 0 chol., 353mg sod., 28g carb. (8g sugars, 9g fiber), 8g pro.
Diabetic Exchanges: 2 starch, 1 lean meat, ½ fat.

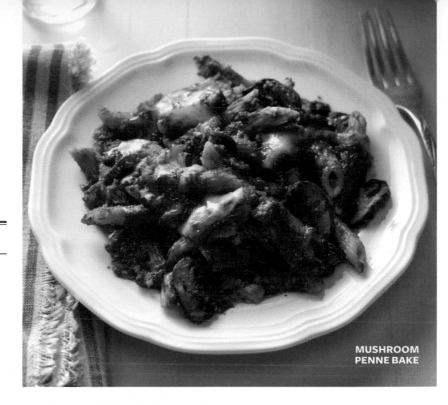

MUSHROOM PENNE BAKE

FAST FIX

BLACK BEANS WITH BELL PEPPERS & RICE

My entire family falls hard for this vegetarian dish every time I make it. It's pretty, quick and has an awesome kick of flavor. For my kids, the more cheese I add, the better.

—**STEPHANIE LAMBERT** MOSELEY, VA

START TO FINISH: 30 MIN.
MAKES: 6 SERVINGS

- 1 tablespoon olive oil
- 1 each medium sweet yellow, orange and red pepper, chopped
- 1 large onion, chopped
- 2 garlic cloves, minced
- 2 cans (15 ounces each) black beans, rinsed and drained
- 1 package (8.8 ounces) ready-to-serve brown rice
- 1½ teaspoons ground cumin
- ½ teaspoon dried oregano
- 1½ cups (6 ounces) shredded Mexican cheese blend, divided
- 3 tablespoons minced fresh cilantro

1. In a large skillet, heat the oil over medium-high heat. Add peppers, onion and garlic; cook and stir 6-8 minutes or until tender. Add beans, rice, cumin and oregano; heat through.

2. Stir in 1 cup cheese; sprinkle with remaining cheese. Remove from heat. Let stand, covered, 5 minutes or until cheese is melted. Sprinkle with cilantro.

Per 1 cup: 347 cal., 12g fat (6g sat. fat), 25mg chol., 477mg sod., 40g carb. (4g sugars, 8g fiber), 15g pro.

Diabetic Exchanges: 2½ starch, 2 lean meat, 1 fat.

MUSHROOM PENNE BAKE

An easy, hearty, delicious meal for a chilly evening, penne's cheesy goodness will have you going for seconds. Serve with salad and garlic bread.

—**SUE ASCHEMEIER** DEFIANCE, OH

PREP: 25 MIN. • **BAKE:** 25 MIN.
MAKES: 8 SERVINGS

- 1 package (12 ounces) whole wheat penne pasta
- 1 tablespoon olive oil
- 1 pound sliced baby portobello mushrooms
- 2 garlic cloves, minced
- 1 jar (24 ounces) marinara sauce
- 1 teaspoon Italian seasoning
- ½ teaspoon salt
- 2 cups reduced-fat ricotta cheese
- 1 cup shredded part-skim mozzarella cheese, divided
- ½ cup grated Parmesan cheese

1. Preheat oven to 350°. In a 6-qt. stockpot, cook pasta according to package directions. Drain and return to pot; cool slightly.

2. In a large skillet, heat oil over medium-high heat; saute mushrooms until tender, 4-6 minutes. Add garlic; cook 1 minute. Stir in marinara sauce and seasonings. Spread half of the mixture into a 13x9-in. baking dish coated with cooking spray.

3. Stir ricotta cheese and ½ cup mozzarella cheese into pasta; spoon over mushroom mixture. Spread with remaining mushroom mixture.

4. Sprinkle with remaining mozzarella cheese and Parmesan cheese. Bake, uncovered, until bubbly, 25-30 minutes.

Per 1 cup: 353 cal., 11g fat (4g sat. fat), 30mg chol., 748mg sod., 44g carb. (10g sugars, 7g fiber), 20g pro.

Diabetic Exchanges: 3 starch, 2 lean meat, 1 fat.

SPINACH & ARTICHOKE PIZZA

My from-scratch pizza has a whole wheat crust flavored with beer and spinach, artichoke hearts, tomatoes and fresh basil for toppings.

—RAYMONDE BOURGEOIS SWASTIKA, ON

PREP: 25 MIN. • **BAKE:** 20 MIN.
MAKES: 6 SLICES

- 1½ to 1¾ cups white whole wheat flour
- 1½ teaspoons baking powder
- ¼ teaspoon salt
- ¼ teaspoon each dried basil, oregano and parsley flakes
- ¾ cup beer or nonalcoholic beer

TOPPINGS
- 1½ teaspoons olive oil
- 1 garlic clove, minced
- 2 cups (8 ounces) shredded Italian cheese blend
- 2 cups fresh baby spinach
- 1 can (14 ounces) water-packed quartered artichoke hearts, drained and coarsely chopped
- 2 medium tomatoes, seeded and coarsely chopped
- 2 tablespoons thinly sliced fresh basil

1. Preheat oven to 425°. In a large bowl, whisk 1½ cups flour, baking powder, salt and dried herbs until blended. Add beer, stirring just until moistened.
2. Turn dough onto a well-floured surface; knead gently 6-8 times, adding additional flour if needed. Press dough to fit a greased 12-in. pizza pan. Pinch edge to form a rim. Bake 8 minutes or until edge is lightly browned.
3. Mix oil and garlic; spread over crust. Sprinkle with ½ cup cheese; layer with spinach, artichoke hearts and tomatoes.

Sprinkle with remaining cheese. Bake 8-10 minutes or until crust is golden and cheese is melted. Sprinkle with sliced fresh basil.

Per slice: 290 cal., 10g fat (6g sat. fat), 27mg chol., 654mg sod., 32g carb. (1g sugars, 5g fiber), 14g pro.
Diabetic Exchanges: 2 starch, 1 medium-fat meat, 1 vegetable.

FAST FIX

RICOTTA-STUFFED PORTOBELLO MUSHROOMS

These mushrooms taste rich, creamy and bright at the same time because of the fresh herbs and tomato. Try them with grilled asparagus!

—TRE BALCHOWSKY SAUSALITO, CA

START TO FINISH: 30 MIN.
MAKES: 6 SERVINGS

- ¾ cup reduced-fat ricotta cheese
- ¾ cup grated Parmesan cheese, divided
- ½ cup shredded part-skim mozzarella cheese
- 2 tablespoons minced fresh parsley
- ⅛ teaspoon pepper
- 6 large portobello mushrooms
- 6 slices large tomato
- ¾ cup fresh basil leaves
- 3 tablespoons slivered almonds or pine nuts, toasted
- 1 small garlic clove
- 2 tablespoons olive oil
- 2 to 3 teaspoons water

1. In a small bowl, mix ricotta cheese, ¼ cup Parmesan cheese, mozzarella cheese, parsley and pepper. Remove and discard stems from mushrooms; with a spoon, scrape and remove gills. Fill caps with ricotta mixture. Top with tomato slices.

2. Grill, covered, over medium heat 8-10 minutes or until mushrooms are tender. Remove from the grill with a metal spatula.
3. Meanwhile, place basil, almonds and garlic in a small food processor; pulse until chopped. Add remaining Parmesan cheese; pulse just until blended. While processing, gradually add the oil and enough water to reach the desired consistency. Spoon the mixture over stuffed mushrooms before serving.
Note: To toast nuts, bake in a shallow pan in a 350° oven for 5-10 minutes or cook in a skillet over low heat until lightly browned, stirring occasionally.
Per mushroom: 201 cal., 13g fat (4g sat. fat), 22mg chol., 238mg sod., 9g carb. (5g sugars, 2g fiber), 12g pro.
Diabetic Exchanges: 1½ fat, 1 medium-fat meat, 1 vegetable.

★ ★ ★ ★ ★ READER REVIEW

"My husband and I both thought these were very good, and we will make then again. I put the mushrooms in a disposable pan, covered with aluminum foil and grilled them for about 13 minutes."

UNCORKED TASTEOFHOME.COM

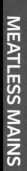

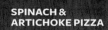

SPINACH &
ARTICHOKE PIZZA

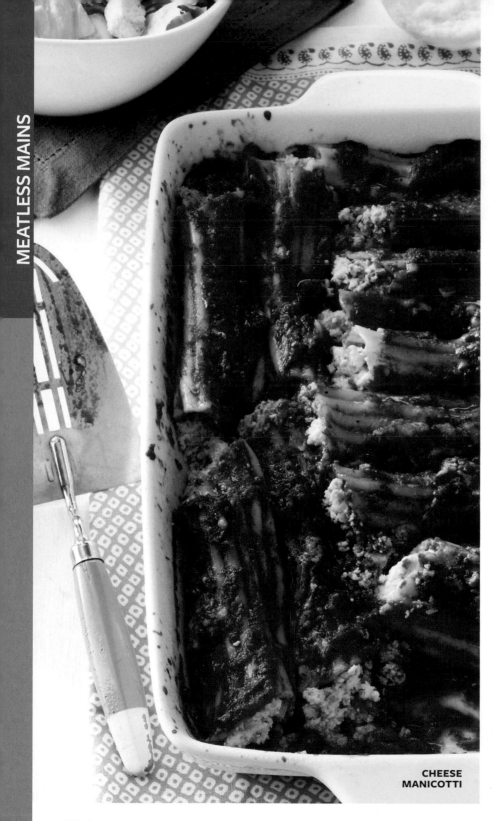

CHEESE MANICOTTI

CHEESE MANICOTTI

Manicotti is the first meal I ever cooked for my husband. All these years later, he still enjoys the dish.

—JOAN HALLFORD
NORTH RICHLAND HILLS, TX

PREP: 25 MIN. • **BAKE:** 1 HOUR
MAKES: 7 SERVINGS

- 1 carton (15 ounces) reduced-fat ricotta cheese
- ½ cup shredded part-skim mozzarella cheese
- 1 small onion, finely chopped
- 1 large egg, lightly beaten
- 2 tablespoons minced fresh parsley
- ½ teaspoon pepper
- ¼ teaspoon salt
- 1 cup grated Parmesan cheese, divided
- 4 cups marinara sauce
- ½ cup water
- 1 package (8 ounces) manicotti shells

1. Preheat oven to 350°. In a small bowl, mix the first seven ingredients; stir in ½ cup Parmesan cheese. In another bowl, mix marinara sauce and water; spread ¾ cup sauce onto bottom of a 13x9-in. baking dish coated with cooking spray. Fill uncooked manicotti shells with ricotta mixture; arrange over sauce. Top with remaining sauce.
2. Bake, covered, 50 minutes or until pasta is tender. Sprinkle with remaining Parmesan cheese. Bake, uncovered, 10-15 minutes longer or until the cheese is melted.
Per 2 stuffed manicotti: 340 cal., 8g fat (5g sat. fat), 60mg chol., 615mg sod., 46g carb. (16g sugars, 4g fiber), 19g pro.
Diabetic Exchanges: 3 starch, 2 lean meat, ½ fat.

BUTTERNUT & PORTOBELLO LASAGNA

Lasagna gets fresh flavor and color when you make it with roasted butternut squash, portobello mushrooms, basil and spinach. We feast on this.

—EDWARD AND DANIELLE WALKER
TRAVERSE CITY, MI

PREP: 1 HOUR
BAKE: 45 MIN. + STANDING
MAKES: 12 SERVINGS

- 1 package (10 ounces) frozen cubed butternut squash, thawed
- 2 teaspoons olive oil
- 1 teaspoon brown sugar
- ¼ teaspoon salt
- ⅛ teaspoon pepper

MUSHROOMS
- 4 large portobello mushrooms, coarsely chopped
- 2 teaspoons balsamic vinegar
- 2 teaspoons olive oil
- ¼ teaspoon salt
- ⅛ teaspoon pepper

SAUCE
- 2 cans (28 ounces each) whole tomatoes, undrained
- 2 teaspoons olive oil
- 2 garlic cloves, minced
- 1 teaspoon crushed red pepper flakes
- ½ cup fresh basil leaves, thinly sliced
- ¼ teaspoon salt
- ⅛ teaspoon pepper

LASAGNA
- 9 no-cook lasagna noodles
- 4 ounces fresh baby spinach (about 5 cups)
- 3 cups part-skim ricotta cheese
- 1½ cups shredded part-skim mozzarella cheese

1. Preheat oven to 350°. In a large bowl, combine the first five ingredients. In another bowl, combine ingredients

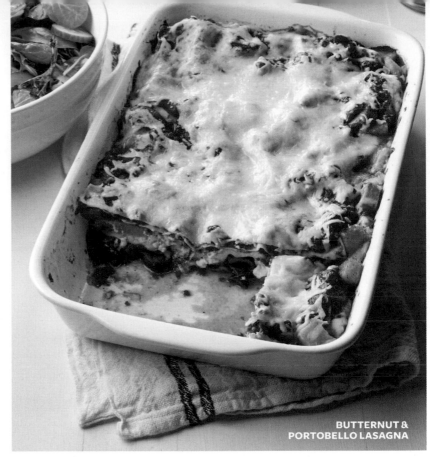

BUTTERNUT & PORTOBELLO LASAGNA

for mushrooms. Transfer vegetables to separate foil-lined 15x10x1-in. baking pans. Roast 14-16 minutes or until tender, stirring occasionally.

2. Meanwhile, for sauce, drain tomatoes, reserving juices; coarsely chop tomatoes. In a large saucepan, heat oil over medium heat. Add garlic and pepper flakes; cook 1 minute longer. Stir in chopped tomatoes, reserved tomato juices, basil, salt and pepper; bring to a boil. Reduce heat; simmer, uncovered, 35-45 minutes or until thickened, stirring occasionally.

3. Spread 1 cup sauce into a greased 13x9-in. baking dish. Layer with three noodles, 1 cup sauce, spinach and mushrooms. Continue layering with three noodles, 1 cup sauce, ricotta cheese and roasted squash. Top with

remaining noodles and sauce. Sprinkle with mozzarella cheese.

4. Bake, covered, 30 minutes. Bake, uncovered, 15-20 minutes longer or until bubbly. Let stand 15 minutes before serving.

Per serving: 252 cal., 10g fat (5g sat. fat), 27mg chol., 508mg sod., 25g carb. (5g sugars, 4g fiber), 15g pro.
Diabetic Exchanges: 2 starch, 1 medium-fat meat, ½ fat.

*
TEST KITCHEN TIP
Before adding any vegetable to your lasagna, it's best to cook it first. Be sure to strain out any excess liquid from the cooking process. Not doing so might make your dish watery.

CHEESY SPINACH-
STUFFED SHELLS

CHEESY SPINACH-STUFFED SHELLS

I'm very proud of this recipe, as it's the first I created as a beginning cook. You can adjust it to your liking by adding more spinach , meat or cheese to it.
—**LACI HOOTEN** MCKINNEY, TX

PREP: 45 MIN. • **BAKE:** 45 MIN.
MAKES: 12 SERVINGS

- 1 package (12 ounces) jumbo pasta shells
- 1 tablespoon butter
- 1 cup sliced mushrooms
- 1 small onion, finely chopped
- 4 garlic cloves, minced
- 2 large eggs, lightly beaten
- 1 carton (15 ounces) part-skim ricotta cheese
- 1 package (10 ounces) frozen chopped spinach, thawed and squeezed dry
- 2 tablespoons minced fresh basil or 2 teaspoons dried basil
- ¼ teaspoon pepper
- 1 can (4¼ ounces) chopped ripe olives
- 1½ cups shredded Italian cheese blend, divided
- 1½ cups shredded part-skim mozzarella cheese, divided
- 1 jar (24 ounces) marinara sauce Additional minced fresh basil, optional

1. Preheat oven to 375°. Cook the pasta shells according to the package directions for al dente. Drain; rinse with cold water.
2. Meanwhile, in a small skillet, heat butter over medium-high heat. Add mushrooms and onion; cook and stir 4-6 minutes or until vegetables are tender. Add garlic; cook 1 minute longer. Remove from heat; cool slightly.
3. In a bowl, mix eggs, ricotta cheese, spinach, basil and pepper. Stir in olives, mushroom mixture and ¾ cup each cheese blend and mozzarella cheese.
4. Spread 1 cup sauce into a 13x9-in. baking dish coated with cooking spray. Fill shells with cheese mixture; place in baking dish, overlapping ends slightly. Spoon remaining sauce over top.
5. Bake, covered, 40-45 minutes or until heated through. Uncover; sprinkle with remaining cheeses. Bake 5 minutes longer or until cheese is melted. Let stand 5 minutes before serving. If desired, sprinkle with additional basil.
Per 3 stuffed shells: 313 cal., 13g fat (7g sat. fat), 65mg chol., 642mg sod., 32g carb. (5g sugars, 3g fiber), 18g pro.
Diabetic Exchanges: 2 starch, 2 medium-fat meat, ½ fat.

GARDEN HARVEST SPAGHETTI SQUASH

In the grocery store one day, I spotted a perfectly ripe spaghetti squash and just had to try it, so I cooked it according to the label. Used in place of pasta and topped it with my favorite vegetables, it became an instant family favorite.
—**VERONICA MCCANN** COLUMBUS, OH

PREP: 30 MIN. • **BAKE:** 35 MIN.
MAKES: 4 SERVINGS

- 1 medium spaghetti squash (about 4 pounds)
- 1 medium sweet red pepper, chopped
- 1 medium red onion, chopped
- 1 small zucchini, chopped
- 1 cup chopped fresh mushrooms
- ½ cup chopped leek (white portion only)
- ½ cup shredded carrots
- 1 tablespoon olive oil
- 1 garlic clove, minced
- 1 can (14½ ounces) stewed tomatoes
- ½ cup tomato paste
- ¼ cup V8 juice
- 1 teaspoon pepper
- ½ teaspoon salt
- 2 cups fresh baby spinach
- 1 tablespoon minced fresh basil
- 2 teaspoons minced fresh oregano
- 2 teaspoons minced fresh thyme
- 1 teaspoon minced fresh rosemary
- ¼ cup grated Parmesan and Romano cheese blend

1. Cut the squash in half lengthwise; discard seeds. Place squash cut side down in a 15x10x1-in. baking pan; add ½ in. of hot water. Bake, uncovered, at 375° for 30-40 minutes. Drain water from the pan; turn squash cut side up. Bake 5 minutes longer or until the squash is tender.
2. Meanwhile, in a Dutch oven, saute the red pepper, onion, zucchini, mushrooms, leek and carrots in oil until tender. Add garlic; cook for 1 minute longer. Add the stewed tomatoes, tomato paste, V8 juice, pepper and salt; bring to a boil. Reduce heat; cover and simmer for 15 minutes. Stir in spinach and herbs; heat through.
3. When squash is cool enough to handle, use a fork to separate strands. Serve with sauce; sprinkle with cheese.
Per 1 cup squash with 1 cup sauce: 270 cal., 8g fat (2g sat. fat), 8mg chol., 751mg sod., 47g carb. (13g sugars, 10g fiber), 10g pro.
Diabetic Exchanges: 3 starch, 1½ fat.

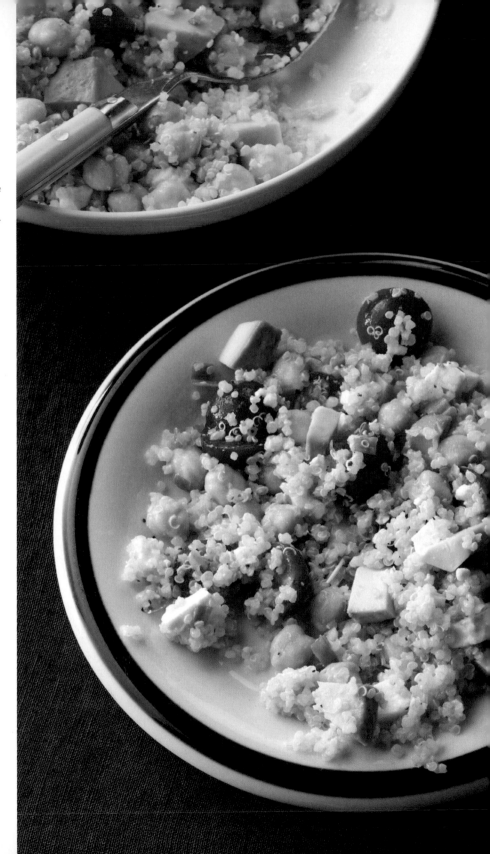

AVOCADO & GARBANZO BEAN QUINOA SALAD

This delicious salad is high in protein and holds well in the fridge for a few days. If you make it ahead, add avocados and tomatoes right before serving.

—**ELIZABETH BENNETT** SEATTLE, WA

PREP: 25 MIN. • **COOK:** 15 MIN.
MAKES: 6 SERVINGS

- 1 cup quinoa, rinsed
- 1 can (15 ounces) garbanzo beans or chickpeas, rinsed and drained
- 2 cups cherry tomatoes, halved
- 1 cup (4 ounces) crumbled feta cheese
- ½ medium ripe avocado, peeled and cubed
- 4 green onions, chopped (about ½ cup)

DRESSING

- 3 tablespoons white wine vinegar
- 1 teaspoon Dijon mustard
- ¼ teaspoon kosher salt
- ¼ teaspoon garlic powder
- ¼ teaspoon freshly ground pepper
- ¼ cup olive oil

1. Cook quinoa according to package directions; transfer to a large bowl and cool slightly.

2. Add beans, tomatoes, cheese, avocado and green onions to quinoa; gently stir to combine. In a small bowl, whisk the first five dressing ingredients. Gradually whisk in oil until blended. Drizzle over salad; gently toss to coat. Refrigerate leftovers.

Note: Look for quinoa in the cereal, rice or organic food aisle.

Per 1⅓ cups: 328 cal., 17g fat (4g sat. fat), 10mg chol., 378mg sod., 34g carb. (3g sugars, 7g fiber), 11g pro.
Diabetic Exchanges: 3 fat, 2 starch, 1 lean meat.

GREEK SALAD PITAS

For a healthy on-the-go meal, combine fresh Greek salad with a zesty chickpea spread. You can also serve the spread as a dip with cut fresh vegetables.
—**NICOLE FILIZETTI** STEVENS POINT, WI

START TO FINISH: 20 MIN.
MAKES: 2 SERVINGS

- ¾ cup canned chickpeas, rinsed and drained
- 2 tablespoons lemon juice
- 1 tablespoon sliced green olives with pimientos
- 1 teaspoon olive oil
- 1 garlic clove, minced
- 1 cup fresh baby spinach
- ¼ cup chopped seeded peeled cucumber
- ¼ cup crumbled feta cheese
- 2 tablespoons chopped marinated quartered artichoke hearts
- 2 tablespoons sliced Greek olives
- ¼ teaspoon dried oregano
- 2 whole wheat pita pocket halves

1. Place the first five ingredients in a food processor; cover and process until smooth. Set aside.
2. In a small bowl, combine spinach, cucumber, cheese, artichokes, olives and oregano.
3. Spread bean mixture into pita halves; add salad. Serve immediately.
Per 1 filled pita half: 292 cal., 12g fat (3g sat. fat), 8mg chol., 687mg sod., 38g carb. (3g sugars, 7g fiber), 10g pro.
Diabetic Exchanges: 2 starch, 1 lean meat, 1 fat.

KALE PESTO FLATBREAD

I'm always making different kinds of flatbreads at home for my wife and me. We love kale, so this recipe just seemed perfect for a quick dinner. It immediately became our favorite flatbread pizza once we tried it. We like to top it with cooked shrimp before baking it, too.
—**ADAM STRICKLAND** BROOKLYN, NY

START TO FINISH: 25 MIN.
MAKES: 4 SERVINGS

- 1 cup chopped fresh kale leaves
- 3 tablespoons shredded Parmesan cheese
- 1 tablespoon chopped walnuts
- 1 tablespoon olive oil
- 1 garlic clove, minced
- ⅛ teaspoon pepper
- 1½ cups reduced-fat ricotta cheese
- 2 whole grain naan flatbreads
- 1 package (8 ounces) frozen artichoke hearts
- 3 pickled hot cherry peppers, chopped
  Thinly sliced fresh basil leaves

1. Preheat oven to 450°. Place first six ingredients in a blender; process until smooth. Add ricotta cheese; pulse just until combined.
2. Place flatbreads on a baking sheet. Spread with kale mixture; top with artichoke hearts. Bake until crust is lightly browned, 10-12 minutes. Top with peppers and basil.
Per ½ flatbread with toppings: 363 cal., 15g fat (5g sat. fat), 30mg chol., 748mg sod., 40g carb. (9g sugars, 7g fiber), 17g pro.
Diabetic Exchanges: 2½ starch, 2 medium-fat meat, 1 fat.

AVOCADO & GARBANZO
BEAN QUINOA SALAD

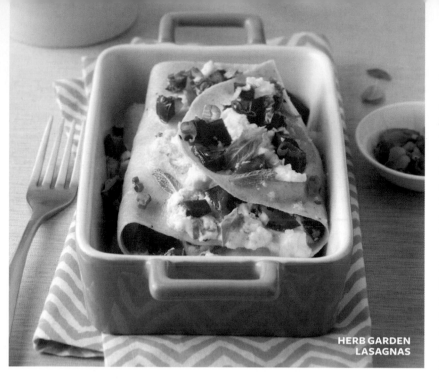

**HERB GARDEN
LASAGNAS**

HERB GARDEN LASAGNAS

*I love the taste and texture of these
homemade noodles and the beautiful
lasagnas they make. A healthy dose of
herbs gives this dish its unique flavor.*
—KATHRYN CONRAD MILWAUKEE, WI

PREP: 45 MIN. + STANDING
BAKE: 30 MIN. • **MAKES:** 6 SERVINGS

- 2 large eggs
- 1 large egg yolk
- ¼ cup water
- 1 tablespoon olive oil
- ½ teaspoon coarsely ground pepper
- ¼ teaspoon salt
- 1½ cups all-purpose flour
- ½ cup semolina flour

FILLING
- 1 cup whole-milk ricotta cheese
- 1 large egg white, lightly beaten
- 2 tablespoons shredded carrot
- 1 tablespoon minced fresh basil
- 1 tablespoon thinly sliced green
  onion
- 1 teaspoon minced fresh mint

- ¼ teaspoon salt
- 1 cup crumbled queso fresco or feta
  cheese, divided
- 4 cups chopped tomatoes (about
  6 medium), divided
  Optional toppings: thinly sliced
  green onion, fresh basil and
  fresh mint

1. In a small bowl, whisk the first six
ingredients. On a clean work surface,
mix all-purpose and semolina flours;
form into a mound. Make a large well in
the center. Pour egg mixture into well.
Using a fork or fingers, gradually mix
flour mixture into egg mixture, forming
a soft dough (dough will be soft and
slightly sticky).

2. Lightly dust work surface with flour;
knead dough gently five times. Divide
into six portions; cover with plastic
wrap. Let rest 30 minutes.

3. In a small bowl, mix the first seven
filling ingredients; stir in ½ cup queso
fresco. Grease six individual 12-oz.

au gratin dishes; place on baking sheets.
Preheat oven to 350°.

4. Fill a Dutch oven three-fourths full
with salted water; bring to a boil. On a
floured surface, roll each portion into a
20x4-in. rectangle, dusting dough with
additional flour as needed.

5. For each lasagna, add one noodle to
boiling water; cook 1-2 minutes or until
al dente. Place one-fifth of the noodle
in bottom of a prepared dish; top with
1 tablespoon of the ricotta mixture and
2 tablespoons tomato. Fold noodle
back to cover filling; repeating three
times, topping and folding the noodle
each time.

6. Sprinkle lasagnas with remaining
queso fresco and tomatoes. Bake,
covered, 30-35 minutes or until heated
through. If desired, sprinkle lasagnas
with additional herbs.

Per 1 individual lasagna: 363 cal., 13g
fat (6g sat. fat), 135mg chol., 343mg
sod., 44g carb. (6g sugars, 3g fiber),
19g pro.
Diabetic Exchanges: 2½ starch,
2 medium-fat meat, 1 vegetable, ½ fat.

✳

TEST KITCHEN TIP
**There's nothing like fresh pasta. The
process may seem intimidating, but
it's actually very easy to do! All you
need is a little time. To get a jump on
it, make dough 2 to 3 days in advance
and store in the refrigerator until you
are ready to roll it out.**

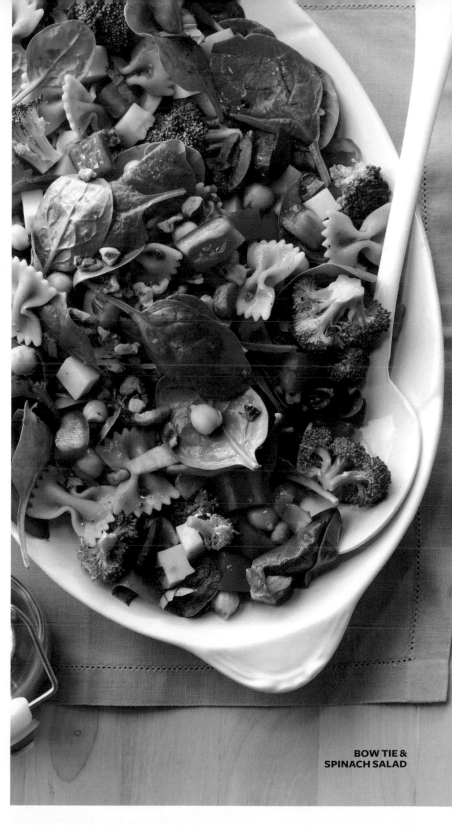

FAST FIX

BOW TIE & SPINACH SALAD

It's easy to change up my salad. Add grilled chicken or black beans.
—JULIE KIRKPATRICK BILLINGS, MT

START TO FINISH: 30 MIN.
MAKES: 6 SERVINGS

- 2 **cups uncooked multigrain bow tie pasta**
- 1 **can (15 ounces) chickpeas, rinsed and drained**
- 6 **cups fresh baby spinach (about 6 ounces)**
- 2 **cups fresh broccoli florets**
- 2 **plum tomatoes, chopped**
- 1 **medium sweet red pepper, chopped**
- ½ **cup cubed part-skim mozzarella cheese**
- ½ **cup pitted Greek olives, halved**
- ¼ **cup minced fresh basil**
- ⅓ **cup reduced-fat sun-dried tomato salad dressing**
- ¼ **teaspoon salt**
- ¼ **cup chopped walnuts, toasted**

1. Cook pasta according to package directions. Drain; transfer to a bowl.
2. Add beans, vegetables, cheese, olives and basil to pasta. Drizzle with dressing and sprinkle with salt; toss to coat. Sprinkle with walnuts.
Note: To toast nuts, bake in a shallow pan in a 350° oven for 5-10 minutes or cook in a skillet over low heat until lightly browned, stirring occasionally.
Per 2 cups: 319 cal., 13g fat (2g sat. fat), 6mg chol., 660mg sod., 39g carb. (6g sugars, 7g fiber), 14g pro.
Diabetic Exchanges: 2 starch, 2 fat, 1 lean meat, 1 vegetable.

BOW TIE & SPINACH SALAD

BUTTERNUT SQUASH
WITH WHOLE GRAINS, PAGE 251

Simply Slow Cooked

If it's comfort food you're craving, look no further than these slow-cooked creations. Simply prep, set and forget. Before you know it, you're ready to serve the ideal family dinner. Main dishes, sides, soups and stews; these hearty recipes are guaranteed to satisfy.

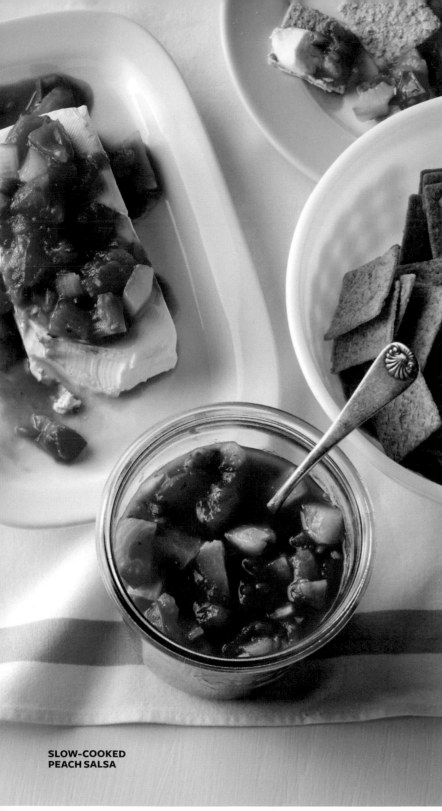

**SLOW-COOKED
PEACH SALSA**

SLOW-COOKED PEACH SALSA

Fresh peaches and tomatoes make my salsa a hands-down winner over store versions. I treat my co-workers to jars of the salsa throughout the year.
—PEGGI STAHNKE CLEVELAND, OH

PREP: 20 MIN.
COOK: 3 HOURS + COOLING
MAKES: 11 CUPS

- 4   pounds tomatoes (about 12 medium), chopped
- 1   medium onion, chopped
- 4   jalapeno peppers, seeded and finely chopped
- ½ to ⅔ cup packed brown sugar
- ¼   cup minced fresh cilantro
- 4   garlic cloves, minced
- 1   teaspoon salt
- 4   cups chopped peeled fresh peaches (about 4 medium), divided
- 1   can (6 ounces) tomato paste

1. In a 5-qt. slow cooker, combine the first seven ingredients; stir in 2 cups peaches. Cook, covered, on low for 3-4 hours or until onion is tender.
2. Stir tomato paste and remaining peaches into the slow cooker. Cool. Transfer to covered containers. (If freezing, use freezer-safe containers and fill containers to within ½ in. of tops.) Refrigerate up to 1 week or freeze up to 12 months. Thaw frozen salsa in refrigerator before serving.
Note: Wear disposable gloves when cutting hot peppers; the oils can burn skin. Avoid touching your face.
Per ¼ cup: 28 cal., 0 fat (0 sat. fat), 0 chol., 59mg sod., 7g carb. (5g sugars, 1g fiber), 1g pro.
Diabetic Exchanges: ½ starch.

SLOW COOKER

TERIYAKI BEEF STEW

In the spirit of the old saying, "Necessity is the mother of invention," I created this sweet-tangy beef recipe— I had a package of stew meat that needed to be used. After spotting a bottle of ginger beer in the fridge, the rest became history. It's always nice to have a new way to serve an affordable cut of meat.

—LESLIE SIMMS SHERMAN OAKS, CA

PREP: 20 MIN. • **COOK:** 6½ HOURS
MAKES: 8 SERVINGS

- 2 pounds beef stew meat
- 1 bottle (12 ounces) ginger beer or ginger ale
- ¼ cup teriyaki sauce
- 2 garlic cloves, minced
- 2 tablespoons sesame seeds
- 2 tablespoons cornstarch
- 2 tablespoons cold water
- 2 cups frozen peas, thawed
  Hot cooked rice, optional

1. In a nonstick skillet, brown beef in batches. Transfer to a 3-qt. slow cooker.
2. In a small bowl, combine the ginger beer, teriyaki sauce, garlic and sesame seeds; pour over beef. Cover and cook on low for 6-8 hours or until the meat is tender.
3. Combine cornstarch and cold water until smooth; gradually stir into stew. Stir in peas. Cover and cook on high for 30 minutes or until thickened. Serve with rice if desired.

Per 1 cup stew without rice: 310 cal., 12g fat (4g sat. fat), 94mg chol., 528mg sod., 17g carb. (9g sugars, 2g fiber), 33g pro.
Diabetic Exchanges: 4 lean meat, 1 starch.

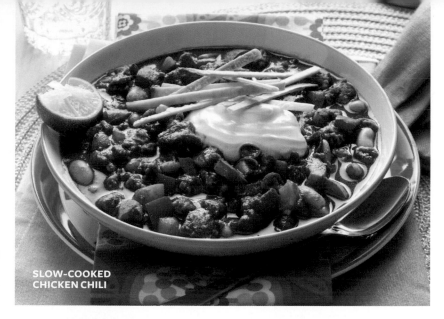

SLOW-COOKED CHICKEN CHILI

SLOW COOKER

SLOW-COOKED CHICKEN CHILI

Lime juice gives this chili a zesty twist, while canned tomatoes and beans make preparation a breeze.

—DIANE RANDAZZO SINKING SPRING, PA

PREP: 25 MIN. • **COOK:** 4 HOURS
MAKES: 6 SERVINGS

- 1 medium onion, chopped
- 1 each medium sweet yellow, red and green pepper, chopped
- 2 tablespoons olive oil
- 3 garlic cloves, minced
- 1 pound ground chicken
- 2 cans (14½ ounces each) diced tomatoes, undrained
- 1 can (15 ounces) cannellini beans, rinsed and drained
- ¼ cup lime juice
- 1 tablespoon all-purpose flour
- 1 tablespoon baking cocoa
- 1 tablespoon ground cumin
- 1 tablespoon chili powder
- 2 teaspoons ground coriander
- 1 teaspoon grated lime peel
- ½ teaspoon salt
- ½ teaspoon garlic pepper blend
- ¼ teaspoon pepper
- 2 flour tortillas (8 inches), cut into ¼-inch strips
- 6 tablespoons reduced-fat sour cream

1. In a large skillet, saute onion and peppers in oil for 7-8 minutes or until crisp-tender. Add garlic; cook 1 minute longer. Add chicken; cook and stir over medium heat for 8-9 minutes or until meat is no longer pink.
2. Transfer to a 3-qt. slow cooker. Stir in the tomatoes, beans, lime juice, flour, cocoa, cumin, chili powder, coriander, lime peel, salt, garlic pepper and pepper.
3. Cover and cook on low for 4-5 hours or until heated through.
4. Place tortilla strips on a baking sheet coated with cooking spray. Bake at 400° for 8-10 minutes or until crisp. Serve chili with sour cream and tortilla strips.

Per 1¼ cups with 10 tortilla strips and 1 tablespoon sour cream: 356 cal., 14g fat (3g sat. fat), 55mg chol., 644mg sod., 39g carb. (5g sugars, 8g fiber), 21g pro.
Diabetic Exchanges: 2 starch, 2 lean meat, 2 vegetable, 1 fat.

SLOW COOKER

GINGER CHICKEN NOODLE SOUP

This is one of my favorite soup recipes to serve in the winter time because it's easy and comforting, and it fills the entire house with a wonderful aroma. My whole family loves it!

—**BRANDY STANSBURY** EDNA, TX

PREP: 15 MIN. • **COOK:** 3½ HOURS
MAKES: 8 SERVINGS

- 1 pound boneless skinless chicken breasts, cubed
- 2 medium carrots, shredded
- 3 tablespoons sherry or reduced-sodium chicken broth
- 2 tablespoons rice vinegar
- 1 tablespoon reduced-sodium soy sauce
- 2 to 3 teaspoons minced fresh gingerroot
- ¼ teaspoon pepper
- 6 cups reduced-sodium chicken broth
- 1 cup water
- 2 cups fresh snow peas, halved
- 2 ounces uncooked angel hair pasta, broken into thirds

1. In a 5-qt. slow cooker, combine the first seven ingredients; stir in broth and water. Cook, covered, on low 3-4 hours or until chicken is tender.

2. Stir in snow peas and pasta. Cook, covered, on low 30 minutes longer or until snow peas and pasta are tender.

Per 1¼ cups: 126 cal., 2g fat (0 sat. fat), 31mg chol., 543mg sod., 11g carb. (3g sugars, 2g fiber), 16g pro.
Diabetic Exchanges: 2 lean meat, 1 starch.

SLOW COOKER

SLOW COOKER SPLIT PEA SOUP

When I have leftover ham in the fridge, I like to make this soup. Just throw the ingredients in the slow cooker, turn it on and walk away until dinner time.

—**PAMELA CHAMBERS** WEST COLUMBIA, SC

PREP: 15 MIN. • **COOK:** 8 HOURS
MAKES: 8 SERVINGS

- 1 package (16 ounces) dried green split peas, rinsed
- 2 cups cubed fully cooked ham
- 1 large onion, chopped
- 1 cup julienned or chopped carrots
- 3 garlic cloves, minced
- ½ teaspoon dried rosemary, crushed
- ½ teaspoon dried thyme
- 1 carton (32 ounces) reduced-sodium chicken broth
- 2 cups water

In a 4- or 5-qt. slow cooker, combine all ingredients. Cover and cook on low for 8-10 hours or until peas are tender.

To freeze: Freeze the cooled soup in freezer containers. To use, thaw soup overnight in the refrigerator. Heat through in a saucepan over medium heat, stirring occasionally.

Per 1 cup: 260 cal., 2g fat (1g sat. fat), 21mg chol., 728mg sod., 39g carb. (7g sugars, 15g fiber), 23g pro.
Diabetic Exchanges: 2½ starch, 2 lean meat.

✱
TEST KITCHEN TIP
Starchy soups can thicken after being stored in the refrigerator overnight. To return your soup to its original consistency, heat slowly over low heat. Add a bit of extra water or chicken stock; stir often to avoid scorching the bottom.

GINGER CHICKEN NOODLE SOUP

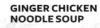

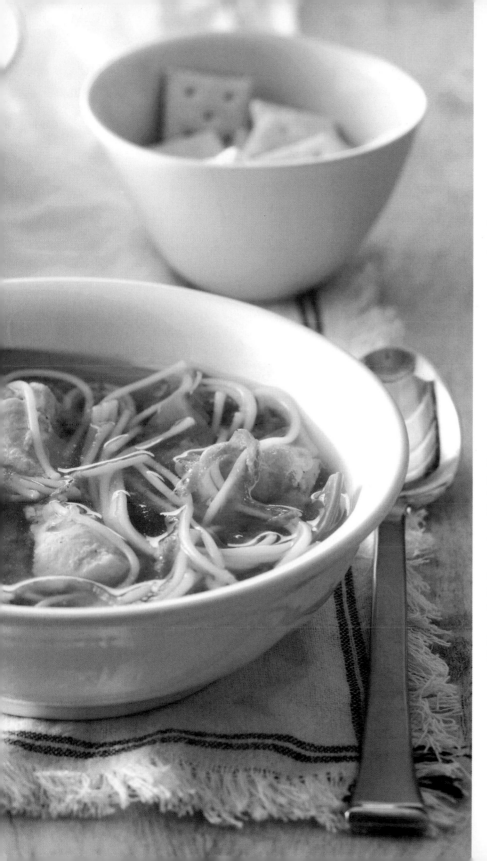

SLOW COOKER 🍲

SLOW COOKER MUSHROOM CHICKEN & PEAS

Some amazingly fresh mushrooms I found at a local farmers market inspired this recipe. When you start with the best ingredients, you can't go wrong.
—**JENN TIDWELL** FAIR OAKS, CA

PREP: 10 MIN. • **COOK:** 3 HOURS 10 MIN.
MAKES: 4 SERVINGS

- 4 **boneless skinless chicken breast halves (6 ounces each)**
- 1 **envelope onion mushroom soup mix**
- 1 **cup water**
- ½ **pound sliced baby portobello mushrooms**
- 1 **medium onion, chopped**
- 4 **garlic cloves, minced**
- 2 **cups frozen peas, thawed**

1. Place chicken in a 3-qt. slow cooker. Sprinkle with soup mix, pressing to help seasonings adhere to chicken. Add water, mushrooms, onion and garlic.
2. Cook, covered, on low 3-4 hours or until chicken is tender (a thermometer inserted in chicken should read at least 165°). Stir in peas; cook, covered, 10 minutes longer or until heated through.
Per 1 chicken breast half with ¾ cup vegetable mixture: 292 cal., 5g fat (1g sat. fat), 94mg chol., 566mg sod., 20g carb. (7g sugars, 5g fiber), 41g pro.
Diabetic Exchanges: 5 lean meat, 1 starch, 1 vegetable.

SLOW COOKER 🍲
MEDITERRANEAN POT ROAST DINNER

My family and I went out to play in the snow all day, and when we came back, supper was waiting to be served! This pot roast is perfect with good dinner rolls or rice.

—**HOLLY BATTISTE** BARRINGTON, NJ

PREP: 30 MIN. • **COOK:** 8 HOURS
MAKES: 8 SERVINGS

- 2 pounds potatoes (about 6 medium), peeled and cut into 2-inch pieces
- 5 medium carrots (about ¾ pound), cut into 1-inch pieces
- 2 tablespoons all-purpose flour
- 1 boneless beef chuck roast (3 to 4 pounds)
- 1 tablespoon olive oil
- 8 large fresh mushrooms, quartered
- 2 celery ribs, chopped
- 1 medium onion, thinly sliced
- ¼ cup sliced Greek olives
- ½ cup minced fresh parsley, divided
- 1 can (14½ ounces) fire-roasted diced tomatoes, undrained
- 1 tablespoon minced fresh oregano or 1 teaspoon dried oregano
- 1 tablespoon lemon juice
- 2 teaspoons minced fresh rosemary or ½ teaspoon dried rosemary, crushed
- 2 garlic cloves, minced
- ¾ teaspoon salt
- ¼ teaspoon pepper
- ¼ teaspoon crushed red pepper flakes, optional

1. Place potatoes and carrots in a 6-qt. slow cooker. Sprinkle the flour over all surfaces of roast. In a large skillet, heat oil over medium-high heat. Brown roast on all sides. Place over vegetables.

2. Add mushrooms, celery, onion, olives and ¼ cup parsley to slow cooker. In a small bowl, mix the remaining ingredients; pour over top.

3. Cook, covered, on low for 8-10 hours or until meat and vegetables are tender. Remove beef. Stir remaining parsley into vegetables. Serve the beef with the vegetables.

Per 5 ounces cooked beef with 1 cup vegetables: 422 cal., 18g fat (6g sat. fat), 111mg chol., 538mg sod., 28g carb. (6g sugars, 4g fiber), 37g pro.
Diabetic Exchanges: 5 lean meat, 1½ starch, 1 vegetable, ½ fat.

SLOW COOKER 🍲
TURKEY STUFFED PEPPERS

Slow cooking can be both delicious and healthy! I created this entree as a lighter alternative to classic stuffed peppers. With 12-hour work shifts as a nurse, I often rely on the slow cooker for feeding my family right.

—**MANDY PEMBERTON**
DENHAM SPRINGS, LA

PREP: 35 MIN. • **COOK:** 4 HOURS
MAKES: 6 SERVINGS

- 2 medium sweet yellow or orange peppers
- 2 medium sweet red peppers
- 2 medium green peppers
- 1 pound lean ground turkey
- 1 small red onion, finely chopped
- 1 small zucchini, shredded
- 2 cups cooked brown rice
- 1 jar (16 ounces) spaghetti sauce, divided
- 1 tablespoon Creole seasoning
- ¼ teaspoon pepper
- 2 tablespoons shredded Parmesan cheese

1. Cut tops from peppers and remove the seeds. Finely chop enough tops to measure 1 cup for filling.

2. In a large skillet, cook turkey, onion and reserved chopped peppers over medium heat for 6-8 minutes or until turkey is no longer pink and vegetables are tender, breaking up turkey into crumbles; drain.

3. Stir in the zucchini; cook and stir about 2 minutes longer. Add the rice, ⅔ cup of the spaghetti sauce, Creole seasoning and pepper.

4. Spread ½ cup spaghetti sauce onto the bottom of a greased 6-qt. slow cooker. Fill peppers with turkey mixture; place over sauce. Pour the remaining spaghetti sauce over peppers; sprinkle with cheese.

5. Cook, covered, on low 4-5 hours or until peppers are tender and filling is heated through.

Note: The following spices may be substituted for 1 teaspoon Creole seasoning: ¼ teaspoon each salt, garlic powder and paprika; and a pinch each of dried thyme, ground cumin and cayenne pepper.

Per 1 stuffed pepper: 290 cal., 10g fat (3g sat. fat), 63mg chol., 818mg sod., 31g carb. (9g sugars, 5g fiber), 19g pro.
Diabetic Exchanges: 3 lean meat, 1½ starch, 1 vegetable.

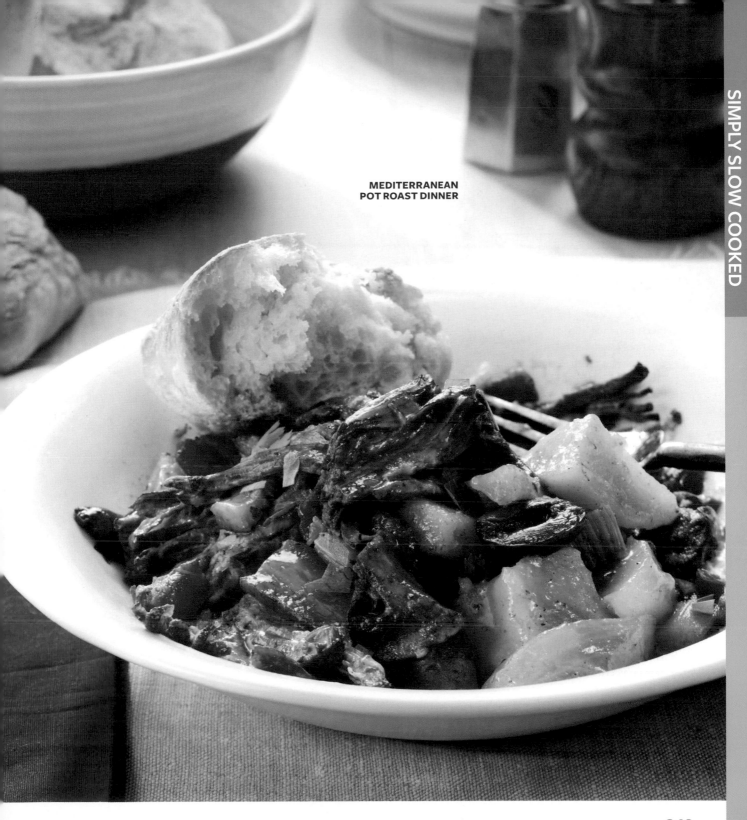

**MEDITERRANEAN
POT ROAST DINNER**

SLOW COOKER

PARSLEY SMASHED POTATOES

I love potatoes but hate the work involved in making mashed potatoes from scratch. So I came up with a simple side dish that was made even easier thanks to my slow cooker. Save the leftover broth for soup the next day.

—KATIE HAGY BLACKSBURG, SC

PREP: 20 MIN. • **COOK:** 6 HOURS
MAKES: 8 SERVINGS

- 16 small red potatoes (about 2 pounds)
- 1 celery rib, sliced
- 1 medium carrot, sliced
- ¼ cup finely chopped onion
- 2 cups chicken broth
- 1 tablespoon minced fresh parsley
- 1½ teaspoons salt, divided
- 1 teaspoon pepper, divided
- 1 garlic clove, minced
- 2 tablespoons butter, melted
  Additional minced fresh parsley

1. Place potatoes, celery, carrot and onion in a 4-qt. slow cooker. In a small bowl, mix broth, parsley, 1 teaspoon salt, ½ teaspoon pepper and garlic; pour over vegetables. Cook, covered, on low 6-8 hours or until potatoes are tender.

2. Transfer potatoes from slow cooker to a 15x10x1-in. pan; discard cooking liquid and vegetables or save for other use. Using bottom of a measuring cup, flatten potatoes slightly. Transfer to a large bowl; drizzle with butter. Sprinkle with remaining salt and pepper; toss to coat. Sprinkle with additional parsley.

Per 2 smashed potatoes: 114 cal., 3g fat (2g sat. fat), 8mg chol., 190mg sod., 20g carb. (2g sugars, 2g fiber), 2g pro.
Diabetic Exchanges: 1 starch, ½ fat.

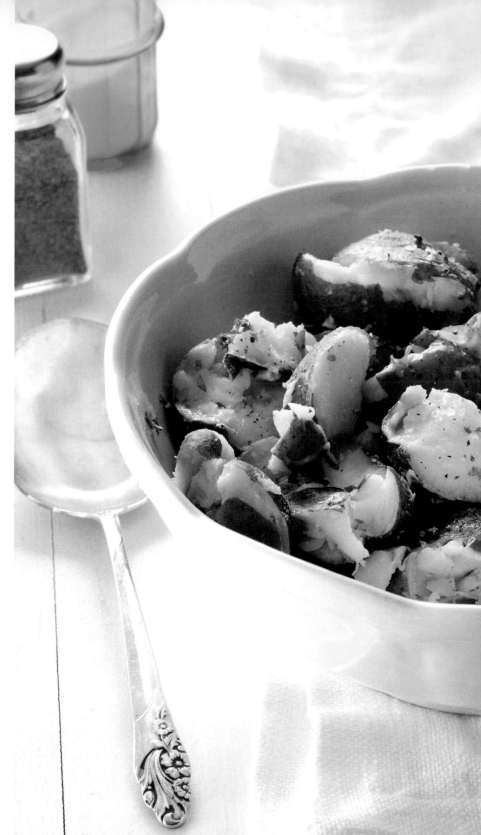

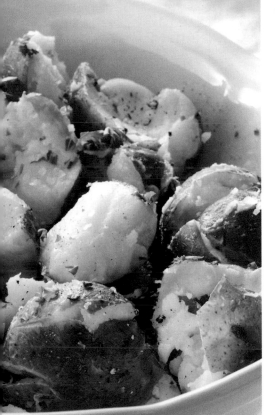

PARSLEY SMASHED POTATOES

SLOW COOKER
BUTTERNUT SQUASH WITH WHOLE GRAINS

Fresh thyme really shines in this hearty slow-cooked side dish featuring tender butternut squash, nutritious whole grain pilaf and vitamin-packed baby spinach.
—*TASTE OF HOME* TEST KITCHEN

PREP: 15 MIN. • **COOK:** 4 HOURS
MAKES: 12 SERVINGS

- 1 medium butternut squash (about 3 pounds), cut into ½-inch cubes
- 1 cup uncooked whole grain brown and red rice blend
- 1 medium onion, chopped
- ½ cup water
- 3 garlic cloves, minced
- 2 teaspoons minced fresh thyme or ½ teaspoon dried thyme
- ½ teaspoon salt
- ¼ teaspoon pepper
- 1 can (14½ ounces) vegetable broth
- 1 package (6 ounces) fresh baby spinach

1. In a 4-qt. slow cooker, combine the first eight ingredients. Stir in broth.
2. Cook, covered, on low 4-5 hours or until grains are tender. Stir in spinach before serving.
Note: This recipe was tested with RiceSelect Royal Blend Whole Grain Texmati Brown & Red Rice with Barley and Rye. Look for it in the rice aisle.
Per ¾ cup: 97 cal., 1g fat (0 sat. fat), 0 chol., 252mg sod., 22g carb. (3g sugars, 4g fiber), 3g pro.
Diabetic Exchanges: 1½ starch.

SLOW COOKER
THAI-STYLE PORK

This creamy pork specialty is from a friend in my cooking club. It's always a favorite.
—**AMY VAN ORMAN** ROCKFORD, MI

PREP: 15 MIN. • **COOK:** 6¼ HOURS
MAKES: 6 SERVINGS

- ¼ cup teriyaki sauce
- 2 tablespoons rice vinegar
- 1 teaspoon crushed red pepper flakes
- 1 teaspoon minced garlic
- 2 pounds boneless pork loin chops
- 1 tablespoon cornstarch
- ¼ cup cold water
- ¼ cup creamy peanut butter
  Hot cooked rice
- ½ cup chopped green onions
- ½ cup dry roasted peanuts
  Lime juice, optional

1. Mix first four ingredients. Place pork chops in a 3-qt. slow cooker; top with sauce. Cook, covered, on low until meat is tender, 6-8 hours.
2. Remove pork and cut into bite-size pieces; keep warm. Transfer cooking juices to a saucepan; bring to a boil. cornstarch and water until smooth; gradually stir into juices. Bring to a boil; cook and stir until thickened, 1-2 minutes. Stir in peanut butter. Add pork.
3. Serve with rice. Sprinkle with green onions and peanuts. If desired, drizzle with lime juice.
Per serving: ⅔ cup: 357 cal., 20g fat (5g sat. fat), 73mg chol., 598mg sod., 9g carb. (3g sugars, 2g fiber), 35g pro.
Diabetic Exchanges: 5 lean meat, 2 fat, ½ starch.

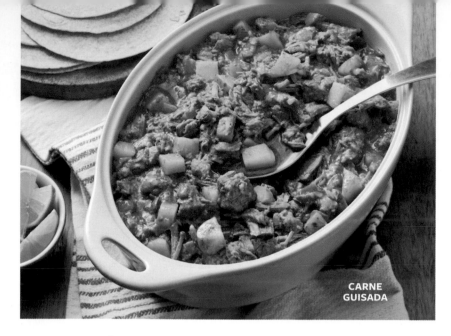

CARNE GUISADA

CARNE GUISADA

After moving temporarily out of state, my boyfriend and I really started to miss the spicy flavors of our Texas home, so we made this recipe often. It goes really well with homemade flour tortillas. We love it over brown rice, too.

—**KELLY EVANS** DENTON, TX

PREP: 25 MIN. • **COOK:** 7 HOURS
MAKES: 12 SERVINGS

- 1 bottle (12 ounces) beer
- ¼ cup all-purpose flour
- 2 tablespoons tomato paste
- 1 jalapeno pepper, seeded and chopped
- 4 teaspoons Worcestershire sauce
- 1 bay leaf
- 2 to 3 teaspoons crushed red pepper flakes
- 2 teaspoons chili powder
- 1½ teaspoons ground cumin
- ½ teaspoon salt
- ½ teaspoon paprika
- 2 garlic cloves, minced
- ½ teaspoon red wine vinegar
  Dash liquid smoke, optional
- 1 boneless pork shoulder butt roast (3 pounds), cut into 2-inch pieces
- 2 large unpeeled red potatoes, chopped
- 1 medium onion, chopped
  Whole wheat tortillas or hot cooked brown rice, lime wedges and chopped fresh cilantro, optional

1. In a 4- or 5-qt. slow cooker, mix first 13 ingredients and, if desired, the liquid smoke. Stir in pork, potatoes and onion. Cook mixture, covered, on low until pork is tender, 7-9 hours.

2. Discard bay leaf; skim fat from cooking juices. Shred pork slightly with two forks. Serve pork with the optional remaining ingredients as desired.

Note: Wear disposable gloves when cutting hot peppers; the oils can burn skin. Avoid touching your face.

Per ⅔ cup: 261 cal., 12g fat (4g sat. fat), 67mg chol., 200mg sod., 16g carb. (3g sugars, 2g fiber), 21g pro.

Diabetic Exchanges: 3 medium-fat meat, 1 starch.

SWEET ONION & RED BELL PEPPER TOPPING

As soon as Vidalia onions hit the market, this is one of the first recipes I make. I use it on hot dogs, bruschetta, cream cheese and crackers. It's so versatile.

—**PAT HOCKETT** OCALA, FL

PREP: 20 MIN. • **COOK:** 4 HOURS
MAKES: 4 CUPS

- 4 large sweet onions, thinly sliced (about 8 cups)
- 4 large sweet red peppers, thinly sliced (about 6 cups)
- ½ cup cider vinegar
- ¼ cup packed brown sugar
- 2 tablespoons canola oil
- 2 tablespoons honey
- 2 teaspoons celery seed
- ¾ teaspoon crushed red pepper flakes
- ½ teaspoon salt

In a 5- or 6-qt. slow cooker, combine all ingredients. Cook, covered, on low 4-5 hours or until the vegetables are tender. Serve with a slotted spoon.

Per ¼ cup: 76 cal., 2g fat (0 sat. fat), 0 chol., 84mg sod., 14g carb. (11g sugars, 2g fiber), 1g pro.

Diabetic Exchanges: 1 starch.

✳

TEST KITCHEN TIP
Aside from soups and slow-cooked meat, you can use your slow cooker to make cheesy dips; mulled wines and beverages; apple butter—even brownies, cakes and puddings.

SLOW COOKER 🍲

ITALIAN CABBAGE SOUP

After doing yard work on a windy day, we love to come in for a light but hearty soup like this one. It's brimming with cabbage, veggies and white beans. Pass the crusty bread.

—**JENNIFER STOWELL** MONTEZUMA, IA

PREP: 15 MIN. • **COOK:** 6 HOURS
MAKES: 8 SERVINGS

- 4 cups chicken stock
- 1 can (6 ounces) tomato paste
- 1 small head cabbage (about 1½ pounds), shredded
- 4 celery ribs, chopped
- 2 large carrots, chopped
- 1 small onion, chopped
- 1 can (15½ ounces) great northern beans, rinsed and drained
- 2 garlic cloves, minced
- 2 fresh thyme sprigs
- 1 bay leaf
- ½ teaspoon salt
   Shredded Parmesan cheese, optional

1. In a 5- or 6-qt. slow cooker, whisk together stock and tomato paste. Stir in the vegetables, beans, garlic and seasonings. Cook, covered, on low until vegetables are tender, 6-8 hours.

2. Remove thyme sprigs and bay leaf. If desired, serve with cheese.

Per 1 cup: 111 cal., 0 fat (0 sat. fat), 0 chol., 537mg sod., 21g carb. (7g sugars, 6g fiber), 8g pro.
Diabetic Exchanges: 1½ starch.

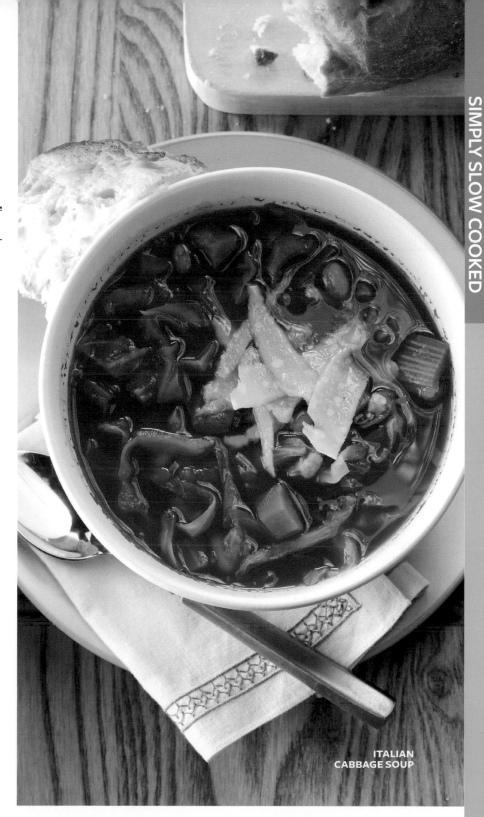

ITALIAN
CABBAGE SOUP

**SLOW COOKER
BEEF TOSTADAS**

SLOW COOKER 🍲
SLOW COOKER BEEF TOSTADAS

I dedicate these slow-simmered tostadas to my husband, the only Italian man I know who can't get enough of Mexican cuisine.

—**TERESA DEVONO** RED LION, PA

PREP: 20 MIN. • **COOK:** 6 HOURS
MAKES: 6 SERVINGS

- 1 **large onion, chopped**
- ¼ **cup lime juice**
- 1 **jalapeno pepper, seeded and minced**
- 1 **serrano pepper, seeded and minced**
- 1 **tablespoon chili powder**
- 3 **garlic cloves, minced**
- ½ **teaspoon ground cumin**
- 1 **beef top round steak (about 1½ pounds)**
- 1 **teaspoon salt**
- ½ **teaspoon pepper**
- ¼ **cup chopped fresh cilantro**
- 12 **corn tortillas (6 inches)**
  Cooking spray

TOPPINGS
- 1½ **cups shredded lettuce**
- 1 **medium tomato, finely chopped**
- ¾ **cup shredded sharp cheddar cheese**
- ¾ **cup reduced-fat sour cream, optional**

1. Place the first seven ingredients in a 3- or 4-qt. slow cooker. Cut steak in half and sprinkle with salt and pepper; add to slow cooker. Cook, covered, on low 6-8 hours or until meat is tender.
2. Remove meat; cool slightly. Shred meat with two forks. Return beef to slow cooker and stir in cilantro; heat through. Spritz both sides of tortillas with cooking spray. Place in a single layer on baking sheets; broil 1-2 minutes on each side or until crisp. Spoon the beef mixture over the tortillas; top with lettuce, tomato, cheese and, if desired, sour cream.

Note: Wear disposable gloves when cutting hot peppers; the oils can burn skin. Avoid touching your face.

Per 2 tostadas: 372 cal., 13g fat (6g sat. fat), 88mg chol., 602mg sod., 30g carb. (5g sugars, 5g fiber), 35g pro.
Diabetic Exchanges: 4 lean meat, 2 starch, ½ fat.

SLOW COOKER 🍲
SPICED CARROTS & BUTTERNUT SQUASH

When I've got a lot going on, my slow cooker is my go-to tool for cooking veggies. Here, the mild sweetness of squash and carrots really is enhanced by hot and spicy seasonings.

—**COURTNEY STULTZ** WEIR, KS

PREP: 15 MIN. • **COOK:** 4 HOURS
MAKES: 6 SERVINGS

- 5 **large carrots, cut into ½-inch pieces (about 3 cups)**
- 2 **cups cubed peeled butternut squash (1-inch pieces)**
- 1 **tablespoon balsamic vinegar**
- 1 **tablespoon olive oil**
- 1 **tablespoon honey**
- 1 **teaspoon ground cinnamon**
- ½ **teaspoon salt**
- ½ **teaspoon ground cumin**
- ¼ **teaspoon chili powder**

Place carrots and squash in a 3-qt. slow cooker. In a small bowl, mix remaining ingredients; drizzle over vegetables and toss to coat. Cook, covered, on low 4-5 hours or until vegetables are tender. Gently stir before serving.

Per ⅔ cup: 85 cal., 3g fat (0 sat. fat), 0 chol., 245mg sod., 16g carb. (8g sugars, 3g fiber), 1g pro.
Diabetic Exchanges: 1 vegetable, ½ starch, ½ fat.

SLOW COOKER 🍲
LENTIL PUMPKIN SOUP

Garlic and ginger brighten up my hearty pumpkin soup. It's just the thing we need on nippy days and nights.

—**LAURA MAGEE** HOULTON, WI

PREP: 15 MIN. • **COOK:** 7 HOURS
MAKES: 6 SERVINGS

- 1 **pound red potatoes (about 4 medium), cut into 1-inch pieces**
- 1 **can (15 ounces) solid-pack pumpkin**
- 1 **cup dried lentils, rinsed**
- 1 **medium onion, chopped**
- 3 **garlic cloves, minced**
- ½ **teaspoon ground ginger**
- ½ **teaspoon pepper**
- ⅛ **teaspoon salt**
- 2 **cans (14½ ounces each) vegetable broth**
- 1½ **cups water**
  Minced fresh cilantro, optional

In a 3- or 4-qt. slow cooker, combine first 10 ingredients. Cook, covered, on low 7-9 hours or until potatoes and lentils are tender. If desired, sprinkle servings with cilantro.

Per 1⅓ cups: 210 cal., 1g fat (0 sat. fat), 0 chol., 463mg sod., 42g carb. (5g sugars, 7g fiber), 11g pro.
Diabetic Exchanges: 3 starch, 1 lean meat.

**ROASTED VEGETABLES
WITH SAGE, PAGE 270**

Savory Side Dishes

It's just not a meal without these supporting players.
Made to go alongside your favorite main dishes,
these scene-stealing sidekicks are chock-full of
healthy vegetables and easy enough to make
any night of the week. Dinner is served!

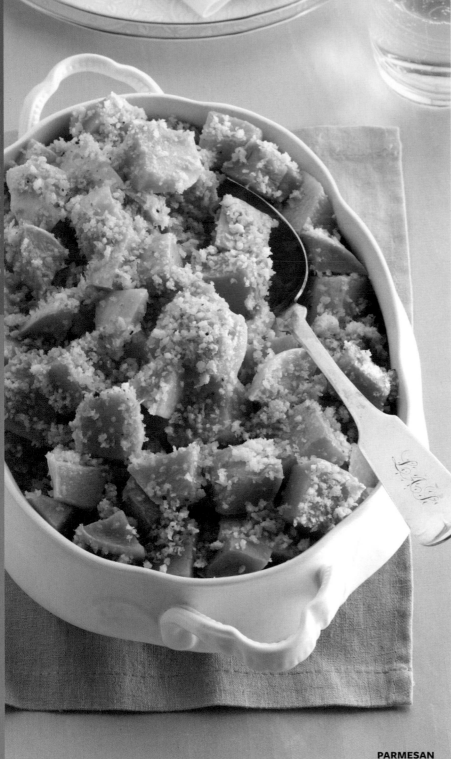

PARMESAN BUTTERNUT SQUASH

(5)INGREDIENTS **FAST FIX**

PARMESAN BUTTERNUT SQUASH

Golden butternut squash sprinkled with Parmesan and breadcrumbs makes a superb side dish we love to share. Using the microwave cuts way down on long roasting time.

—JACKIE O'CALLAGHAN
WEST LAFAYETTE, IN

START TO FINISH: 25 MIN.
MAKES: 8 SERVINGS

- 1 medium butternut squash (about 3 pounds), peeled and cut into 1-inch cubes
- 2 tablespoons water
- ½ cup panko (Japanese) bread crumbs
- ½ cup grated Parmesan cheese
- ¼ teaspoon salt
- ⅛ teaspoon pepper

1. Place squash and water in a large microwave-safe bowl. Microwave, covered, on high 15-17 minutes or until tender; drain.

2. Preheat broiler. Transfer squash to a greased 15x10x1-in. baking pan. Toss bread crumbs with cheese, salt and pepper; sprinkle over squash. Broil 3-4 in. from heat 1-2 minutes or until topping is golden brown.

Note: This recipe was tested in a 1,100-watt microwave.

Per ¾ cup: 112 cal., 2g fat (1g sat. fat), 4mg chol., 168mg sod., 23g carb. (5g sugars, 6g fiber), 4g pro.
Diabetic Exchanges: 1½ starch.

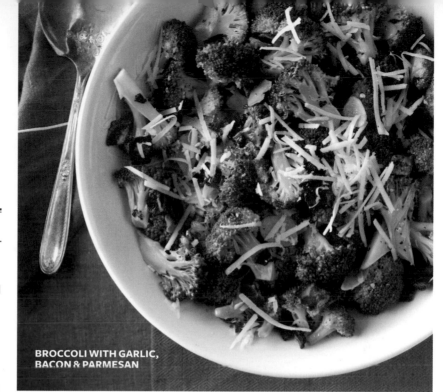

BROCCOLI WITH GARLIC, BACON & PARMESAN

⑤ INGREDIENTS | FAST FIX
TOMATO-ONION GREEN BEANS

Fresh green beans are the star of this healthy side. Serve them with grilled chicken, pork tenderloin or seafood for a delicious ending to a busy day.
—**DAVID FEDER** BUFFALO GROVE, IL

START TO FINISH: 30 MIN.
MAKES: 6 SERVINGS

- 2 **tablespoons olive oil**
- 1 **large onion, finely chopped**
- 1 **pound fresh green beans, trimmed**
- 3 **tablespoons tomato paste**
- ½ **teaspoon salt**
- 2 **tablespoons minced fresh parsley**

1. In a large skillet, heat the oil over medium-high heat. Add chopped onion; cook until tender and lightly browned, stirring occasionally.

2. Meanwhile, place green beans in a large saucepan; add water to cover. Bring to a boil. Cook, covered, for 5-7 minutes or until crisp-tender. Drain; add to onion. Stir in tomato paste and salt; heat through. Sprinkle with parsley.

Per ⅔ cup: 81 cal., 5g fat (1g sat. fat), 0 chol., 208mg sod., 9g carb. (4g sugars, 3g fiber), 2g pro.
Diabetic Exchanges: 1 vegetable, 1 fat.

✳

DID YOU KNOW?
Instead of snapping off the ends of each green bean like Grandma did, trim a bunch in seconds. Gather beans in a small pile, lining up the tips on one side. Cut off tips with a single slice using a chef's knife. Flip the pile over and do the same on the other side.

⑤ INGREDIENTS | FAST FIX
BROCCOLI WITH GARLIC, BACON & PARMESAN

My approach to cooking fresh broccoli is to infuse it with savory garlic and smoky bacon. A few simple ingredients are all it takes to make this ordinary veggie irresistible.
—**ERIN CHILCOAT** CENTRAL ISLIP, NY

START TO FINISH: 30 MIN.
MAKES: 8 SERVINGS

- 1 **teaspoon salt**
- 2 **bunches broccoli (about 3 pounds), stems removed, cut into florets**
- 6 **thick-sliced bacon strips, chopped**
- 2 **tablespoons olive oil**
- 6 **to 8 garlic cloves, thinly sliced**
- ½ **teaspoon crushed red pepper flakes**
- ¼ **cup shredded Parmesan cheese**

1. Fill a 6-qt. stockpot two-thirds full with water; add salt and bring to a boil over high heat. In batches, add broccoli and cook for 2-3 minutes or until the broccoli turns bright green; remove with a slotted spoon.

2. In a large skillet, cook the bacon over medium heat until crisp, stirring occasionally. Remove with a slotted spoon; drain on paper towels. Discard the drippings, reserving 1 tablespoon in pan.

3. Add oil to the drippings; heat over medium heat. Add garlic and pepper flakes; cook and stir 2-3 minutes or until the garlic is fragrant (do not allow to brown). Add broccoli; cook until broccoli is tender, stirring occasionally. Stir in bacon; sprinkle with cheese.

Per ¾ cup: 155 cal., 10g fat (3g sat. fat), 11mg chol., 371mg sod., 11g carb. (3g sugars, 4g fiber), 8g pro.
Diabetic Exchanges: 2 fat, 1 vegetable.

⟨5⟩INGREDIENTS **FAST FIX▸**

BRUSSELS SPROUTS WITH BACON & GARLIC

When we have company, these sprouts are my go-to side dish because they look and taste fantastic. Fancy them up a notch with pancetta instead of bacon.
—**MANDY RIVERS** LEXINGTON, SC

START TO FINISH: 30 MIN.
MAKES: 12 SERVINGS

- 2 pounds fresh Brussels sprouts (about 10 cups)
- 8 bacon strips, coarsely chopped
- 3 garlic cloves, minced
- ¾ cup chicken broth
- ½ teaspoon salt
- ¼ teaspoon pepper

1. Trim Brussels sprouts. Cut sprouts lengthwise in half; cut crosswise into thin slices. In a 6-qt. stockpot, cook bacon over medium heat until crisp, stirring occasionally. Add garlic; cook 30 seconds longer. Remove with a slotted spoon; drain on paper towels.

2. Add Brussels sprouts to bacon drippings; cook and stir 4-6 minutes or until sprouts begin to brown lightly. Stir in broth, salt and pepper; cook, covered, 4-6 minutes longer or until Brussels sprouts are tender. Stir in bacon mixture.

Per ¾ cup: 109 cal., 8g fat (3g sat. fat), 13mg chol., 300mg sod., 7g carb. (2g sugars, 3g fiber), 5g pro.
Diabetic Exchanges: 1½ fat, 1 vegetable.

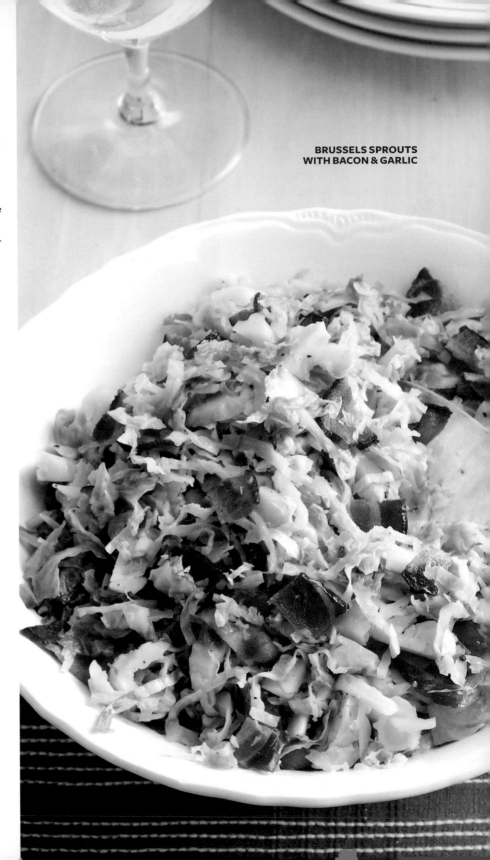

BRUSSELS SPROUTS WITH BACON & GARLIC

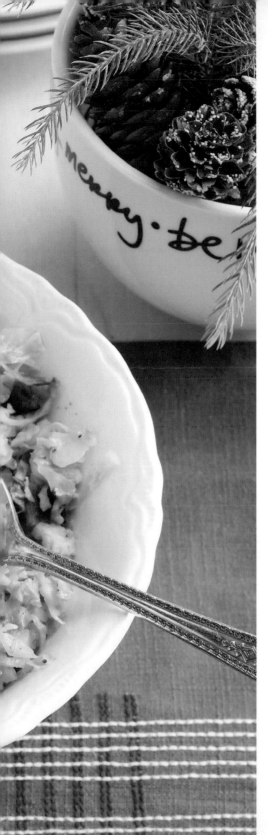

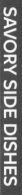

BEET & SWEET POTATO FRIES

Instead of offering traditional french fries, try these oven-baked root vegetables as a flavorful side dish.
—**MARIE RIZZIO** INTERLOCHEN, MI

PREP: 15 MIN. • **BAKE:** 20 MIN.
MAKES: 5 SERVINGS (½ CUP SAUCE)

- ½ cup reduced-fat mayonnaise
- 1 teaspoon pink peppercorns, crushed
- ½ teaspoon green peppercorns, crushed
- ½ teaspoon coarsely ground pepper, divided
- 1 large sweet potato (about 1 pound)
- 2 tablespoons olive oil, divided
- ½ teaspoon sea salt, divided
- 2 large fresh beets (about 1 pound)

1. In a small bowl, combine the mayonnaise, peppercorns and ¼ teaspoon ground pepper. Cover and refrigerate until serving.
2. Peel and cut sweet potato in half widthwise; cut each half into ½-in. strips. Place in a small bowl. Add 1 tablespoon oil, ¼ teaspoon salt and ⅛ teaspoon pepper; toss to coat. Spread onto a parchment paper-lined baking sheet.
3. Peel and cut beets in half; cut into ½-in. strips. Transfer to the same bowl; add the remaining oil, salt and pepper. Toss to coat. Spread onto another parchment paper-lined baking sheet.
4. Bake vegetables, uncovered, at 425° for 20-30 minutes or until tender, turning once. Serve with a dollop of peppercorn mayonnaise.
Per serving: 226 cal., 14g fat (2g sat. fat), 8mg chol., 455mg sod., 25g carb. (14g sugars, 4g fiber), 3g pro.
Diabetic Exchanges: 2 starch, 2 fat.

GOLDEN ZUCCHINI PANCAKES

If your garden is overflowing with zucchini this time of year, make these incredible pancakes to use it up. We squeeze the zucchini well before using to remove excess moisture.
—**TERRY ANN DOMINGUEZ** SILVER CITY, NM

PREP: 15 MIN.
COOK: 10 MIN./BATCH
MAKES: 8 ZUCCHINI PANCAKES

- 3 cups shredded zucchini
- 2 large eggs
- 2 garlic cloves, minced
- ¾ teaspoon salt
- ½ teaspoon pepper
- ¼ teaspoon dried oregano
- ½ cup all-purpose flour
- ½ cup finely chopped sweet onion
- 1 tablespoon butter
  Marinara sauce, warmed, optional

1. Place zucchini in a colander to drain; squeeze well to remove excess liquid. Pat dry.
2. In a large bowl, whisk eggs, garlic, salt, pepper and oregano until blended. Stir in flour just until moistened. Fold in zucchini and onion.
3. Lightly grease a griddle with butter; heat over medium heat. Drop the zucchini mixture by ¼ cupfuls onto griddle; flatten to ½-in. thickness (3-in. diameter). Cook 4-5 minutes on each side or until golden brown. If desired, serve with marinara sauce.
Per 2 pancakes: 145 cal., 6g fat (3g sat. fat), 101mg chol., 510mg sod., 18g carb. (3g sugars, 2g fiber), 6g pro.
Diabetic Exchanges: 1 starch, 1 fat.

ROASTED GREEN VEGETABLE MEDLEY

Roasting vegetables like broccoli, green beans and Brussels sprouts adds to their deliciousness, and almost any veggie combo works.

—**SUZAN CROUCH** GRAND PRAIRIE, TX

PREP: 15 MIN. • **BAKE:** 20 MIN.
MAKES: 12 SERVINGS (¾ CUP EACH)

- 2 cups fresh broccoli florets
- 1 pound thin fresh green beans, trimmed and cut into 2-inch pieces
- 10 small fresh mushrooms, halved
- 8 fresh Brussels sprouts, halved
- 2 medium carrots, cut into ¼-inch slices
- 1 medium onion, sliced
- 3 to 5 garlic cloves, thinly sliced
- 4 tablespoons olive oil, divided
- ½ cup grated Parmesan cheese
- 3 tablespoons julienned fresh basil leaves, optional
- 2 tablespoons minced fresh parsley
- 2 tablespoons lemon juice
- 1 tablespoon grated lemon peel
- ¼ teaspoon salt
- ¼ teaspoon pepper

1. Preheat oven to 425°. Place the first seven ingredients in a large bowl; drizzle with 2 tablespoons oil and toss to coat. Divide between two 15x10x1-in. baking pans coated with cooking spray. Roast vegetables for 20-25 minutes or until tender, stirring occasionally.
2. Transfer to a large serving bowl. In a small bowl, mix the remaining oil with the remaining ingredients; add to the vegetables and toss to combine.
Per ¾ cup: 87 cal., 6g fat (1g sat. fat), 3mg chol., 68mg sod., 7g carb. (3g sugars, 3g fiber), 3g pro.
Diabetic Exchanges: 1 vegetable, 1 fat.

FAST FIX ▶

ORZO WITH PEPPERS & SPINACH

The bright colors from chopped bell peppers in this dish are eye-catching. They're also a good source of vitamin C, which helps the body absorb iron and other nutrients and fight infection. Try it with other fresh veggies for a change.

—**TAMMI KETTENBACH** JERSEYVILLE, IL

START TO FINISH: 30 MIN.
MAKES: 6 SERVINGS

- 1 cup uncooked orzo pasta (about 8 ounces)
- 1 tablespoon olive oil
- 1 medium sweet orange pepper, chopped
- 1 medium sweet red pepper, chopped
- 1 medium sweet yellow pepper, chopped
- 1 cup sliced fresh mushrooms
- 3 garlic cloves, minced
- ½ teaspoon Italian seasoning
- ¼ teaspoon salt
- ¼ teaspoon pepper
- 2 cups fresh baby spinach
- ½ cup grated Parmesan cheese

1. Cook orzo according to package directions; drain.
2. Meanwhile, in large skillet, heat oil over medium-high heat; saute peppers and mushrooms until tender. Add garlic and seasonings; cook and stir 1 minute.
3. Stir in the spinach until wilted. Stir in orzo and cheese; heat through.
Orzo with Mushrooms: Omit the peppers, spinach and cheese. Use ½ pound thinly sliced assorted fresh mushrooms, such as portobello, button and/or shiitake. With the mushrooms, saute ¾ pound fresh snow peas. Sprinkle dish with ½ cup toasted pine nuts.

Per ¾ cup: 196 cal., 5g fat (1g sat. fat), 6mg chol., 232mg sod., 30g carb. (4g sugars, 2g fiber), 7g pro.
Diabetic Exchanges: 1½ starch, 1 vegetable, 1 fat.

HERBED POTATO PACKET

Every year, my father and I plant a garden together. We like to use the herbs from our garden, but you can use ⅓ teaspoon of each dried herb that you don't have available fresh.

—**BERNADETTE BENNETT** WACO, TX

PREP: 15 MIN. • **GRILL:** 25 MIN.
MAKES: 4 SERVINGS

- 1 pound baby red potatoes (about 16), halved
- ¼ cup cranberry juice
- 2 tablespoons butter, cubed
- 1 teaspoon each minced fresh dill, oregano, rosemary and thyme
- ½ teaspoon salt
- ⅛ teaspoon pepper

1. In a large bowl, combine all the ingredients; place on a piece of heavy-duty foil (about 18x12-in. rectangle). Fold foil around mixture, sealing tightly.
2. Grill, covered, over medium heat 25-30 minutes or until potatoes are tender. Open foil carefully to allow steam to escape.
Per ¾ cup: 117 cal., 6g fat (4g sat. fat), 15mg chol., 351mg sod., 15g carb. (3g sugars, 1g fiber), 2g pro.
Diabetic Exchanges: 1 starch, 1 fat.

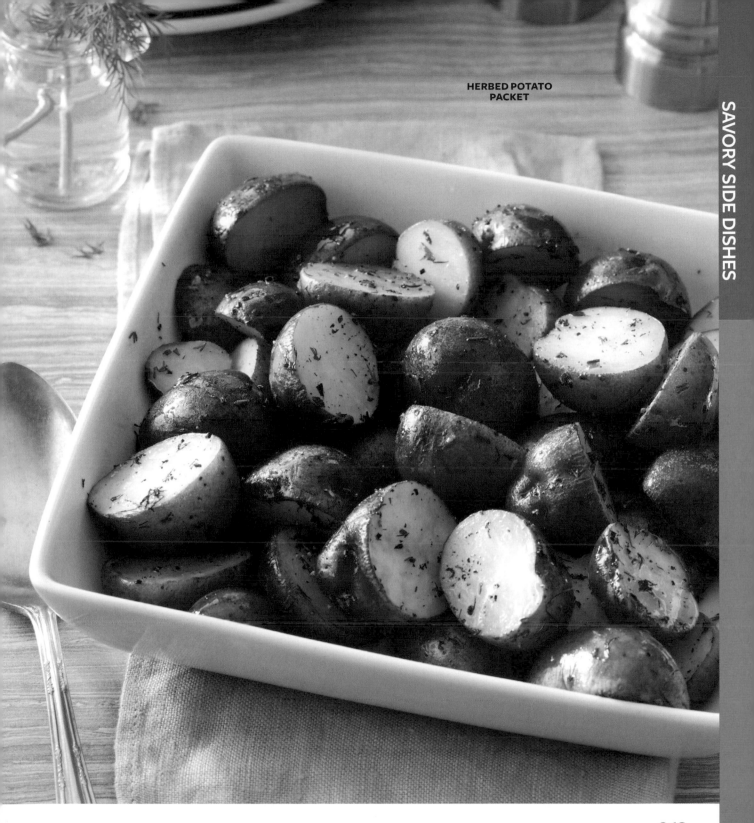

HERBED POTATO
PACKET

RICH & CREAMY PARMESAN MASHED POTATOES

GARLIC-HERB PATTYPAN SQUASH

The first time I planted a garden, I harvested summer squash and cooked it with garlic and herbs. Now I like to use pattypan squash.

—KAYCEE MASON SILOAM SPRINGS, AR

START TO FINISH: 25 MIN.
MAKES: 4 SERVINGS

- 5 cups halved small pattypan squash (about 1¼ pounds)
- 1 tablespoon olive oil
- 2 garlic cloves, minced
- ½ teaspoon salt
- ¼ teaspoon dried oregano
- ¼ teaspoon dried thyme
- ¼ teaspoon pepper
- 1 tablespoon minced fresh parsley

Preheat oven to 425°. Place squash in a greased 15x10x1-in. baking pan. Mix oil, garlic, salt, oregano, thyme and pepper; drizzle over squash. Toss to coat. Roast 15-20 minutes or until tender, stirring occasionally. Sprinkle with parsley.

Per ⅔ cup: 58 cal., 3g fat (0 sat. fat), 0 chol., 296mg sod., 6g carb. (3g sugars, 2g fiber), 2g pro.

Diabetic Exchanges: 1 vegetable, ½ fat.

✱
TEST KITCHEN TIP
You can often find pattypan squash at your local farmers market. Quite a versatile veggie, its mild texture and interesting shape makes it a summertime favorite. Aside from roasting them, try grilling, stuffing, steaming, sauteing and even pickling pattypans. Their skins are thin so there's no need for peeling.

⑤ INGREDIENTS

RICH & CREAMY PARMESAN MASHED POTATOES

For special occasions, like my husband's birthday dinners, I mash my potatoes with cream cheese, sour cream and Parmesan. It's divine comfort food.

—JO ANN BURRINGTON OSCEOLA, IN

PREP: 15 MIN. • **COOK:** 25 MIN.
MAKES: 6 SERVINGS

- 2 pounds red potatoes, cut into ½-inch cubes (about 6 cups)
- 1 cup chicken broth
- 4 ounces reduced-fat cream cheese
- ½ cup reduced-fat sour cream
- ¼ cup grated Parmesan cheese
- ¾ teaspoon salt
  Butter and additional grated Parmesan cheese, optional

1. Place potatoes in a large saucepan; add broth. Bring to a boil. Reduce heat; simmer, covered, 15-20 minutes or until potatoes are tender. Uncover; cook 4-6 minutes longer or until broth is almost evaporated, stirring occasionally.
2. Reduce heat to low; stir in cream cheese until melted. Mash potatoes slightly, gradually adding sour cream, Parmesan cheese and salt; heat mixture through. If desired, serve with butter and additional Parmesan cheese.

Per ⅔ cup: 199 cal., 7g fat (4g sat. fat), 24mg chol., 612mg sod., 26g carb. (4g sugars, 3g fiber), 8g pro.

Diabetic Exchanges: 2 starch, 1½ fat.

⑤ INGREDIENTS

BASIL GRILLED CORN ON THE COB

Corn on the cob is a most cherished Midwestern comfort food. It's amazing when grilled, and my recipe adds a few unexpected ingredients to make it taste even better.

—**CAITLIN DAWSON** MONROE, OH

PREP: 15 MIN. + SOAKING
GRILL: 20 MIN. • **MAKES:** 4 SERVINGS

- 4 **medium ears sweet corn**
- 4 **teaspoons butter, melted**
- ¾ **teaspoon salt**
- ¼ **teaspoon pepper**
- 16 **fresh basil leaves**
- ½ **medium lemon**
- 2 **teaspoons minced fresh cilantro**
  Additional butter, optional

1. Place corn in a 6-qt. stockpot; cover with cold water. Soak 20 minutes; drain. Carefully peel back corn husks to within 1 in. of bottoms; remove silk. Brush butter over corn; sprinkle with salt and pepper. Press four basil leaves onto each cob. Rewrap corn in husks; secure with kitchen string.

2. Grill corn, covered, over medium heat 20-25 minutes or until tender, turning often. Cut string and peel back husks; discard basil leaves. Squeeze lemon juice over corn; sprinkle with cilantro. If desired, spread the corn with additional butter.

Per ear of corn: 125 cal., 5g fat (3g sat. fat), 10mg chol., 489mg sod., 20g carb. (7g sugars, 2g fiber), 4g pro.
Diabetic Exchanges: 1 starch, 1 fat.

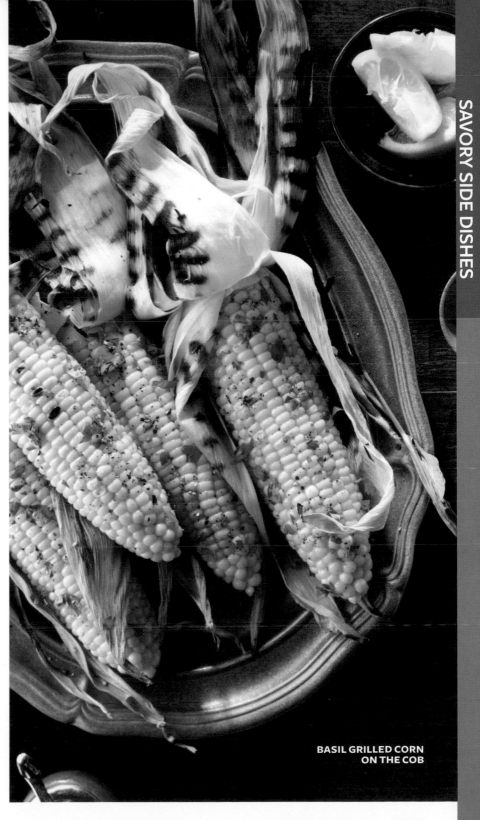

BASIL GRILLED CORN ON THE COB

GRILLED VEGGIES WITH MUSTARD VINAIGRETTE

I make this healthy and inviting side dish whenever my friends come over for a cookout. The honeyed vinaigrette lets the veggies shine.
—SHELLY GRAVER LANSDALE, PA

PREP: 20 MIN. • **GRILL:** 15 MIN.
MAKES: 10 SERVINGS (¾ CUP EACH)

- ¼ cup red wine vinegar
- 1 tablespoon Dijon mustard
- 1 tablespoon honey
- ½ teaspoon salt
- ⅛ teaspoon pepper
- ¼ cup canola oil
- ¼ cup olive oil

VEGETABLES

- 2 large sweet onions
- 2 medium zucchini
- 2 yellow summer squash
- 2 large sweet red peppers, halved and seeded
- 1 bunch green onions, trimmed
  Cooking spray

1. In a small bowl, whisk the first five ingredients. Gradually whisk in the oils until blended.
2. Peel and quarter each sweet onion, leaving root ends intact. Cut zucchini and yellow squash lengthwise into ½-in.-thick slices. Lightly spritz onions, zucchini, yellow squash and remaining vegetables with cooking spray, turning to coat all sides.
3. Grill sweet onions, covered, over medium heat 15-20 minutes until tender, turning occasionally. Grill zucchini, squash and peppers, covered, over medium heat 10-15 minutes or until crisp-tender and lightly charred, turning once. Grill the green onions, covered, 2-4 minutes or until lightly charred, turning once.
4. Cut vegetables into bite-size pieces; place in a large bowl. Add ½ cup vinaigrette and toss to coat. Serve with remaining vinaigrette.

Per ¾ cup: 155 cal., 12g fat (1g sat. fat), 0 chol., 166mg sod., 13g carb. (8g sugars, 2g fiber), 2g pro.
Diabetic Exchanges: 2½ fat, 1 vegetable, ½ starch.

⑤ INGREDIENTS **FAST FIX**

SMOKY CAULIFLOWER

Smoked Spanish paprika gives a simple side of cauliflower a bit more depth of flavor. We're fans of roasted veggies of any kind, and this one is a favorite.
—JULIETTE MULHOLLAND CORVALLIS, OR

START TO FINISH: 30 MIN.
MAKES: 8 SERVINGS

- 1 large head cauliflower, broken into 1-inch florets (about 9 cups)
- 2 tablespoons olive oil
- 1 teaspoon smoked paprika
- ¾ teaspoon salt
- 2 garlic cloves, minced
- 2 tablespoons minced fresh parsley

1. Place cauliflower florets in a large bowl. Combine the oil, paprika and salt. Drizzle over cauliflower; toss to coat. Transfer to a 15x10x1-in. baking pan. Bake, uncovered, at 450° for about 10 minutes.
2. Stir in garlic. Bake 10-15 minutes longer or until cauliflower is tender and lightly browned, stirring occasionally. Sprinkle with parsley.

Per ¾ cup: 58 cal., 4g fat (0 sat. fat), 0 chol., 254mg sod., 6g carb. (3g sugars, 3g fiber), 2g pro.
Diabetic Exchanges: 1 vegetable, ½ fat.

GRILLED VEGGIES WITH MUSTARD VINAIGRETTE

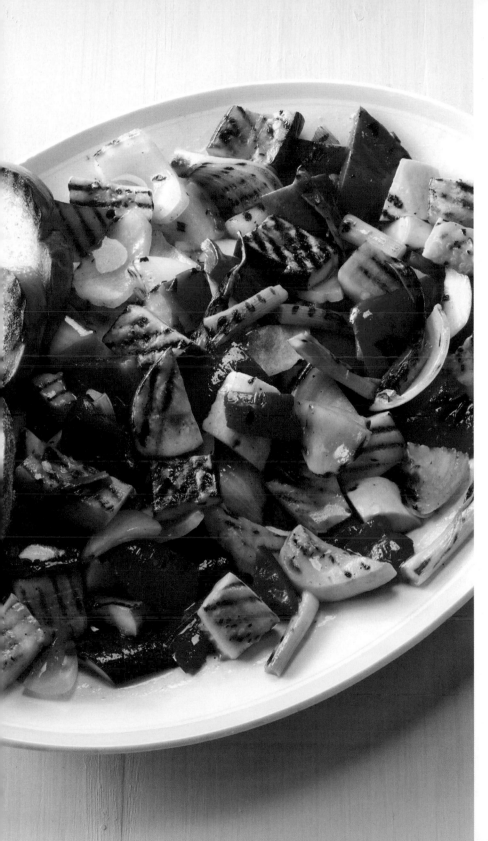

⑤INGREDIENTS **FAST FIX▶**

WARM TASTY GREENS WITH GARLIC

My farm box had too many greens, so I had to use them up. This tasty idea uses kale, tomatoes and garlic in a dish that quickly disappears.

—MARTHA NETH AURORA, CO

START TO FINISH: 30 MIN.
MAKES: 4 SERVINGS

- 1 **pound kale, trimmed and torn (about 20 cups)**
- 2 **tablespoons olive oil**
- ¼ **cup chopped oil-packed sun-dried tomatoes**
- 5 **garlic cloves, minced**
- 2 **tablespoons minced fresh parsley**
- ¼ **teaspoon salt**

1. In a 6-qt. stockpot, bring 1 in. of water to a boil. Add kale; cook, covered, 10-15 minutes or until tender. Remove with a slotted spoon; discard the cooking liquid.

2. In same pot, heat oil over medium heat. Add tomatoes and garlic; cook and stir 1 minute. Add kale, parsley and salt; heat through, stirring occasionally.

Per ⅔ cup: 137 cal., 9g fat (1g sat. fat), 0 chol., 216mg sod., 14g carb. (0 sugars, 3g fiber), 4g pro.
Diabetic Exchanges: 2 vegetable, 2 fat.

✱

DID YOU KNOW?
Kale is a nutritional powerhouse. Chock-full of vitamins K, A, C and B-6, it's also rich in manganese, copper, iron, omega-3 and omega-6 fatty acids, and antioxidants. Saute or boil mature kale to tenderize or use fresh baby kale raw in salads.

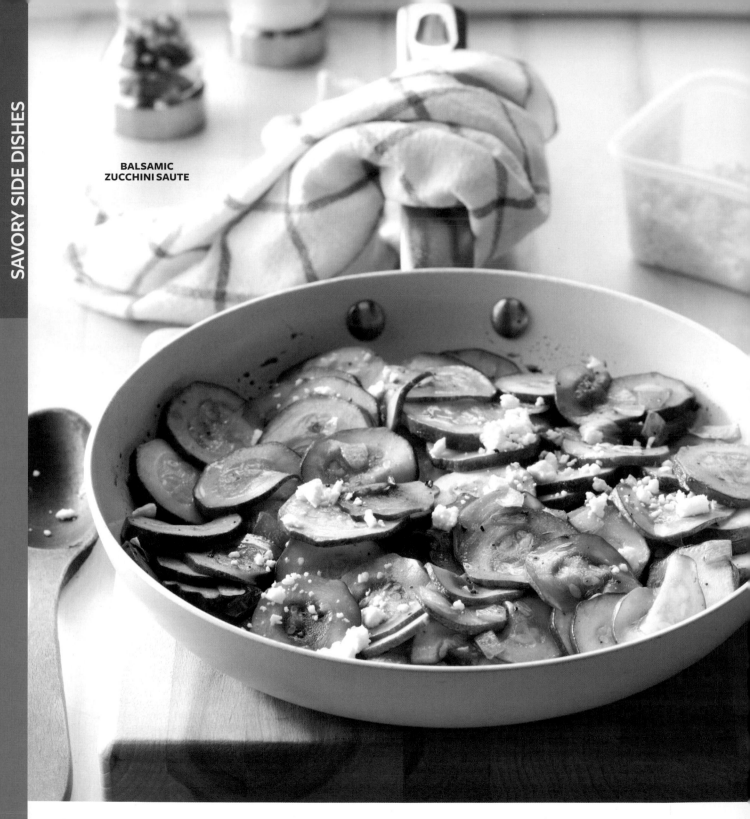

BALSAMIC
ZUCCHINI SAUTE

(5)INGREDIENTS FAST FIX

BALSAMIC ZUCCHINI SAUTE

This fast vegetarian dish with a little feta cheese is flavorful and only uses a few ingredients, making it easy to whip up while your entree is cooking.

—ELIZABETH BRAMKAMP GIG HARBOR, WA

START TO FINISH: 20 MIN.
MAKES: 4 SERVINGS

- 1 tablespoon olive oil
- 3 medium zucchini, cut into thin slices
- ½ cup chopped sweet onion
- ½ teaspoon salt
- ½ teaspoon dried rosemary, crushed
- ¼ teaspoon pepper
- 2 tablespoons balsamic vinegar
- ⅓ cup crumbled feta cheese

In a large skillet, heat oil over medium-high heat; saute zucchini and onion until crisp-tender, 6-8 minutes. Stir in the seasonings. Add vinegar; cook and stir 2 minutes. Top with cheese.

Per ½ cup: 94 cal., 5g fat (2g sat. fat), 5mg chol., 398mg sod., 9g carb. (6g sugars, 2g fiber), 4g pro.
Diabetic Exchanges: 1 vegetable, 1 fat.

✳
TEST KITCHEN TIP
When selecting vegetables to prepare, buy ones that are in season. They are fresher, so they taste better. Every day after picking, veggies lose more nutrients, so fresher is probably healthier, too. Produce that's in season is often less expensive, especially when there is ample local supply.

(5)INGREDIENTS FAST FIX

GREEN BEANS WITH SHALLOTS

Frozen green beans make this recipe ultra quick for a busy night. It's a simple, nutritious solution for any meal.

—LINDA RABBITT CHARLES CITY, IA

START TO FINISH: 15 MIN.
MAKES: 4 SERVINGS

- 1 package (12 ounces) frozen whole green beans
- 1¾ cups sliced fresh mushrooms
- 2 shallots, chopped
- 1 tablespoon olive oil
- ½ teaspoon salt
- ½ teaspoon dill weed
- ½ teaspoon pepper

1. Cook green beans according to package directions.

2. Meanwhile, in a large skillet, saute mushrooms and shallots in oil until tender. Remove from the heat. Add the green beans, salt, dill and pepper; toss to coat.

Per ¾ cup: 83 cal., 4g fat (0 sat. fat), 0 chol., 299mg sod., 10g carb. (3g sugars, 3g fiber), 2g pro.
Diabetic Exchanges: 2 vegetable, ½ fat.

FAST FIX

MASHED PEPPERY TURNIPS

I was trying to use up a turnip bumper crop from our garden—and also lighten up one of our favorite dishes—when I created this recipe. Replacing some potatoes with turnips made a low-carb side that we like even better!

—COURTNEY STULTZ WEIR, KS

START TO FINISH: 30 MIN.
MAKES: 4 SERVINGS

- 4 medium turnips (about 1 pound), peeled and cut into 1¼-in. pieces
- 1 large potato (about ¾ pound), peeled and cut into 1¼-in. pieces
- 2 tablespoons reduced-fat cream cheese
- 1 tablespoon butter
- 1 tablespoon minced fresh parsley
- 1 teaspoon sea salt
- ½ teaspoon garlic powder
- ¼ teaspoon pepper
- ⅛ teaspoon chili powder
- ⅛ teaspoon ground chipotle pepper

1. Place turnips, potato and enough water to cover in a large saucepan; bring to a boil. Reduce heat; cook, uncovered, until tender, 15-20 minutes. Drain; return to pan.

2. Mash vegetables to the desired consistency. Stir in remaining items.

Per ¾ cup: 140 cal., 5g fat (3g sat. fat), 13mg chol., 608mg sod., 23g carb. (5g sugars, 3g fiber), 3g pro.
Diabetic Exchanges: 1½ starch, 1 fat.

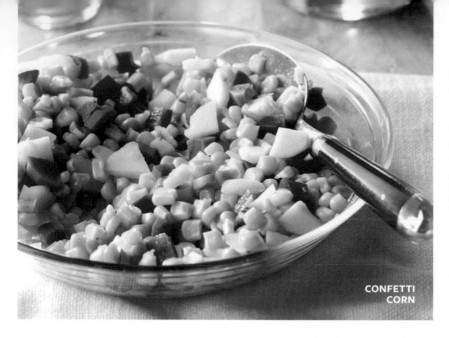

CONFETTI CORN

ROASTED VEGETABLES WITH SAGE

When I can't decide what veggie I want to serve, I just roast a bunch. That's how we boost veggie love at our house.
—**BETTY FULKS** ONIA, AR

PREP: 20 MIN. • **BAKE:** 35 MIN.
MAKES: 8 SERVINGS

- 5 cups cubed peeled butternut squash
- ½ pound fingerling potatoes (about 2 cups)
- 1 cup fresh Brussels sprouts, halved
- 1 cup fresh baby carrots
- 3 tablespoons butter
- 1 tablespoon minced fresh sage or 1 teaspoon dried sage leaves
- 1 garlic clove, minced
- ½ teaspoon salt

1. Preheat oven to 425°. Place vegetables in a large bowl. In a microwave, melt butter; stir in remaining ingredients. Add to vegetables and toss to coat.
2. Transfer to a greased 15x10x1-in. baking pan. Roast 35-45 minutes or until tender, stirring occasionally.
Per ¾ cup: 122 cal., 5g fat (3g sat. fat), 11mg chol., 206mg sod., 20g carb. (4g sugars, 3g fiber), 2g pro.
Diabetic Exchanges: 1 starch, 1 fat.

---

⑤ INGREDIENTS **FAST FIX ▶**
CONFETTI CORN

This easy corn dish is sure to dress up almost any entree. Tender corn is paired with the crunch of water chestnuts, red pepper and chopped carrot in a side that's pretty and pleasing.
—**GLENDA WATTS** CHARLESTON, IL

START TO FINISH: 15 MIN.
MAKES: 4 SERVINGS

- ¼ cup chopped carrot
- 1 tablespoon olive oil
- 2¾ cups fresh or frozen corn, thawed
- ¼ cup chopped water chestnuts
- ¼ cup chopped sweet red pepper

In a large skillet, saute the carrot in oil until crisp-tender. Stir in the corn, water chestnuts and red pepper; heat until warmed through.
Per ¾ cup: 140 cal., 4g fat (1g sat. fat), 0 chol., 7mg sod., 26g carb. (3g sugars, 3g fiber), 4g pro.
Diabetic Exchanges: 1½ starch, ½ fat.

---

⑤ INGREDIENTS **FAST FIX ▶**
ROASTED BROCCOLI & CAULIFLOWER

When we make a time-consuming entree, we also do a quick broccoli and cauliflower side. The veggies are a good fit when you're watching calories.
—**DEBRA TOLBERT** DEVILLE, LA

START TO FINISH: 25 MIN.
MAKES: 8 SERVINGS

- 4 cups fresh cauliflowerets
- 4 cups fresh broccoli florets
- 10 garlic cloves, peeled and halved
- 2 tablespoons olive oil
- ½ teaspoon salt
- ½ teaspoon pepper

Preheat oven to 425°. In a large bowl, combine all ingredients; toss to coat. Transfer to two greased 15x10x1-in. baking pans. Roast 15-20 minutes or until tender.
Per ¾ cup: 58 cal., 4g fat (1g sat. fat), 0 chol., 173mg sod., 6g carb. (2g sugars, 2g fiber), 2g pro.
Diabetic Exchanges: 1 vegetable, ½ fat.

⑤ INGREDIENTS **FAST FIX**

PESTO PASTA & POTATOES

Although this healthy pasta dish is pretty simple to begin with, the cooking method makes it even simpler: You can throw the green beans and pasta into one big pot.

—**LAURA FLOWERS** MOSCOW, ID

START TO FINISH: 30 MIN.
MAKES: 12 SERVINGS

- 1½ pounds small red potatoes, halved
- 12 ounces uncooked whole grain spiral pasta
- 3 cups cut fresh or frozen green beans
- 1 jar (6½ ounces) prepared pesto
- 1 cup grated Parmigiano-Reggiano cheese

1. Place potatoes in a large saucepan; add water to cover. Bring to a boil. Reduce heat; cook, uncovered, until tender, 8-10 minutes. Drain; transfer to a large bowl.

2. Meanwhile, cook pasta according to package directions, adding green beans during the last 5 minutes of cooking. Drain, reserving ¾ cup pasta water, and add to potatoes. Toss with the pesto, cheese blend and enough pasta water to moisten.

Per ¾ cup: 261 cal., 10g fat (3g sat. fat), 11mg chol., 233mg sod., 34g carb. (2g sugars, 5g fiber), 11g pro.
Diabetic Exchanges: 2 starch, 2 fat.

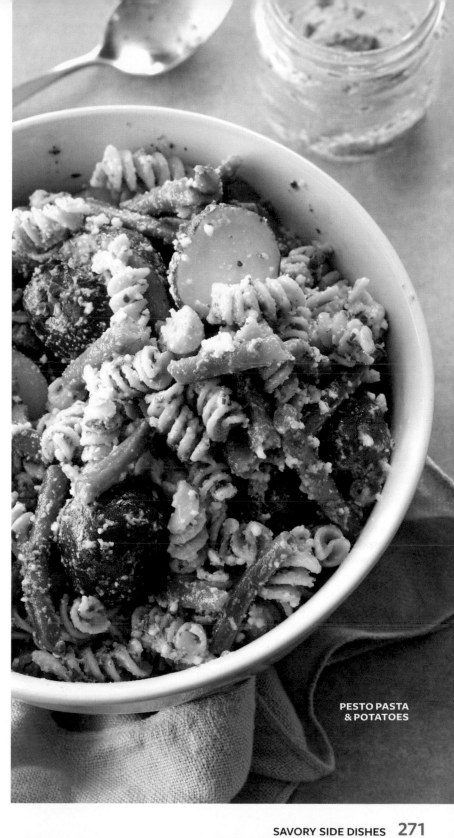

PESTO PASTA & POTATOES

FAST FIX

HONEY & GINGER GLAZED CARROTS

For weeknights and special events alike, we make sweet and tangy carrots flavored with ginger, lemon and honey. You could substitute pecans for the almonds or opt to leave the nuts out. The dish is also tasty made ahead and reheated in the oven.

—LAURA MIMS LITTLE ELM, TX

START TO FINISH: 25 MIN.
MAKES: 6 SERVINGS

- 1½ pounds fresh carrots, sliced
- ½ cup golden raisins
- 3 tablespoons honey
- 2 tablespoons butter
- 2 tablespoons lemon juice
- 1½ teaspoons ground ginger
- ½ teaspoon salt
- ½ cup slivered almonds, toasted

1. Place carrots in a large saucepan; add water to cover. Bring to a boil. Cook, covered, 6-8 minutes or until crisp-tender. Drain and return to pan.
2. Add raisins, honey, butter, lemon juice, ginger and salt; cook and stir 4-5 minutes longer or until carrots are tender. Just before serving, sprinkle with almonds.

Note: To toast nuts, bake in a shallow pan in a 350° oven for 5-10 minutes or cook in a skillet over low heat until lightly browned, stirring occasionally.

Per ⅔ cup: 204 cal., 9g fat (3g sat. fat), 10mg chol., 307mg sod., 32g carb. (22g sugars, 5g fiber), 4g pro.
Diabetic Exchanges: 2 vegetable, 1½ fat, 1 starch.

⑤INGREDIENTS   FAST FIX

SAUTEED RADISHES WITH GREEN BEANS

I'd heard that you don't cook radishes, but I found a cookbook from the 1950s that disagreed—and now cooking them is popular again. Green or wax beans and toasted nuts round out the dish.

—PAM KAISER MANSFIELD, MO

START TO FINISH: 20 MIN.
MAKES: 4 SERVINGS

- 1 tablespoon butter
- ½ pound fresh green or wax beans, trimmed
- 1 cup thinly sliced radishes
- ½ teaspoon sugar
- ¼ teaspoon salt
- 2 tablespoons pine nuts, toasted

1. In a large skillet, heat butter over medium-high heat. Add the beans; cook and stir 3-4 minutes or until beans are crisp-tender.
2. Add radishes; cook 2-3 minutes longer or until vegetables are tender, stirring occasionally. Stir in sugar and salt; sprinkle with nuts.

Note: To toast nuts, bake in a shallow pan in a 350° oven for 5-10 minutes or cook in a skillet over low heat until lightly browned, stirring occasionally.

Per ½ cup: 75 cal., 6g fat (2g sat. fat), 8mg chol., 177mg sod., 5g carb. (2g sugars, 2g fiber), 2g pro.
Diabetic Exchanges: 1 vegetable, 1 fat.

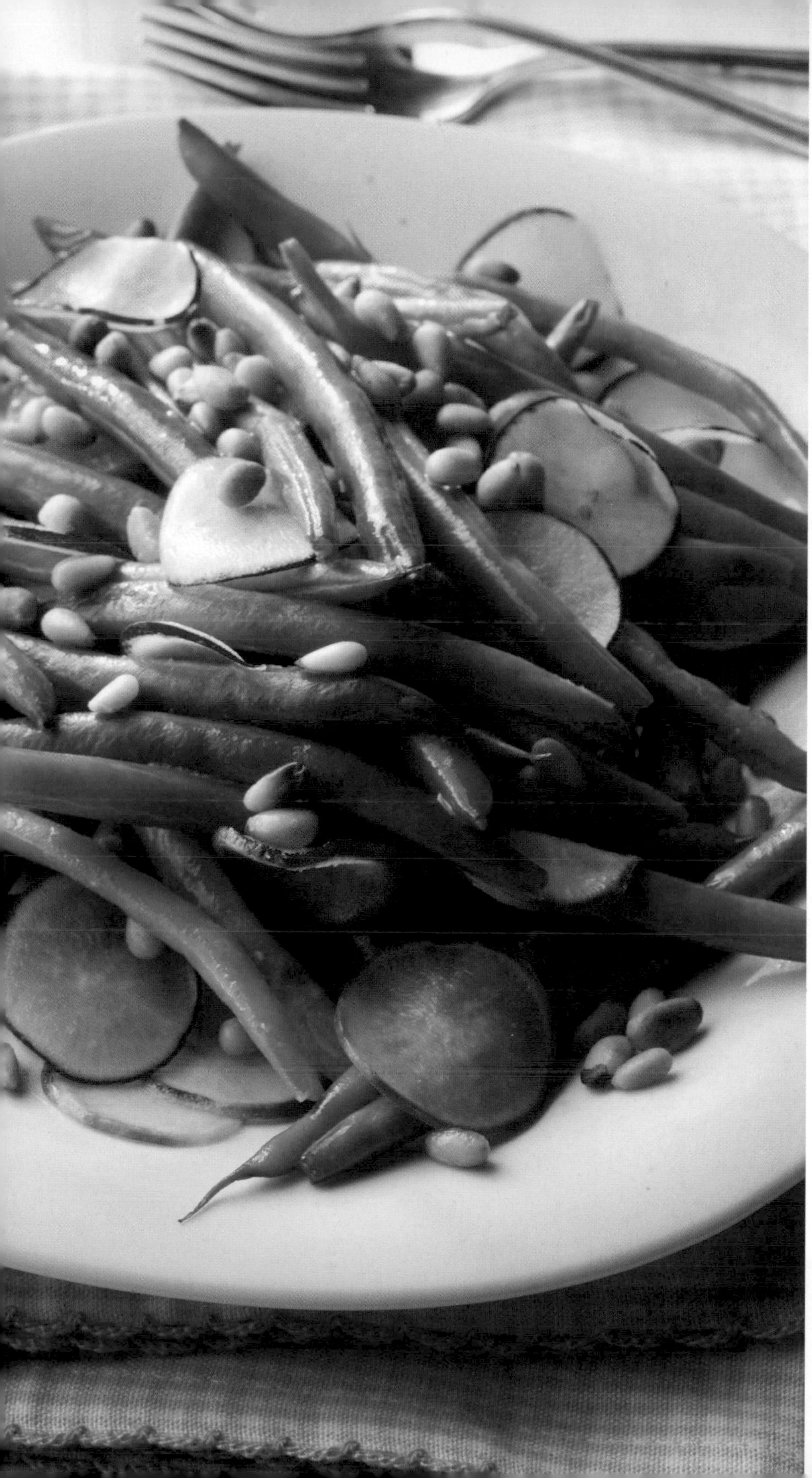

FAST FIX ▸

SQUASH & MUSHROOM MEDLEY

Bring the taste of summer to your dinner table with an easy zucchini and summer squash dish. It's a delight with so many main dishes.

—HEATHER ESPOSITO ROME, NY

START TO FINISH: 20 MIN.
MAKES: 5 SERVINGS

- 1 **large yellow summer squash, chopped**
- 1 **large zucchini, chopped**
- 1 **medium onion, chopped**
- 2 **teaspoons butter**
- 1 **can (7 ounces) mushroom stems and pieces, drained**
- 2 **garlic cloves, minced**
- ¼ **teaspoon salt**
- ⅛ **teaspoon pepper**

In a large skillet, saute the summer squash, zucchini and onion in butter until tender. Add the mushrooms, garlic, salt and pepper; saute 2-3 minutes longer or until heated through.
Per 1 cup: 58 cal., 2g fat (1g sat. fat), 4mg chol., 283mg sod., 9g carb. (5g sugars, 3g fiber), 3g pro.
Diabetic Exchanges: 1 vegetable, ½ fat.

★ ★ ★ ★ ★ **READER REVIEW**

"I have made it twice already. Everyone loves it. Goes great with any grilled meat and reheats well in the micro for a light lunch!"

KAROLK TASTEOFHOME.COM

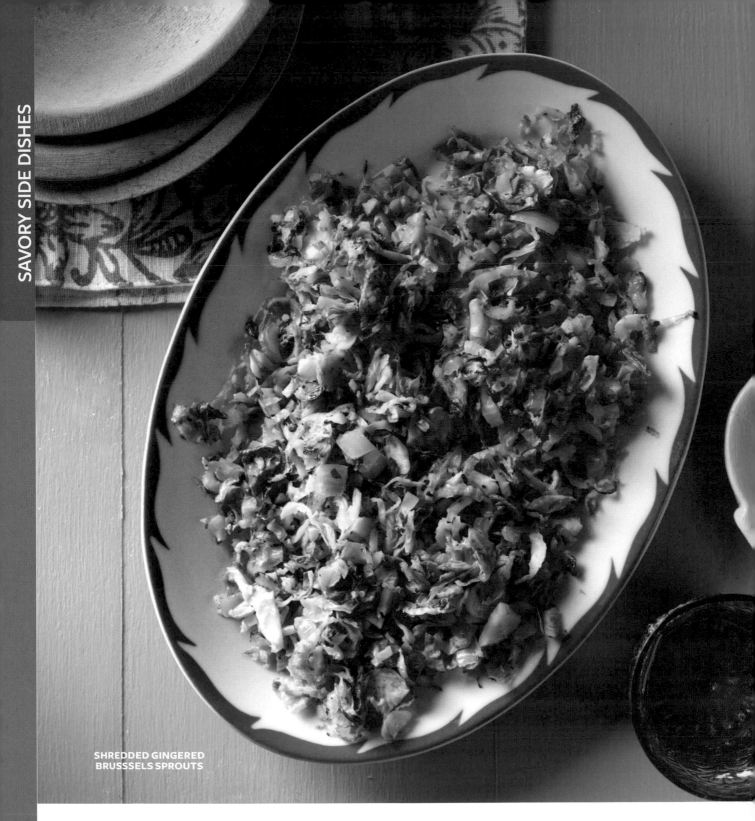

SHREDDED GINGERED
BRUSSSELS SPROUTS

(5) INGREDIENTS FAST FIX

SHREDDED GINGERED BRUSSELS SPROUTS

If you have folks who usually turn away from Brussels sprouts, have them try these. Then expect lots of requests for second helpings.

—JAMES SCHEND PLEASANT PRAIRIE, WI

START TO FINISH: 25 MIN.
MAKES: 6 SERVINGS

- 1 pound fresh Brussels sprouts (about 5½ cups)
- 1 tablespoon olive oil
- 1 small onion, finely chopped
- 1 tablespoon minced fresh gingerroot
- 1 garlic clove, minced
- ½ teaspoon salt
- 2 tablespoons water
- ¼ teaspoon pepper

1. Trim Brussels sprouts. Cut sprouts lengthwise in half; cut crosswise into thin slices.
2. Place a large skillet over medium-high heat. Add Brussels sprouts; cook and stir 2-3 minutes or until sprouts begin to brown lightly. Add oil and toss to coat. Stir in onion, ginger, garlic and salt. Add water; reduce heat to medium and cook, covered, 1-2 minutes or until vegetables are tender. Stir in pepper.
Per ¾ cup: 56 cal., 2g fat (0 sat. fat), 0 chol., 214mg sod., 8g carb. (2g sugars, 3g fiber), 2g pro.
Diabetic Exchanges: 1 vegetable, ½ fat.

(5) INGREDIENTS

TWO-TONE POTATO WEDGES

Better than french fries, these tasty potatoes have just the right touch of garlic and Parmesan cheese. This is the only way my daughter will eat sweet potatoes, and she loves 'em!

—MARIA NICOLAU SCHUMACHER LARCHMONT, NY

PREP: 10 MIN. • **BAKE:** 40 MIN.
MAKES: 4 SERVINGS

- 2 medium potatoes
- 1 medium sweet potato
- 1 tablespoon olive oil
- ¼ teaspoon salt
- ¼ teaspoon pepper
- 1 tablespoon grated Parmesan cheese
- 2 garlic cloves, minced

1. Cut each potato and sweet potato into eight wedges; place in a large resealable plastic bag. Add the oil, salt and pepper; seal bag and shake to coat. Arrange in a single layer in a 15x10x1-in. baking pan coated with cooking spray.
2. Bake, uncovered, at 425° for about 20 minutes. Turn potatoes; sprinkle with cheese and garlic. Bake 20-25 minutes longer or until golden brown.
Per 6 potato wedges: 151 cal., 4g fat (1g sat. fat), 1mg chol., 176mg sod., 27g carb. (4g sugars, 3g fiber), 3g pro.
Diabetic Exchanges: 1½ starch, 1 fat.

FAST FIX

PUMPKIN & CAULIFLOWER GARLIC MASH

I wanted healthy alternatives to my family's favorite recipes. Pumpkin, cauliflower and thyme are an amazing combination. You'll never miss those plain old mashed potatoes.

—KARI WHEATON SOUTH BELOIT, IL

START TO FINISH: 25 MIN.
MAKES: 6 SERVINGS

- 1 medium head cauliflower, broken into florets (about 6 cups)
- 3 garlic cloves
- ⅓ cup spreadable cream cheese
- 1 can (15 ounces) solid-pack pumpkin
- 1 tablespoon minced fresh thyme
- 1 teaspoon salt
- ¼ teaspoon cayenne pepper
- ¼ teaspoon pepper

1. Place 1 in. of water in a large saucepan; bring to a boil. Add cauliflower and garlic cloves; cook, covered, 8-10 minutes or until tender. Drain; transfer to a food processor.
2. Add remaining ingredients; process until smooth. Return to pan; heat through, stirring occasionally.
Per ⅔ cup: 87 cal., 4g fat (2g sat. fat), 9mg chol., 482mg sod., 12g carb. (5g sugars, 4g fiber), 4g pro.
Diabetic Exchanges: 1 vegetable, ½ starch, ½ fat.

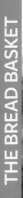

WILD RICE BREAD
WITH SUNFLOWER
SEEDS, PAGE 279

The Bread Basket

There's nothing quite like the aroma of bread baking
in the oven. Bake up a wholesome batch in your own
kitchen today with these easy recipes for loaves,
rolls and muffins. Your family is sure to love the
heartwarming flavor of your handiwork!

BANANA WHEAT BREAD

A subtle banana flavor comes through in this moist whole wheat loaf. Flecked with poppy seeds, the sweet slices are wonderful warm or toasted and spread with butter.

—**LOUISE MYERS** POMEROY, OH

PREP: 15 MIN. • **BAKE:** 4 HOURS
MAKES: 1 LOAF (1½ POUNDS, 16 SLICES)

- ¾ cup water (70° to 80°)
- ¼ cup honey
- 1 large egg, lightly beaten
- 4½ teaspoons canola oil
- ½ teaspoon vanilla extract
- 1 medium ripe banana, sliced
- 2 teaspoons poppy seeds
- 1 teaspoon salt
- 1¾ cups bread flour
- 1½ cups whole wheat flour
- 2¼ teaspoons active dry yeast

In a bread machine pan, place all the ingredients in the order suggested by manufacturer. Select the basic bread setting. Choose crust color and loaf size if available. Bake according to the bread machine directions (check the dough after about 5 minutes of mixing; add 1 to 2 tablespoons of water or flour if needed).

To freeze: Freeze the sliced loaf in resealable plastic freezer bag. To use, thaw at room temperature.

Note: We recommend you do not use a bread machine's time-delay feature for this recipe.

Per slice: 125 cal., 2g fat (0 sat. fat), 13mg chol., 153mg sod., 24g carb. (6g sugars, 2g fiber), 4g pro.
Diabetic Exchanges: 1½ starch, ½ fat.

BANANA WHEAT BREAD

WILD RICE BREAD WITH SUNFLOWER SEEDS

Every chance I got I skipped the boring school cafeteria meals and headed to my grandma's house for lunch. The ingredients in this hearty loaf reflect northeastern Minnesota, where she spent most of her life. It's good plain, but try it in your holiday stuffing, too.

—**CRYSTAL SCHLUETER** NORTHGLENN, CO

PREP: 35 MIN. + RISING • **BAKE:** 35 MIN.
MAKES: 2 LOAVES (16 SLICES EACH)

- 2 packages (¼ ounce each) active dry yeast
- 1 cup warm water (110° to 115°)
- 1 package (8.8 ounces) ready-to-serve long grain and wild rice
- 1 cup plus 1 tablespoon unsalted sunflower kernels, divided
- 1 cup warm fat-free milk (110° to 115°)
- ⅓ cup honey or molasses
- ¼ cup butter, softened
- 2 tablespoons ground flaxseed
- 2 teaspoons salt
- 3 cups whole wheat flour
- 2¾ to 3¼ cups all-purpose flour
- 1 large egg white, lightly beaten
- 1 tablespoon toasted wheat germ, optional

1. In a small bowl, dissolve yeast in warm water. In a large bowl, combine rice, 1 cup sunflower kernels, milk, honey, butter, flaxseed, salt, yeast mixture, whole wheat flour and 1 cup all-purpose flour; beat on medium speed until combined. Stir in enough remaining flour to form a stiff dough (dough will be sticky).

2. Turn dough onto a floured surface; knead until elastic, about 6-8 minutes. Place in a greased bowl, turning once to grease the top. Cover with plastic wrap and let dough rise in a warm place until doubled, about 1¼ hours.

3. Punch down dough. Turn onto a lightly floured surface; divide in half. Roll each half into a 12x8-in. rectangle. Roll up jelly-roll style, starting with a short side; pinch seam and ends to seal. Place each in a 9x5-in. loaf pan coated with cooking spray, seam side down.

4. Cover with kitchen towels; let the loaves rise in a warm place until almost doubled, about 45 minutes. Preheat oven to 375°.

5. Brush loaves with egg white; sprinkle with remaining sunflower kernels and, if desired, wheat germ. Bake for 35-45 minutes or until dark golden brown. Cool in pans 5 minutes. Remove to a wire rack to cool.

Per slice without wheat germ:
142 cal., 4g fat (1g sat. fat), 4mg chol., 205mg sod., 23g carb. (4g sugars, 2g fiber), 4g pro.
Diabetic Exchanges: 1½ starch, ½ fat.

✳

TEST KITCHEN TIP
Seeds add both crunch and fiber to bread. Good options include sunflower, sesame, pumpkin, poppy and flaxseed. (Flaxseed is usually ground to make more nutrients available.) For more flavor, lightly toast seeds on a baking sheet before adding to the dough or sprinkling on top of your loaf.

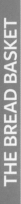

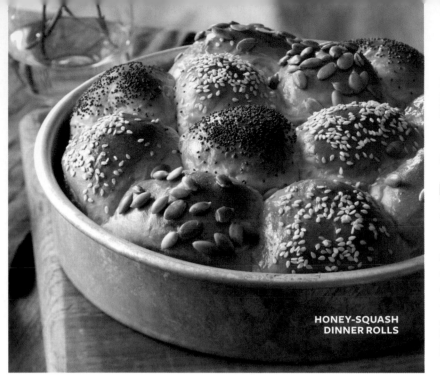

HONEY-SQUASH DINNER ROLLS

HONEY-SQUASH DINNER ROLLS

These puffy dinner rolls take on rich color when you add winter squash to the dough. Any squash variety works. I've even used cooked carrots.
—**MARCIA WHITNEY** GAINESVILLE, FL

PREP: 40 MIN. + RISING • **BAKE:** 20 MIN.
MAKES: 2 DOZEN

- 2 packages (¼ ounce each) active dry yeast
- 2 teaspoons salt
- ¼ teaspoon ground nutmeg
- 6 to 6½ cups all-purpose flour
- 1¼ cups 2% milk
- ½ cup butter, cubed
- ½ cup honey
- 1 package (12 ounces) frozen mashed winter squash, thawed (about 1⅓ cups)
- 1 large egg, lightly beaten
  Poppy seeds, salted pumpkin seeds or pepitas, or sesame seeds

1. In a large bowl, mix the yeast, salt, nutmeg and 3 cups flour. In a small saucepan, heat milk, butter and honey to 120°-130°. Add to dry ingredients; beat on medium speed 2 minutes. Add squash; beat on high 2 minutes. Stir in enough remaining flour to form a soft dough (dough will be sticky).

2. Turn dough onto a floured surface; knead until smooth and elastic, about 6-8 minutes. Place in a greased bowl, turning once to grease the top. Cover with plastic wrap and let rise in a warm place until doubled, about 1 hour.

3. Punch down dough. Turn onto a lightly floured surface; divide and shape into 24 balls. Divide balls between two greased 9-in. round baking pans. Cover with kitchen towels; let rise in a warm place until doubled, about 45 minutes.

4. Preheat oven to 375°. Brush tops with beaten egg; sprinkle with seeds. Bake 20-25 minutes or until dark golden brown. Cover loosely with foil during the last 5-7 minutes if needed to prevent overbrowning. Remove from pans to wire racks; serve warm.

Per roll: 186 cal., 5g fat (3g sat. fat), 19mg chol., 238mg sod., 32g carb. (6g sugars, 1g fiber), 4g pro.
Diabetic Exchanges: 2 starch, 1 fat.

FAST FIX

TENDER WHOLE WHEAT MUFFINS

Want oven-baked treats but need something light? Simple whole wheat muffins are wonderful paired with soup or spread with a little jam for breakfast.
—**KRISTINE CHAYES** SMITHTOWN, NY

START TO FINISH: 30 MIN.
MAKES: 10 MUFFINS

- 1 cup all-purpose flour
- 1 cup whole wheat flour
- 2 tablespoons sugar
- 2½ teaspoons baking powder
- 1 teaspoon salt
- 1 large egg
- 1¼ cups milk
- 3 tablespoons butter, melted

1. Preheat the oven to 400°. In a large bowl, whisk the flours, sugar, baking powder and salt. In another bowl, whisk egg, milk and melted butter until blended. Add to flour mixture; stir just until moistened.

2. Fill greased muffin cups three-fourths full. Bake 15-17 minutes or until a toothpick inserted in center comes out clean. Cool for 5 minutes before removing from pan to a wire rack. Serve muffins warm.

Per muffin: 152 cal., 5g fat (3g sat. fat), 35mg chol., 393mg sod., 22g carb. (4g sugars, 2g fiber), 5g pro.
Diabetic Exchanges: 1½ starch, 1 fat.

DOUBLE BERRY QUICK BREAD

Healthy, fast and easy! This bread is a favorite of mine when prep time is tight and I have small amounts of different kinds of berries to use up.

—JENNIFER CODUTO KENT, OH

PREP: 15 MIN. • **BAKE:** 50 MIN. + COOLING
MAKES: 1 LOAF (12 SLICES)

- 1½ cups all-purpose flour
- ½ cup whole wheat flour
- ½ cup sugar
- 1½ teaspoons baking powder
- ½ teaspoon salt
- ¼ teaspoon baking soda
- 2 large egg whites
- 1 large egg
- ½ cup fat-free milk
- ½ cup reduced-fat sour cream
- ¼ cup unsweetened applesauce
- ¼ cup canola oil
- 2 teaspoons vanilla extract
- 1 cup fresh raspberries
- 1 cup fresh blackberries

1. Preheat oven to 375°. In a large bowl, whisk the first six ingredients. In another bowl, whisk egg whites, egg, milk, sour cream, applesauce, oil and vanilla until blended. Add to the flour mixture; stir just until moistened. Gently fold in berries.

2. Transfer batter to a 9x5-in. loaf pan coated with cooking spray. Bake about 50-60 minutes or until a toothpick inserted in the center comes out clean. Cool in pan 10 minutes before removing to a wire rack to cool.

Per slice: 188 cal., 6g fat (1g sat. fat), 19mg chol., 201mg sod., 28g carb. (11g sugars, 2g fiber), 5g pro.
Diabetic Exchanges: 2 starch, 1 fat.

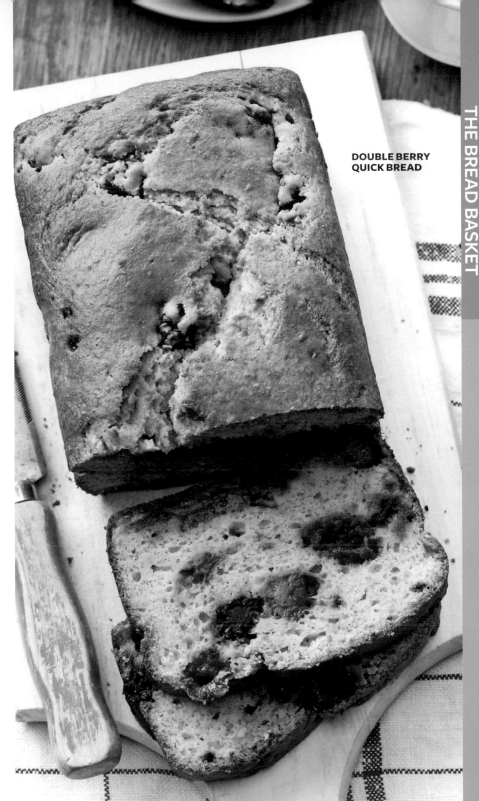

DOUBLE BERRY QUICK BREAD

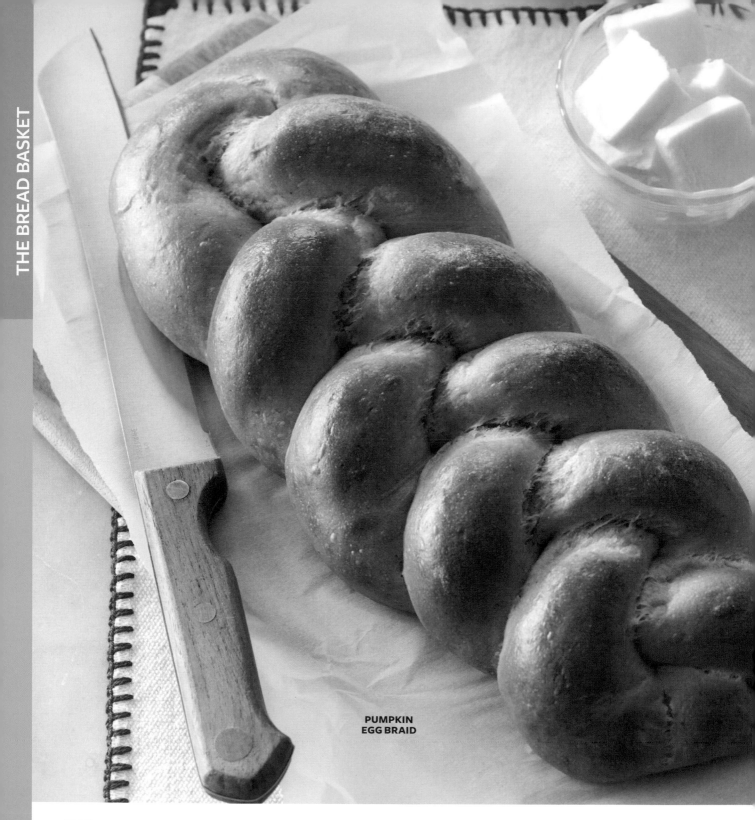

**PUMPKIN
EGG BRAID**

BLUEBERRY-BRAN MUFFINS

I've only had one truly outstanding bran muffin at a restaurant, so I wanted to create an awesome version I could enjoy at home. These came about by trial and error. They are moist, healthy—full of grains and fruits— and so tasty!

—NANCY RENS PRESCOTT, AZ

PREP: 25 MIN. • **BAKE:** 20 MIN.
MAKES: 1½ DOZEN

- 1½ cups bran flakes
- ⅓ cup boiling water
- 1 cup whole wheat flour
- 1 cup all-purpose flour
- ¾ cup packed brown sugar
- ⅓ cup quick-cooking oats
- ¾ teaspoon baking powder
- ½ teaspoon baking soda
- ½ teaspoon salt
- 1 large egg
- 1 cup buttermilk
- ½ cup unsweetened applesauce
- 2 tablespoons molasses
- ¾ cup fresh or frozen blueberries
- ¾ cup pitted dried plums, coarsely chopped
- ¼ cup slivered almonds
- 2 tablespoons honey

1. Preheat oven to 375°. In a small bowl, combine bran flakes and boiling water; set aside.
2. Whisk together flours, brown sugar, oats, baking powder, baking soda and salt. In another bowl, whisk together the egg, buttermilk, applesauce and molasses; stir in bran mixture. Add to the dry ingredients, stirring just until moistened. Fold in blueberries, plums and almonds.
3. Coat muffin cups with cooking spray; fill three-fourths full. Drizzle with honey. Bake until a toothpick inserted in center comes out clean, 18-20 minutes. Cool for 5 minutes before removing from pans to wire racks. Serve warm.
Note: If using frozen blueberries, do not thaw to avoid discoloring the batter.
Per muffin: 155 cal., 2g fat (0 sat. fat), 12mg chol., 166mg sod., 33g carb. (17g sugars, 2g fiber), 3g pro.
Diabetic Exchanges: 2 starch.

PUMPKIN EGG BRAID

I developed this bread to celebrate our two favorite holidays, Thanksgiving and Hanukkah. Try it with flavored butters, and use leftovers for French toast.

—SARA MELLAS HARTFORD, CT

PREP: 30 MIN. + RISING • **BAKE:** 20 MIN.
MAKES: 1 LOAF (12 SLICES)

- 1 package (¼ ounce) active dry yeast
- 3 tablespoons warm water (110° to 115°)
- ½ cup canned pumpkin
- 1 large egg
- 2 tablespoons light brown sugar
- 2 tablespoons butter, softened
- 1 teaspoon pumpkin pie spice
- ½ teaspoon salt
- 2 to 2½ cups bread flour

EGG WASH

- 1 large egg
- 1 tablespoon water

1. In a small bowl, dissolve yeast in warm water. In a large bowl, combine pumpkin, egg, brown sugar, butter, pie spice, salt, yeast mixture and 1 cup of flour; beat on medium speed until smooth. Stir in enough remaining flour to form a soft dough (the dough will be sticky).
2. Turn dough onto a floured surface; knead until smooth and elastic, about 6-8 minutes. Place in a greased bowl, turning once to grease the top. Cover with plastic wrap and let rise in a warm place until doubled, about 1 hour.
3. Punch down dough. Turn onto a lightly floured surface; divide into thirds. Roll each into a 16-in. rope. Place ropes on a greased baking sheet and braid. Pinch ends to seal; tuck under.
4. Cover with a kitchen towel; let rise in a warm place until almost doubled, about 45 minutes. Preheat the oven to 350°.
5. For egg wash, in a small bowl, whisk egg and water until blended; brush over loaf. Bake 20-25 minutes or until golden brown. Remove from pan to a wire rack to cool.
Per slice: 126 cal., 3g fat (2g sat. fat), 36mg chol., 129mg sod., 20g carb. (3g sugars, 1g fiber), 4g pro.
Diabetic Exchanges: 1 starch, ½ fat.

★ ★ ★ ★ ★ **READER REVIEW**

"I made this yesterday and it was wonderful. The aroma was so enticing, I could hardly wait for the bread to cool down enough to be able to slice it. Once I did, it disappeared fast. Family loved it. Thanks for sharing."

MAGGIE5047 TASTEOFHOME.COM

YOGURT YEAST ROLLS

Present these fluffy, golden rolls at a potluck and people will snap them up in a hurry. It's a nice contribution because rolls are easy to transport, don't need slicing, and one batch goes a long way.

—CAROL FORCUM MARION, IL

PREP: 30 MIN. + RISING • **BAKE:** 15 MIN.
MAKES: 2 DOZEN

- 1½ cups whole wheat flour
- 3¾ cups all-purpose flour, divided
- 2 packages (¼ ounce each) active dry yeast
- 2 teaspoons salt
- ½ teaspoon baking soda
- 1½ cups (12 ounces) plain yogurt
- ½ cup water
- 3 tablespoons butter
- 2 tablespoons honey
  Additional melted butter, optional

1. In a large bowl, combine the whole wheat flour, ½ cup all-purpose flour, yeast, salt and baking soda. In a saucepan over low heat, heat yogurt, water, butter and honey to 120°-130°. Pour over dry ingredients; blend well. Beat on medium speed for 3 minutes. Add enough remaining all-purpose flour to form a soft dough.

2. Turn onto a lightly floured surface; knead until smooth and elastic, about 6-8 minutes. Place in a greased bowl, turning once to grease top. Cover and let rise in a warm place until doubled, about 1 hour.

3. Punch dough down. Turn onto a lightly floured surface; divide into 24 portions. Roll each into a 10-in. rope. Shape rope into an S, then coil each end until it touches the center. Place 3 in. apart on greased baking sheets. Cover and let rise until doubled, for about 30 minutes. Preheat oven to 400°.

4. Bake until golden brown, about 15 minutes. If desired, brush tops with additional butter while warm. Remove from pans to wire racks to cool.

Per roll: 115 cal., 2g fat (1g sat. fat), 6mg chol., 245mg sod., 21g carb. (3g sugars, 1g fiber), 3g pro.
Diabetic Exchanges: 1½ starch, ½ fat.

HERB QUICK BREAD

This simple loaf is especially good with soups and stews, but slices are also tasty alongside green salads. The herbs make it a flavorful bread any time of the year.

—DONNA ROBERTS MANHATTAN, KS

PREP: 15 MIN. • **BAKE:** 40 MIN. + COOLING
MAKES: 1 LOAF (16 SLICES)

- 3 cups all-purpose flour
- 3 tablespoons sugar
- 1 tablespoon baking powder
- 3 teaspoons caraway seeds
- ½ teaspoon salt
- ½ teaspoon ground nutmeg
- ½ teaspoon dried thyme
- 1 large egg
- 1 cup fat-free milk
- ⅓ cup canola oil

1. Preheat oven to 350°. In a large bowl, whisk together the first seven ingredients. In another bowl, whisk together egg, milk and oil. Add to flour mixture; stir just until moistened.

2. Transfer to a 9x5-in. loaf pan coated with cooking spray. Bake until a toothpick inserted in center comes out clean, 40-50 minutes. Cool in pan about 10 minutes before removing to a wire rack to cool.

Per slice: 147 cal., 5g fat (1g sat. fat), 12mg chol., 160mg sod., 21g carb. (3g sugars, 1g fiber), 3g pro.
Diabetic Exchanges: 1½ starch, 1 fat.

**YOGURT
YEAST ROLLS**

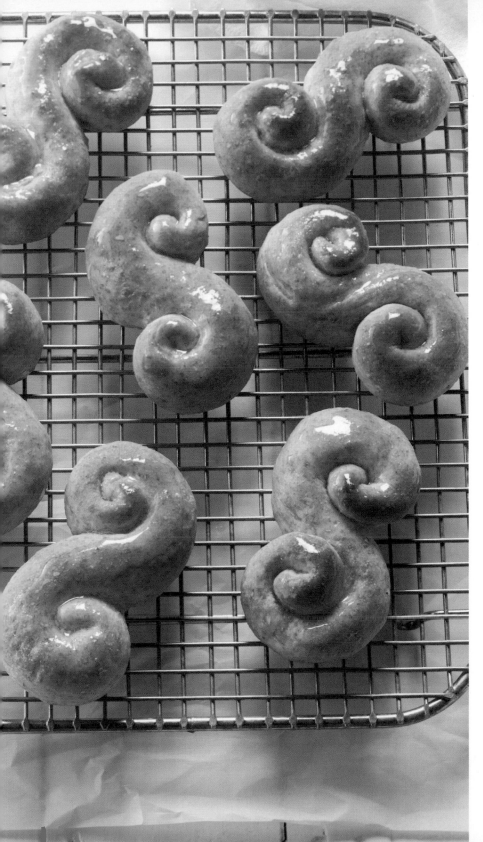

WHOLESOME BANANA BREAD

To make homemade breakfast food more healthy, I cut a lot of fat out of my regular banana bread recipe. Even with less fat, this bread turns out moist and delicious every time.

—**SARAH BIALOCK** YUMA, AZ

PREP: 15 MIN. • **BAKE:** 30 MIN. + COOLING
MAKES: 2 MINI LOAVES (6 SLICES EACH)

- 2 tablespoons butter, softened
- ⅓ cup packed brown sugar
- 1 large egg
- ½ cup mashed ripe banana
- 2 tablespoons unsweetened applesauce
- ½ teaspoon vanilla extract
- ¾ cup all-purpose flour
- 2 tablespoons whole wheat flour
- 1½ teaspoons ground flaxseed
- 1 teaspoon ground cinnamon
- ½ teaspoon baking soda
- ½ teaspoon ground nutmeg
- ⅛ teaspoon salt

1. In a large bowl, cream butter and brown sugar until light and fluffy. Add egg; beat well. Beat in the banana, applesauce and vanilla. Combine the remaining ingredients; add to the creamed mixture.

2. Transfer to two 5¾x3x2-in. loaf pans coated with cooking spray. Bake at 350° for 25-30 minutes or until a toothpick inserted in the center comes out clean. Cool for 10 minutes before removing from pans to wire racks.

Per slice: 91 cal., 3g fat (1g sat. fat), 23mg chol., 99mg sod., 16g carb. (7g sugars, 1g fiber), 2g pro.
Diabetic Exchanges: 1 starch, ½ fat.

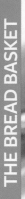

VEGGIE CORN MUFFINS

VEGGIE CORN MUFFINS

I make a game of adding at least one new healthy ingredient to all my recipes. My family appreciates the results.
—PEGGIE BROTT DAHLONEGA, GA

START TO FINISH: 30 MIN.
MAKES: 1 DOZEN

- 1 cup yellow cornmeal
- ½ cup all-purpose flour
- ½ cup whole wheat flour
- 1 teaspoon baking powder
- ¾ teaspoon salt
- 1 large egg
- 1 cup unsweetened almond milk
- ¼ cup canola oil
- ¼ cup honey
- ½ cup finely shredded carrot
- ½ cup finely chopped green pepper

1. Preheat oven to 400°. Coat 12 muffin cups with cooking spray.

2. Whisk together cornmeal, flours, baking powder and salt. In another bowl, whisk together egg, milk, oil and honey. Add to cornmeal mixture; stir just until moistened. Fold in vegetables. Fill prepared cups two-thirds full.

3. Bake until a toothpick inserted in center comes out clean, 12-15 minutes. Cool 5 minutes before removing from pan to a wire rack. Serve warm.

To freeze: Freeze cooled muffins in resealable plastic freezer bags. To use, microwave each muffin on high until warmed, 30-45 seconds.

Per muffin: 159 cal., 6g fat (1g sat. fat), 16mg chol., 207mg sod., 25g carb. (6g sugars, 2g fiber), 3g pro. **Diabetic Exchanges:** 1½ starch, 1 fat.

CHOCOLATE CHOCOLATE CHIP MUFFINS

These extra-chocolaty muffins feature nutritious ingredients like whole wheat flour and applesauce to make a lighter muffin. Because they are so delicious and surprisingly healthy, we even serve them for breakfast at the school where I work.

—THERESA HARRINGTON SHERIDAN, WY

PREP: 20 MIN. • **BAKE:** 20 MIN./BATCH
MAKES: 32 MUFFINS

- 2½ cups all-purpose flour
- 1¾ cups whole wheat flour
- 1¾ cups packed brown sugar
- ½ cup baking cocoa
- 1¼ teaspoons salt
- 1 teaspoon baking powder
- 1 teaspoon baking soda
- 2 large egg whites
- 1 large egg
- 2 cups unsweetened applesauce
- 1¾ cups fat-free milk
- 2 tablespoons canola oil
- 2½ teaspoons vanilla extract
- 1¼ cups semisweet chocolate chips

1. Preheat the oven to 350°. Whisk together first seven ingredients. In another bowl, whisk together egg whites, egg, applesauce, milk, oil and vanilla; add to the dry ingredients, stirring just until moistened. Fold in chocolate chips.

2. Coat muffin cups with cooking spray; fill three-fourths full with batter. Bake until a toothpick inserted in center comes out clean, 18-20 minutes. Cool 5 minutes before removing from pans to wire racks. Serve warm.

Per muffin: 161 cal., 3g fat (1g sat. fat), 7mg chol., 150mg sod., 31g carb. (18g sugars, 2g fiber), 3g pro.
Diabetic Exchanges: 2 starch, 1 fat.

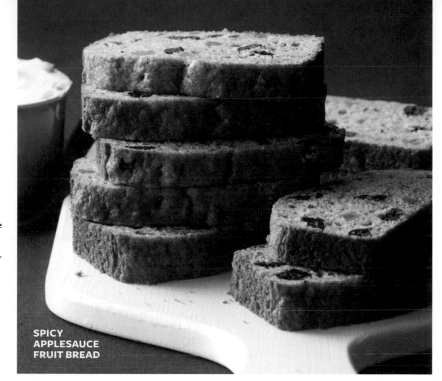

SPICY APPLESAUCE FRUIT BREAD

SPICY APPLESAUCE FRUIT BREAD

I've had this fruity loaf in my recipe collection forever. Depending on the season, I tweak the spices and fruit. If you don't like citron use something else.

—DAWN E. LOWENSTEIN HUNTINGDON VALLEY, PA

PREP: 20 MIN. • **BAKE:** 30 MIN. + COOLING
MAKES: 2 LOAVES (12 SLICES EACH)

- 2 cups plus 2 tablespoons all-purpose flour, divided
- 2 teaspoons baking powder
- 1 teaspoon salt
- 1 teaspoon ground cinnamon
- 1 teaspoon ground nutmeg
- ½ teaspoon ground allspice
- ½ teaspoon ground cloves
- ½ teaspoon baking soda
- 2 large eggs
- 1¼ cups unsweetened applesauce
- ¾ cup sugar
- ¼ cup packed brown sugar
- ¼ cup butter, melted
- 1 tablespoon grated orange peel
- ½ cup dried cranberries or raisins
- ½ cup chopped candied citron

1. Preheat oven to 350°. In a large bowl, whisk 2 cups flour, baking powder, salt, spices and baking soda. In another bowl, whisk eggs, applesauce, sugars, melted butter and orange peel until blended. Add to flour mixture; stir just until moistened. In a small bowl, toss cranberries and candied citron with remaining flour; fold into batter.

2. Transfer to two greased 8x4-in. loaf pans. Bake 30-35 minutes or until a toothpick inserted in center comes out clean. Cool in pans 10 minutes before removing to wire racks to cool.

Per slice: 126 cal., 3g fat (1g sat. fat), 21mg chol., 194mg sod., 25g carb. (15g sugars, 1g fiber), 2g pro.
Diabetic Exchanges: 1½ starch, ½ fat.

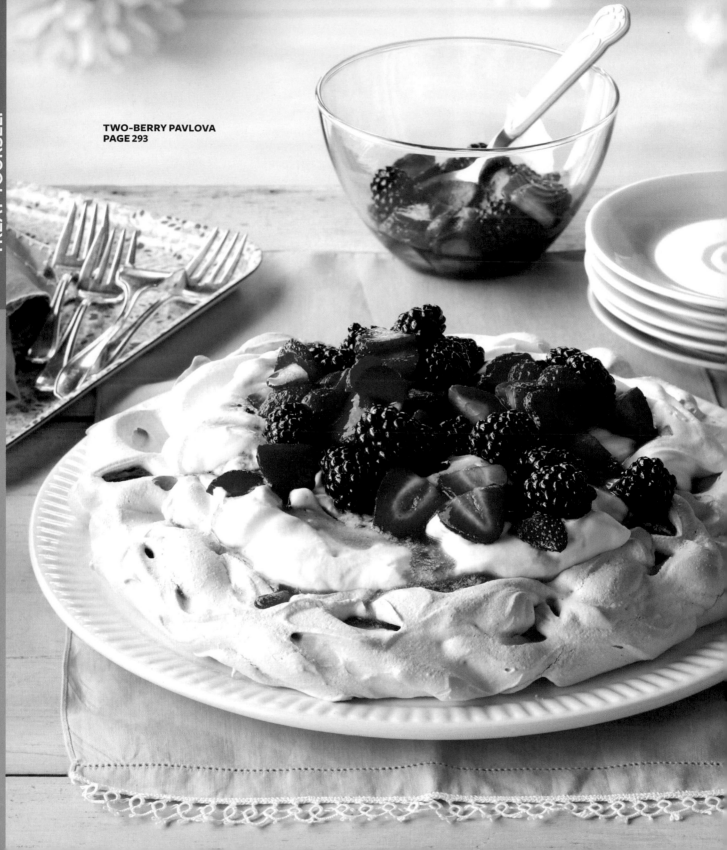

TWO-BERRY PAVLOVA
PAGE 293

Treat Yourself

It's a misconception that people on a diabetic diet can't enjoy dessert. Like everything else, it's all about making the right choices. These lightened-up recipes for cookies, cakes and more help you satisfy that sweet tooth while staying on top of your healthy habits.

CREAM CHEESE SWIRL BROWNIES

I'm a chocolate lover, and this treat has satisfied my cravings many times. No one guesses the brownies are light because their chewy texture and rich chocolate taste can't be beat.

—HEIDI JOHNSON WORLAND, WY

PREP: 20 MIN. • **BAKE:** 25 MIN.
MAKES: 1 DOZEN

- 3 large eggs, divided
- 6 tablespoons reduced-fat butter, softened
- 1 cup sugar, divided
- 3 teaspoons vanilla extract
- ½ cup all-purpose flour
- ¼ cup baking cocoa
- 1 package (8 ounces) reduced-fat cream cheese

1. Preheat oven to 350°. Separate two eggs, putting each white in a separate bowl (discard yolks or save for another use); set aside. In a small bowl, beat butter and ¾ cup sugar until crumbly. Beat in the whole egg, one egg white and vanilla until well combined. Combine flour and cocoa; gradually add to egg mixture until blended. Pour into a 9-in. square baking pan coated with cooking spray; set aside.

2. In a small bowl, beat cream cheese and remaining sugar until smooth. Beat in second egg white. Drop by rounded tablespoonfuls over the batter; cut through batter with a knife to swirl.

3. Bake 25-30 minutes or until set and edges pull away from sides of pan. Cool on a wire rack.

Per brownie: 172 cal., 8g fat (5g sat. fat), 36mg chol., 145mg sod., 23g carb. (18g sugars, 0 fiber), 4g pro.
Diabetic Exchanges: 1½ starch, 1½ fat.

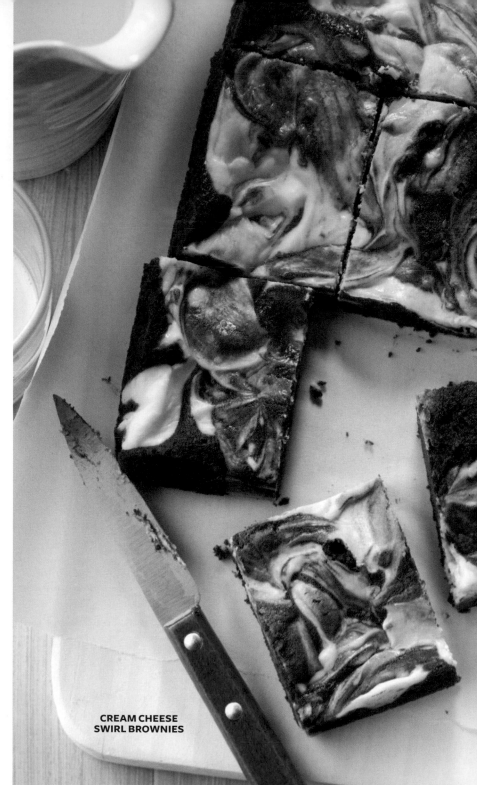

CREAM CHEESE
SWIRL BROWNIES

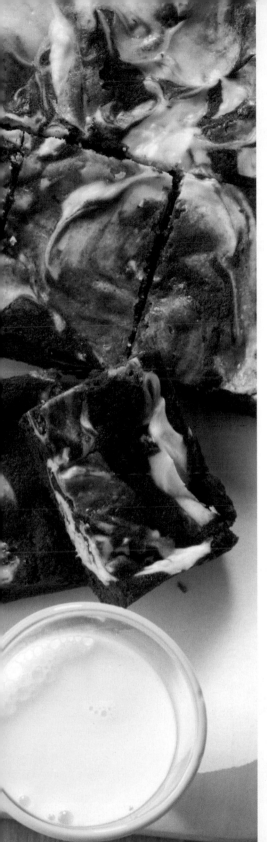

BUTTERMILK PEACH ICE CREAM

My mother's family owned peach orchards in Missouri. I live in Tennessee, a top consumer of buttermilk. This summery ice cream combines my past and present.

—KIM HIGGINBOTHAM KNOXVILLE, TN

PREP: 15 MIN. + CHILLING
PROCESS: 30 MIN./BATCH + FREEZING
MAKES: 2 QUARTS

- 2 pounds ripe peaches (about 7 medium), peeled and quartered
- ½ cup sugar
- ½ cup packed brown sugar
- 1 tablespoon lemon juice
- 1 teaspoon vanilla extract
  Pinch salt
- 2 cups buttermilk
- 1 cup heavy whipping cream

1. Place peaches in a food processor; process until smooth. Add sugars, lemon juice, vanilla and salt; process until blended.

2. In a bowl, mix buttermilk and cream. Stir in the peach mixture. Refrigerate, covered, 1 hour or until cold.

3. Fill cylinder of ice cream maker no more than two-thirds full. Freeze according to manufacturer's directions, refrigerating any remaining mixture to process later. Transfer ice cream to freezer containers, allowing headspace for expansion. Freeze 2-4 hours or until firm. Let ice cream stand at room temperature 10 minutes before serving.

Per ½ cup: 137 cal., 6g fat (4g sat. fat), 22mg chol., 75mg sod., 20g carb. (19g sugars, 1g fiber), 2g pro.
Diabetic Exchanges: 1 starch, 1 fat.

FAST FIX

SAUCY SPICED PEARS

We serve these tangy, saucy pears over angel food cake, pound cake or with a little yogurt or vanilla ice cream. Sprinkle with a favorite topping.

—JOY ZACHARIA CLEARWATER, FL

START TO FINISH: 20 MIN.
MAKES: 4 SERVINGS

- ½ cup orange juice
- 2 tablespoons butter
- 2 tablespoons sugar
- 2 teaspoons lemon juice
- 1 teaspoon vanilla extract
- 1 teaspoon ground ginger
- ¼ teaspoon ground cinnamon
- ⅛ teaspoon salt
- ⅛ teaspoon ground allspice
- ⅛ teaspoon cayenne pepper, optional
- 3 large Bosc pears (about 1¾ pounds), cored, peeled and sliced
  Thinly sliced fresh mint leaves, optional

1. In a large skillet, combine the first nine ingredients and, if desired, cayenne. Cook over medium-high heat 1-2 minutes or until butter is melted, stirring occasionally.

2. Add pears; bring to a boil. Reduce heat to medium; cook, uncovered, 3-4 minutes or until sauce is slightly thickened and pears are crisp-tender, stirring occasionally. Cool slightly. If desired, top with mint.

Per ¾ cup: 192 cal., 6g fat (4g sat. fat), 15mg chol., 130mg sod., 36g carb. (26g sugars, 5g fiber), 1g pro.
Diabetic Exchanges: 1 starch, 1 fruit, 1 fat.

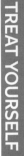

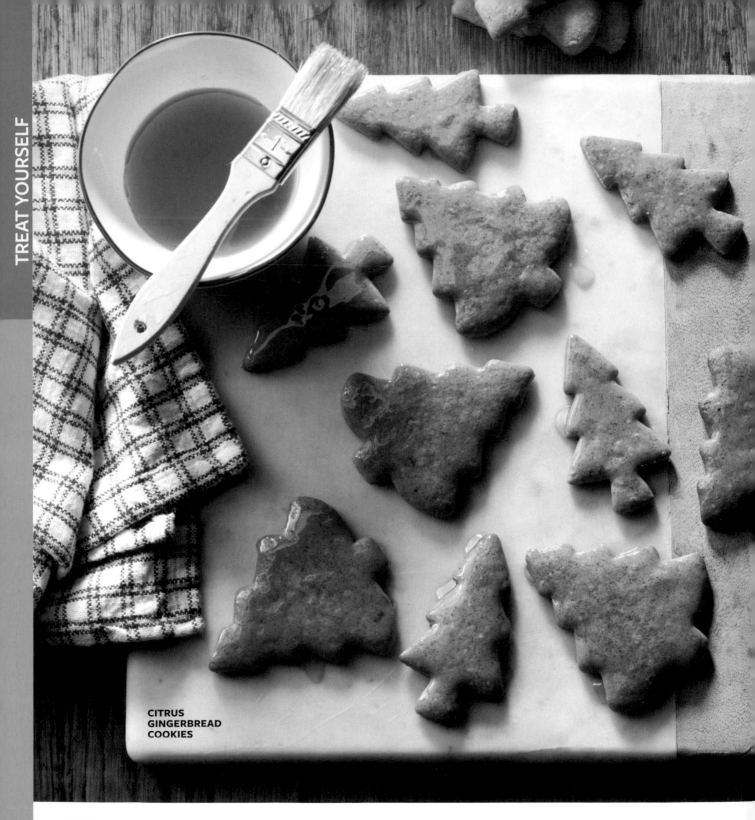

CITRUS
GINGERBREAD
COOKIES

CITRUS GINGERBREAD COOKIES

Orange and lemon zest give gingerbread cutouts a refreshing twist. Brushing a honey glaze over the top adds a subtle shine and extra touch of sweetness.

—**MONIQUE HOOKER** DESOTO, WI

PREP: 40 MIN. + CHILLING
BAKE: 10 MIN./BATCH + COOLING
MAKES: 6 DOZEN

- ¾ cup sugar
- ½ cup honey
- ½ cup molasses
- ½ cup unsalted butter, cubed
- 1 large egg
- 3½ cups all-purpose flour
- ¼ cup ground almonds
- 2 teaspoons baking powder
- 2 teaspoons grated lemon peel
- 2 teaspoons grated orange peel
- 1 teaspoon each ground cardamom, ginger, nutmeg, cinnamon and cloves

GLAZE

- ½ cup honey
- 2 tablespoons water

1. In a large saucepan, combine sugar, honey and molasses. Bring to a boil; remove from heat. Let stand about 20 minutes. Stir in butter; let stand 20 minutes longer.

2. Beat in egg. In another bowl, whisk flour, almonds, baking powder, lemon peel, orange peel and spices; gradually beat into sugar mixture. Refrigerate, covered, 8 hours or overnight.

3. Preheat oven to 375°. On a lightly floured surface, divide dough into three portions. Roll each portion to ¼-in. thickness. Cut with a floured 2-in. tree-shaped cookie cutter. Place 2 in. apart on baking sheets coated with cooking spray.

4. Bake 7-8 minutes or until lightly browned. Cool on pans 1 minute. Remove cookies to wire racks to cool completely. In a small bowl, mix glaze ingredients; brush over cookies. Let stand until set.

Note: Dough can be made 2 days in advance. Simply wrap in plastic wrap and place in a resealable bag. Store in the refrigerator.

To freeze: Freeze undecorated cookies in freezer containers. To use, thaw in covered containers and decorate as directed.

Per cookie: 66 cal., 2g fat (1g sat. fat), 6mg chol., 13mg sod., 12g carb. (7g sugars, 0 fiber), 1g pro.

Diabetic Exchanges: 1 starch, ½ fat.

TWO-BERRY PAVLOVA

Here's an airy dessert that I tried in Ireland. My kids love to build their own Pavlova with their favorite fruits.

—**NORMA STEVENSON** EAGAN, MN

PREP: 20 MIN. + STANDING
BAKE: 45 MIN. + COOLING
MAKES: 12 SERVINGS

- 4 large egg whites
- ½ teaspoon cream of tartar
- 1 cup sugar
- 1 tablespoon cornstarch
- 1 teaspoon lemon juice

TOPPINGS

- 2 cups fresh blackberries
- 2 cups sliced fresh strawberries
- ¼ cup plus 3 tablespoons sugar, divided
- 1¼ cups heavy whipping cream

1. Place egg whites in a large bowl; let stand at room temperature 30 minutes. Meanwhile, line a baking sheet with parchment paper; draw a 10-in. circle on paper. Invert paper.

2. Preheat oven to 300°. Add cream of tartar to egg whites; beat on medium speed until soft peaks form. Gradually add sugar, 1 tablespoon at a time, beating on high after each addition until sugar is dissolved. Continue beating until stiff glossy peaks form. Fold in cornstarch and lemon juice.

3. Spoon meringue onto prepared pan; with the back of a spoon, shape into a 10-in. circle, forming a shallow well in the center. Bake 45-55 minutes or until meringue is set and dry. Turn off oven (do not open oven door); leave meringue in oven 1 hour. Remove from oven; cool completely on baking sheet.

4. To serve, toss berries with ¼ cup sugar in a small bowl; let stand about 10 minutes. Meanwhile, in a large bowl, beat cream until it begins to thicken. Add remaining sugar; beat until soft peaks form.

5. Remove meringue from parchment paper; place on a serving plate. Spoon the whipped cream over top, forming a slight well in the center. Top with the berries.

Per serving: 208 cal., 9g fat (6g sat. fat), 34mg chol., 29mg sod., 30g carb. (27g sugars, 2g fiber), 2g pro.

Diabetic Exchanges: 2 starch, 2 fat.

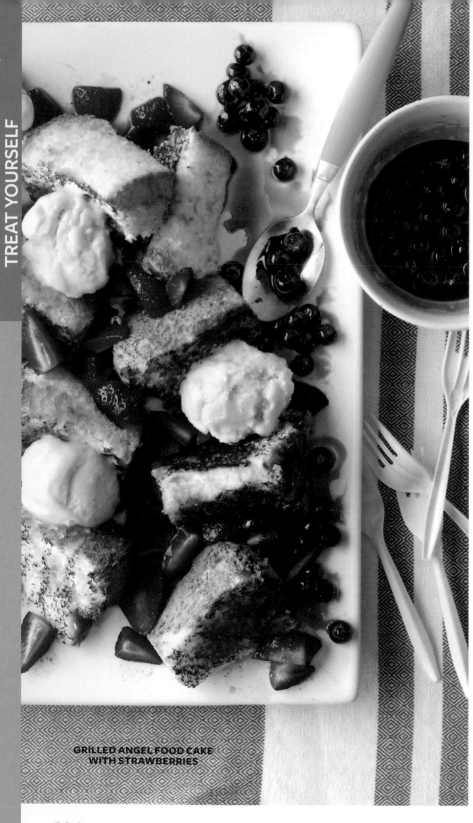

GRILLED ANGEL FOOD CAKE WITH STRAWBERRIES

(5)INGREDIENTS **FAST FIX**

GRILLED ANGEL FOOD CAKE WITH STRAWBERRIES

One night I goofed, accidentally using the balsamic butter I save for grilling chicken on my pound cake. What a delicious mistake that my entire family loved! For a patriotic look, add a drizzle of blueberry syrup.

—TAMMY HATHAWAY
FREEMAN TOWNSHIP, ME

START TO FINISH: 15 MIN.
MAKES: 8 SERVINGS

2 cups sliced fresh strawberries
2 teaspoons sugar
3 tablespoons butter, melted
2 tablespoons balsamic vinegar
8 slices angel food cake (about 1 ounce each)
Reduced-fat vanilla ice cream and blueberries in syrup, optional

1. In a bowl, toss strawberries with sugar. In another bowl, mix butter and vinegar; brush over cut sides of cake.
2. On a greased rack, grill cake, uncovered, over medium heat about 1-2 minutes on each side or until golden brown. Serve cake with the strawberries and, if desired, the ice cream and syrup.
Per 1 cake slice with ¼ cup strawberries without ice cream and syrup: 132 cal., 5g fat (3g sat. fat), 11mg chol., 247mg sod., 22g carb. (4g sugars, 1g fiber), 2g pro.
Diabetic Exchanges: 1½ starch, 1 fat.

PEANUT BUTTER SNACK BARS

Store-bought granola bars are full of sugar, so I came up with this nutritious version that my kids love. We like to bring these snacks on road trips.

—**NETTIE HOGAN** WADSWORTH, OH

PREP: 25 MIN. + COOLING
MAKES: 3 DOZEN

- 3¼ cups Kashi Heart to Heart honey toasted oat cereal
- 2¾ cups old-fashioned oats
- 1 cup unblanched almonds
- ½ cup sunflower kernels
- ¼ cup ground flaxseed
- ¼ cup uncooked oat bran cereal
- ¼ cup wheat bran
- ¼ cup whole flaxseed
- 3 tablespoons sesame seeds
- 2 cups creamy peanut butter
- 1½ cups honey
- 1 teaspoon vanilla extract

1. In a large bowl, combine the first nine ingredients. In a small saucepan, combine peanut butter and honey. Cook over medium heat until peanut butter is melted, stirring occasionally. Remove from the heat. Stir in vanilla. Pour over cereal mixture; mix well.

2. Transfer to a greased 15x10x1-in. baking pan; gently press into pan. Cool completely. Cut into bars. Store in an airtight container.

Note: Look for oat bran cereal near the hot cereals or in the natural foods section of the supermarket.

Per bar: 215 cal., 12g fat (2g sat. fat), 0 chol., 87mg sod., 24g carb. (14g sugars, 3g fiber), 7g pro.
Diabetic Exchanges: 1½ starch, 1 high-fat meat.

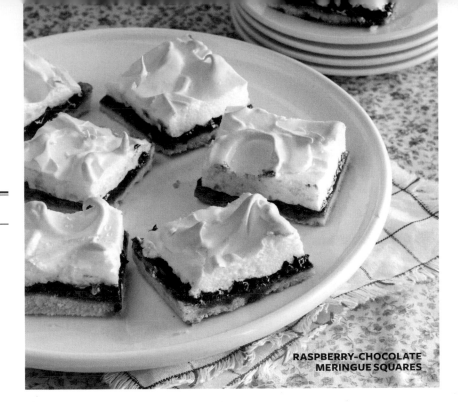

RASPBERRY-CHOCOLATE MERINGUE SQUARES

RASPBERRY-CHOCOLATE MERINGUE SQUARES

My family loves all sorts of cookies, like this luscious treat with a buttery crust, raspberry jam, chocolate and meringue. Bake it for a buffet, party or treat.

—**NANCY HEISHMAN** LAS VEGAS, NV

PREP: 15 MIN. • **BAKE:** 20 MIN. + COOLING
MAKES: 9 SERVINGS

- 3 large egg whites, divided
- ¼ cup butter, softened
- ¼ cup confectioners' sugar
- 1 cup all-purpose flour
- ¼ cup sugar
- ½ cup seedless raspberry jam
- 3 tablespoons miniature semisweet chocolate chips

1. Preheat oven to 350°. Place two egg whites in a small bowl; let stand at room temperature 30 minutes. Meanwhile, in a large bowl, cream the butter and confectioners' sugar until light and fluffy. Beat in remaining egg white; gradually add flour to creamed mixture, mixing well.

2. Press into a greased 8-in. square baking pan. Bake 9-11 minutes or until lightly browned. Increase oven setting to 400°.

3. With clean beaters, beat reserved egg whites on medium speed until foamy. Gradually add the sugar, 1 tablespoon at a time, beating on high after each addition until sugar is dissolved. Continue beating until stiff glossy peaks form. Spread jam over crust; sprinkle with chocolate chips. Spread meringue over top.

4. Bake 8-10 minutes or until meringue is lightly browned. Cool completely in pan on a wire rack.

Per bar: 198 cal., 6g fat (4g sat. fat), 14mg chol., 60mg sod., 33g carb. (22g sugars, 1g fiber), 3g pro.
Diabetic Exchanges: 2 starch, 1 fat.

(5) INGREDIENTS

CHOCOLATE-DIPPED STRAWBERRY MERINGUE ROSES

Eat these kid-friendly treats as is, or crush them into a bowl of strawberries and whipped cream. Readers of my blog, utry.it, went nuts when I posted that idea!

—AMY TONG ANAHEIM, CA

PREP: 25 MIN.
BAKE: 40 MIN. + COOLING
MAKES: 3½ DOZEN

  3 **large egg whites**
 ¼ **cup sugar**
 ¼ **cup freeze-dried strawberries**
  1 **package (3 ounces) strawberry gelatin**
 ½ **teaspoon vanilla extract, optional**
  1 **cup 60% cacao bittersweet chocolate baking chips, melted**

1. Place egg whites in a large bowl; let stand at room temperature 30 minutes. Preheat oven to 225°.
2. Place sugar and strawberries in a food processor; process until powdery. Add gelatin; pulse to blend.
3. Beat egg whites on medium speed until foamy, adding vanilla if desired. Gradually add gelatin mixture, 1 tablespoon at a time, beating on high after each addition until sugar is dissolved. Continue beating until stiff glossy peaks form.
4. Cut a small hole in the tip of a pastry bag or in a corner of a food-safe plastic bag; insert a #1M star tip. Transfer meringue to bag. Pipe 2-in. roses 1½ in. apart onto parchment paper-lined baking sheets.
5. Bake 40-45 minutes or until set and dry. Turn off oven (do not open oven door); leave meringues in oven 1½ hours. Remove from oven; cool completely on baking sheets.
6. Remove meringues from paper. Dip bottoms in melted chocolate; allow excess to drip off. Place on waxed paper; let stand until set, about 45 minutes. Store in an airtight container at room temperature.

Per cookie: 33 cal., 1g fat (1g sat. fat), 0 chol., 9mg sod., 6g carb. (5g sugars, 0 fiber), 1g pro.
Diabetic Exchanges: ½ starch.

BAKED ELEPHANT EARS

My mother-in-law handed down this recipe from her mother. They're a special treat—even better, I think, than those at a carnival or festival.

—DELORES BAETEN DOWNERS GROVE, IL

PREP: 35 MIN. + CHILLING • **BAKE:** 10 MIN.
MAKES: 2 DOZEN

  1 **package (¼ ounce) active dry yeast**
 ¼ **cup warm water (110° to 115°)**
  2 **cups all-purpose flour**
4½ **teaspoons sugar**
 ½ **teaspoon salt**
 ⅓ **cup cold butter, cubed**
 ⅓ **cup fat-free milk**
  1 **large egg yolk**
FILLING
  2 **tablespoons butter, softened**
 ½ **cup sugar**
  2 **teaspoons ground cinnamon**
CINNAMON SUGAR
 ½ **cup sugar**
 ¾ **teaspoon ground cinnamon**

1. In a small bowl, dissolve yeast in warm water. In a large bowl, mix flour, sugar and salt; cut in butter until crumbly. Stir milk and egg yolk into yeast mixture; add to flour mixture, stirring to form a stiff dough (dough will be sticky). Cover with plastic wrap and refrigerate 2 hours.
2. Preheat oven to 375°. Turn dough onto a lightly floured surface; roll dough into an 18x10-in. rectangle. Spread with softened butter to within ¼ in. of edges. Mix sugar and cinnamon; sprinkle over butter. Roll up jelly-roll style, starting with a long side; pinch seam to seal. Cut crosswise into 24 slices. Cover slices with plastic wrap until ready to flatten.
3. In a small bowl, mix ingredients for cinnamon sugar. Place a 6-in.-square piece of waxed paper on a work surface; sprinkle with ½ teaspoon cinnamon sugar. Top with one slice of dough; sprinkle dough with an additional ½ teaspoon cinnamon sugar. Roll dough to a 4-in. circle. Using waxed paper, flip dough onto a baking sheet coated with cooking spray. Repeat with remaining ingredients, placing slices 2 in. apart. Bake 7-9 minutes or until golden brown. Cool on wire racks.

Per elephant ear: 109 cal., 4g fat (2g sat. fat), 18mg chol., 76mg sod., 18g carb. (9g sugars, 0 fiber), 1g pro.
Diabetic Exchanges: 1 starch, ½ fat,

✳

DID YOU KNOW?
Also called "beaver tails" or simply "fried dough," elephant ears are popular fair food. Another favorite is funnel cakes. What's the difference? While elephant ears are large pieces of dough that are flattened and fried, funnel cakes are made by piping long strands of dough into hot oil.

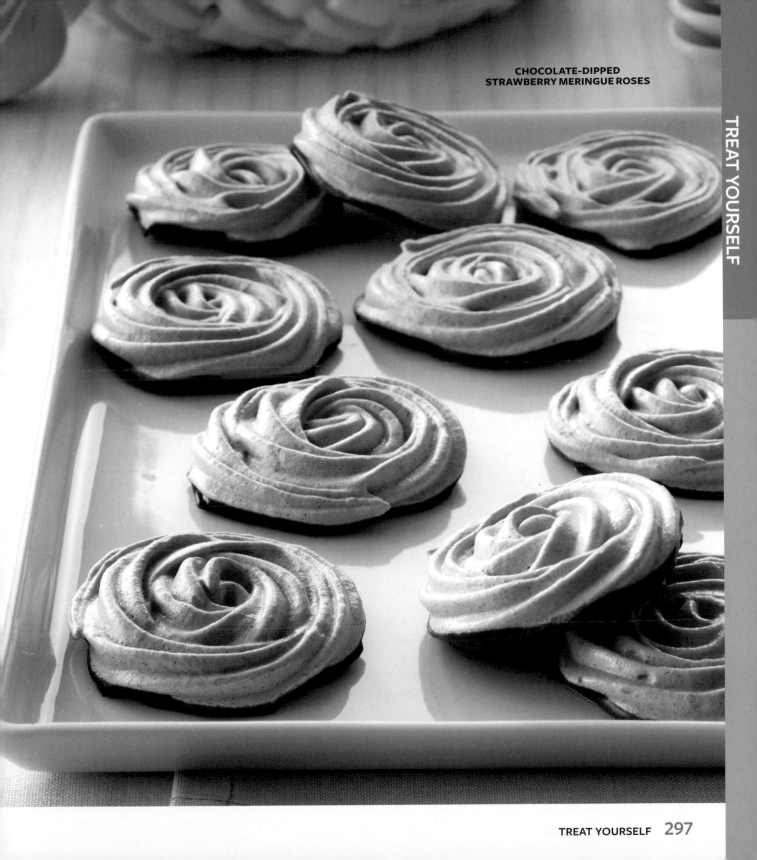

**CHOCOLATE-DIPPED
STRAWBERRY MERINGUE ROSES**

LEMON CUPCAKES WITH STRAWBERRY FROSTING

I sometimes call these my Triple Lemon Whammy Cupcakes because they take full advantage of vibrant citrus flavor. Strawberries really nudge this dessert over the top!

—**EMMA SISK** PLYMOUTH, MN

PREP: 20 MIN.
BAKE: 25 MIN. + COOLING
MAKES: 2 DOZEN

- 1 package white cake mix (regular size)
- ¼ cup lemon curd
- 3 tablespoons lemon juice
- 3 teaspoons grated lemon peel
- ½ cup butter, softened
- 3½ cups confectioners' sugar
- ¼ cup seedless strawberry jam
- 2 tablespoons 2% milk
- 1 cup sliced fresh strawberries

1. Line 24 muffin cups with paper liners. Prepare cake mix batter according to package directions, decreasing water by 1 tablespoon and adding lemon curd, lemon juice and lemon peel before mixing batter. Fill the prepared cups about two-thirds full. Bake and cool cupcakes as the package directs.

2. In a large bowl, beat the butter, confectioners' sugar, jam and milk until smooth. Frost cooled cupcakes; top with strawberries. Refrigerate leftovers.

Per cupcake: 219 cal., 7g fat (3g sat. fat), 13mg chol., 171mg sod., 23g carb. (29g sugars, 0 fiber), 1g pro.
Diabetic Exchanges: 1½ starch, 1½ fat.

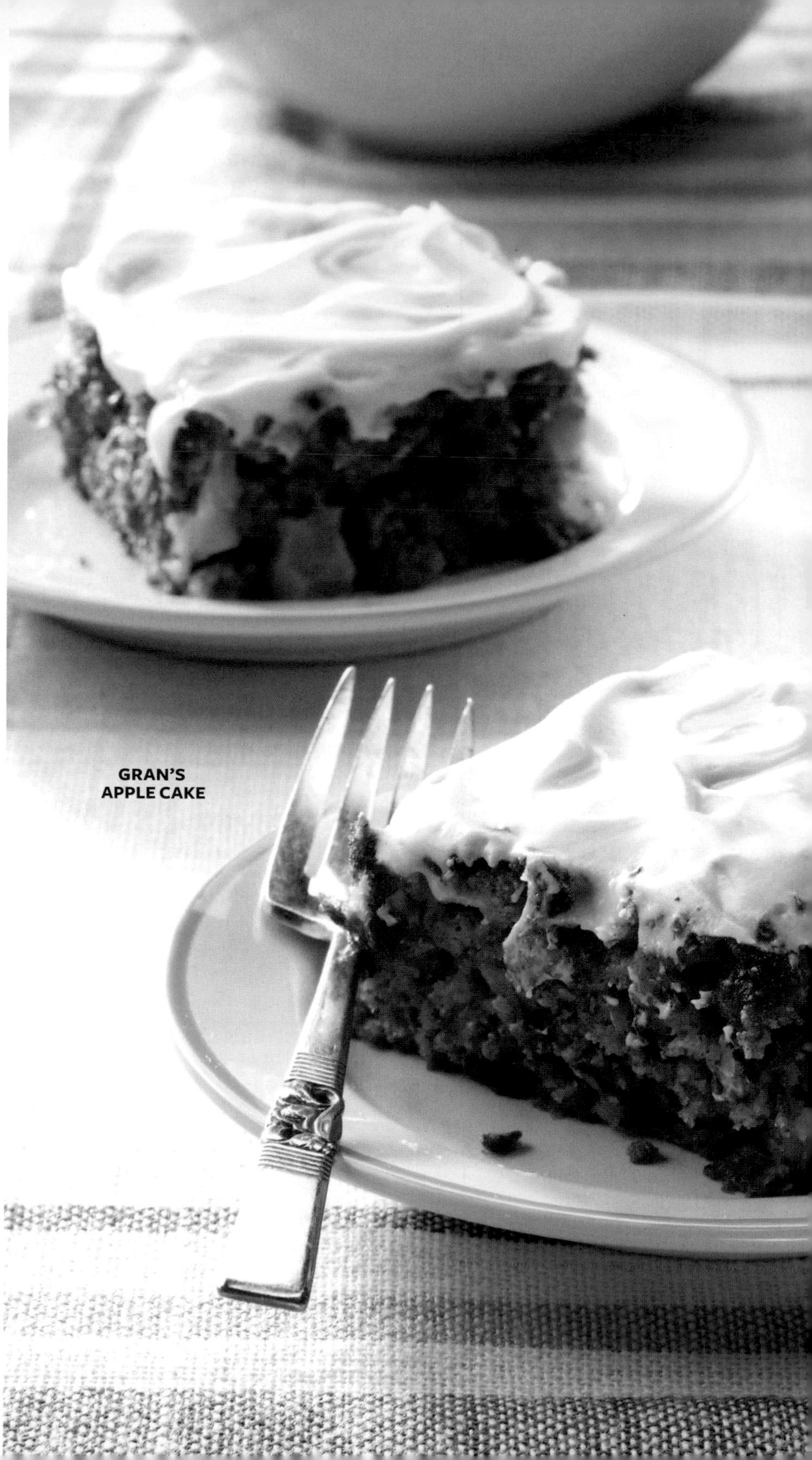

GRAN'S APPLE CAKE

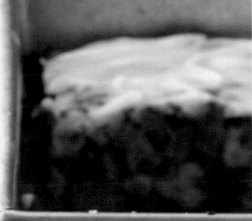

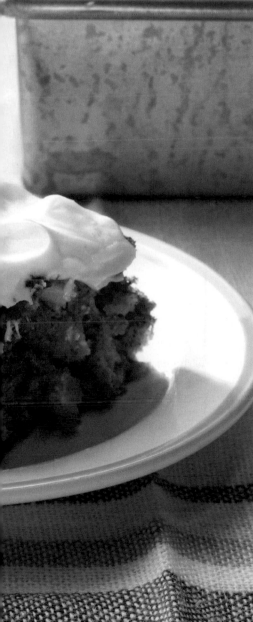

GRAN'S APPLE CAKE

My grandmother occasionally brought over a wonderful cake warm from the oven. The spicy apple flavor combined with the sweet cream cheese frosting made this dessert a treasured recipe. Even though I've lightened it up, it's still a family favorite.

—LAURIS CONRAD TURLOCK, CA

PREP: 20 MIN. • **BAKE:** 35 MIN. + COOLING
MAKES: 18 SERVINGS

- 1⅔ cups sugar
- 2 large eggs
- ½ cup unsweetened applesauce
- 2 tablespoons canola oil
- 2 teaspoons vanilla extract
- 2 cups all-purpose flour
- 2 teaspoons baking soda
- 2 teaspoons ground cinnamon
- ¾ teaspoon salt
- 6 cups chopped peeled tart apples
- ½ cup chopped pecans

FROSTING
- 4 ounces reduced-fat cream cheese
- 2 tablespoons butter, softened
- 1 teaspoon vanilla extract
- 1 cup confectioners' sugar

1. Preheat oven to 350°. Coat a 13x9-in. baking pan with cooking spray.
2. In a large bowl, beat sugar, eggs, applesauce, oil and vanilla until well blended. In another bowl, whisk flour, baking soda, cinnamon and salt; gradually beat into sugar mixture. Fold in apples and pecans.
3. Transfer to prepared pan. Bake 35-40 minutes or until top is golden brown and a toothpick inserted in center comes out clean. Cool completely in pan on a wire rack.
4. In a small bowl, beat cream cheese, butter and vanilla until smooth. Gradually beat in confectioners' sugar (mixture will be soft). Spread over cake. Refrigerate leftovers.

Per piece: 241 cal., 7g fat (2g sat. fat), 29mg chol., 284mg sod., 42g carb. (30g sugars, 1g fiber), 3g pro.
Diabetic Exchanges: 2 starch, 1-½ fat, 1 fruit.

★ ★ ★ ★ ★ **READER REVIEW**

"This is a delicious cake. Our favorite! I used Chehalis apples from our tree, and it turned out moist and full of apple flavor. The cream cheese frosting is yummy, too."

CHERIE_HILL TASTEOFHOME.COM

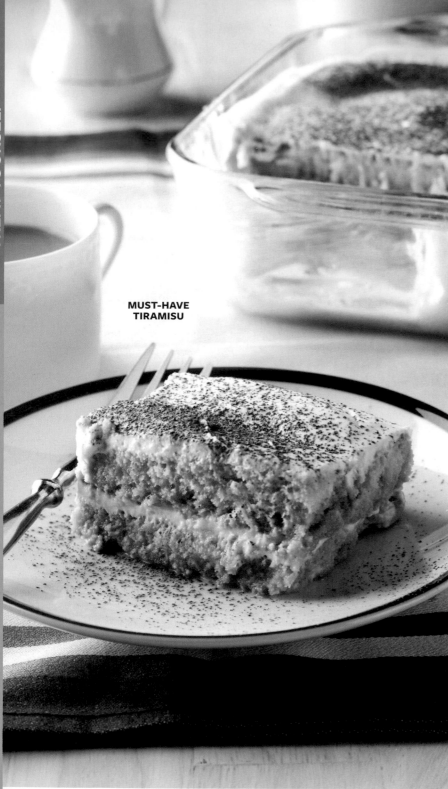

MUST-HAVE TIRAMISU

MUST-HAVE TIRAMISU

This is the perfect guilt-free version of a classic dessert. My friends even say that they prefer my healthy recipe over traditional tiramisu.

—**ALE GAMBINI** BEVERLY HILLS, CA

PREP: 25 MIN. + CHILLING
MAKES: 9 SERVINGS

½ cup heavy whipping cream
2 cups (16 ounces) vanilla yogurt
1 cup fat-free milk
½ cup brewed espresso or strong coffee, cooled
24 crisp ladyfinger cookies
    Baking cocoa
    Fresh raspberries, optional

1. In a small bowl, beat cream until stiff peaks form; fold in yogurt. Spread ½ cup cream mixture onto bottom of an 8-in. square dish.

2. In a shallow dish, mix milk and espresso. Quickly dip 12 ladyfingers into coffee mixture, allowing excess to drip off. Arrange in dish in a single layer, breaking to fit as needed. Top with half of the remaining cream mixture; dust with cocoa. Repeat layers.

3. Refrigerate, covered, at least 2 hours before serving. If desired, serve with the raspberries.

Per piece without raspberries:
178 cal., 6g fat (4g sat. fat), 45mg chol., 82mg sod., 25g carb. (18g sugars, 0 fiber), 5g pro.
Diabetic Exchanges: 1 starch, 1 fat, ½ fat-free milk.

SUPER SPUD BROWNIES

These moist and cake-like brownies came from my mom's old cookbook. Mashed potatoes may seem like an unusual ingredient, but this recipe took first place at a local festival.

—MARLENE GERER DENTON, MT

PREP: 15 MIN. • **BAKE:** 25 MIN.
MAKES: 16 SERVINGS

- ¾ cup mashed potatoes
- ½ cup sugar
- ½ cup packed brown sugar
- ½ cup canola oil
- 2 large eggs, lightly beaten
- 1 teaspoon vanilla extract
- ½ cup all-purpose flour
- ⅓ cup cocoa powder
- ½ teaspoon baking powder
- ⅛ teaspoon salt
- ½ cup chopped pecans, optional
  Confectioners' sugar

1. In a large bowl, combine the mashed potatoes, sugars, oil, eggs and vanilla. Combine the flour, cocoa, baking powder and salt; gradually add to potato mixture. Fold in pecans if desired. Transfer to a greased 9-in. square baking pan.

2. Bake at 350° for 23-27 minutes or until toothpick inserted near the center comes out clean. Cool on a wire rack. Dust with confectioners' sugar.

Per brownie without nuts: 150 cal., 8g fat (1g sat. fat), 27mg chol., 68mg sod., 19g carb. (13g sugars, 0 fiber), 2g pro.
Diabetic Exchanges: 1½ fat, 1 starch.

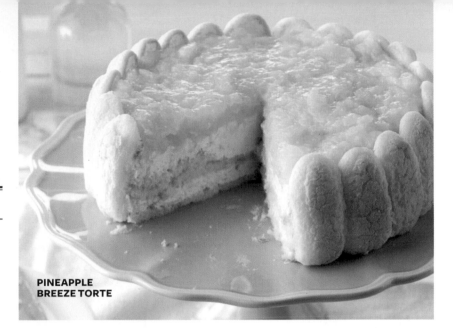

PINEAPPLE BREEZE TORTE

PINEAPPLE BREEZE TORTE

This lovely torte features ladyfingers, a creamy filling and a crushed pineapple topping. It's a special treat for my large family and a must at Christmas.

—BARBARA JOYNER FRANKLIN, VA

PREP: 25 MIN. + CHILLING
COOK: 5 MIN. + COOLING
MAKES: 12 SERVINGS

- 3 packages (3 ounces each) soft ladyfingers, split

FILLING

- 1 package (8 ounces) fat-free cream cheese
- 3 ounces cream cheese, softened
- ⅓ cup sugar
- 2 teaspoons vanilla extract
- 1 carton (8 ounces) frozen reduced-fat whipped topping, thawed

TOPPING

- ⅓ cup sugar
- 3 tablespoons cornstarch
- 1 can (20 ounces) unsweetened crushed pineapple, undrained

1. Line bottom and sides of an ungreased 9-In. springform pan with ladyfinger halves; reserve remaining ladyfingers for layering.

2. Beat cream cheeses, sugar and vanilla until smooth; fold in whipped topping. Spread half of the mixture over bottom ladyfingers. Layer with the remaining ladyfingers, overlapping as needed. Spread with the remaining filling. Refrigerate, covered, while preparing topping.

3. In a small saucepan, mix sugar and cornstarch; stir in pineapple. Bring to a boil over medium heat, stirring constantly; cook and stir until thickened, 1-2 minutes. Cool the mixture completely.

4. Spread topping gently over torte. Refrigerate, covered, until set, at least 4 hours. Remove rim from pan.

Per slice: 243 cal., 7g fat (5g sat. fat), 87mg chol., 156mg sod., 39g carb. (27g sugars, 1g fiber), 6g pro.
Diabetic Exchanges: 2 starch, 1½ fat, ½ fruit.

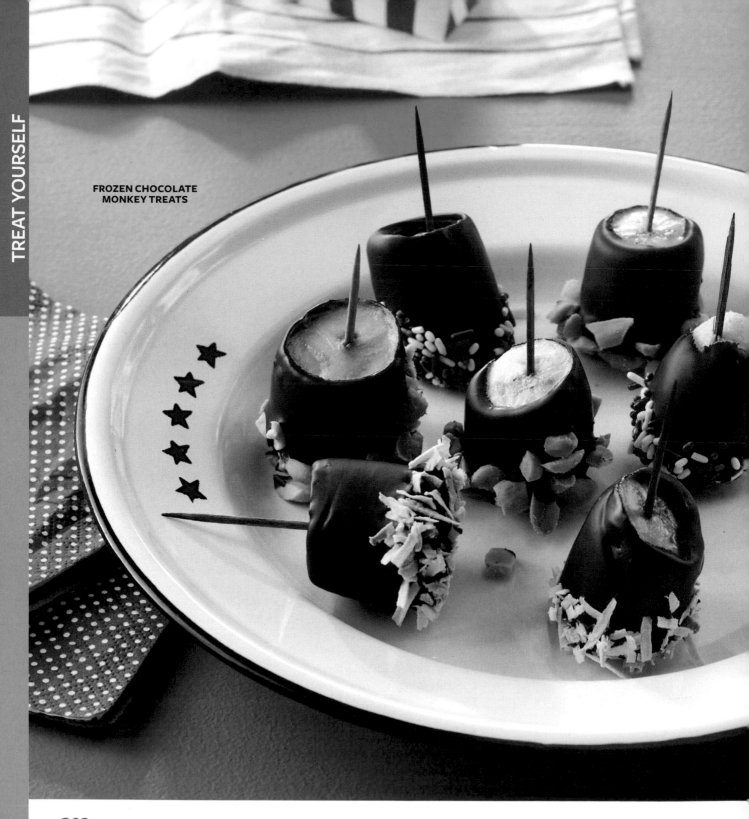

**FROZEN CHOCOLATE
MONKEY TREATS**

[5] INGREDIENTS
FROZEN CHOCOLATE MONKEY TREATS

Everyone needs a fun, friendly way for kids young and old to play with food. When you coat bananas in chocolate and dip them into peanuts, sprinkles or coconut, you get nutty, yummy bites.
—SUSAN HEIN BURLINGTON, WI

PREP: 20 MIN. + FREEZING
MAKES: 1½ DOZEN

- 3 medium bananas
- 1 cup (6 ounces) dark chocolate chips
- 2 teaspoons shortening
  Toppings: chopped peanuts, toasted flaked coconut and/or colored jimmies

1. Cut each banana into six pieces (about 1 in.). Insert a toothpick into each piece; transfer to a waxed paper-lined baking sheet. Freeze until completely firm, about 1 hour.

2. In a microwave, melt chocolate and shortening; stir until smooth. Dip banana pieces in chocolate mixture; allow excess to drip off. Dip in toppings as desired; return to baking sheet. Freeze 30 minutes before serving.

Note: To toast coconut, bake in a shallow pan in a 350° oven for about 5-10 minutes or cook in a skillet over low heat until golden brown, stirring occasionally.

Per treat without toppings: 72 cal., 4g fat (2g sat. fat), 0 chol., 0 sod., 10g carb. (7g sugars, 1g fiber), 1g pro.
Diabetic Exchanges: 1 fat, ½ starch.

STRAWBERRY POT STICKERS

My wife and daughter love this unusual dessert. I combined my favorite flavors—strawberries with chocolate and cinnamon—with my favorite dim sum dish to create this surprise combo.
—RICK BROWNE RIDGEFIELD, WA

PREP: 30 MIN. + COOLING
COOK: 10 MIN./BATCH
MAKES: 32 POT STICKERS (⅔ CUP SAUCE)

- 3 ounces milk chocolate, chopped
- ¼ cup half-and-half cream
- 1 teaspoon butter
- 1 teaspoon vanilla extract
- ¼ teaspoon ground cinnamon

POT STICKERS

- 2 cups chopped fresh strawberries
- 3 ounces milk chocolate, chopped
- 1 tablespoon brown sugar
- ¼ teaspoon ground cinnamon
- 32 pot sticker or gyoza wrappers
- 1 large egg, lightly beaten
- 2 tablespoons canola oil, divided
- ½ cup water, divided

1. Place chocolate in a small bowl. In a small saucepan, bring cream and butter just to a boil. Pour over chocolate; whisk until smooth. Stir in vanilla and cinnamon. Cool to room temperature, stirring occasionally.

✱

TEST KITCHEN TIP
Have leftover pot sticker wrappers? Have fun experimenting with other sweet sensations. Try spiced apples, bananas and cream cheese, Nutella and raspberries, or mascarpone and apricots. Dust with powdered or cinnamon sugar—or create a sweet dipping sauce to serve on the side.

2. For pot stickers, in a small bowl, toss strawberries and chopped chocolate with brown sugar and cinnamon. Place 1 tablespoon mixture in center of 1 gyoza wrapper. (Cover remaining wrappers with a damp paper towel until ready to use.)

3. Moisten wrapper edge with egg. Fold wrapper over filling; seal edges, pleating the front side several times to form a pleated pouch. Repeat with remaining wrappers and filling. Stand pot stickers on a work surface to flatten bottoms; curve slightly to form crescent shapes, if desired.

4. In a large skillet, heat 1 tablespoon oil over medium-high heat. Arrange half of the pot stickers, flat side down, in concentric circles in pan; cook 1-2 minutes or until bottoms are golden brown. Add ¼ cup water; bring to a simmer. Cook, covered, 3-5 minutes or until water is almost absorbed and wrappers are tender.

5. Cook, uncovered, 1 minute or until bottoms are crisp and the water is completely evaporated. Repeat with remaining pot stickers. Serve the pot stickers with chocolate sauce.

Per 1 pot sticker with 1 teaspoon sauce: 58 cal., 3g fat (1g sat. fat), 6mg chol., 18mg sod., 8g carb. (4g sugars, 0 fiber), 1g pro.
Diabetic Exchanges: ½ starch, ½ fat.

BANANA-PINEAPPLE CREAM PIES

RASPBERRY-BANANA SOFT SERVE

(5) INGREDIENTS

When I make this ice cream, I mix bananas for their ripeness. Very ripe ones add more banana flavor; less ripe ones have a fluffier texture.

—**MELISSA HANSEN** MILWAUKEE, WI

PREP: 10 MIN. + FREEZING
MAKES: 2½ CUPS

- 4 medium ripe bananas
- ½ cup fat-free plain yogurt
- 1 to 2 tablespoons maple syrup
- ½ cup frozen unsweetened raspberries
  Fresh raspberries, optional

1. Thinly slice bananas; transfer to a large resealable plastic freezer bag. Arrange slices in a single layer; freeze overnight.

2. Pulse bananas in a food processor until finely chopped. Add yogurt, maple syrup and raspberries. Process just until smooth, scraping sides as needed. Serve immediately, adding fresh berries if desired.

Per ½ cup: 104 cal., 0 fat (0 sat. fat), 1mg chol., 15mg sod., 26g carb. (15g sugars, 2g fiber), 2g pro.
Diabetic Exchanges: 1 fruit, ½ starch.

BANANA-PINEAPPLE CREAM PIES

My mother gave me this simple and delicious recipe years ago. Because it makes two pies, it's perfect for a potluck. I've never met anyone who didn't like it!

—**ROBYN APPENZELLER** PORTSMOUTH, VA

PREP: 15 MIN. + CHILLING
MAKES: 2 PIES (8 SERVINGS EACH)

- ¼ cup cornstarch
- ¼ cup sugar
- 1 can (20 ounces) unsweetened crushed pineapple, undrained
- 3 medium bananas, sliced
  Two 9-inch graham cracker crusts (about 6 ounces each)
- 1 carton (8 ounces) frozen whipped topping, thawed

1. In a large saucepan, combine cornstarch and sugar. Stir in pineapple until blended. Bring to a boil; cook and stir 1-2 minutes or until thickened.

2. Arrange bananas over bottom of each crust; spread the pineapple mixture over tops. Refrigerate at least 1 hour before serving. Top with the whipped topping.

Per slice: 205 cal., 8g fat (3g sat. fat), 0 chol., 122mg sod., 33g carb. (23g sugars, 1g fiber), 1g pro.
Diabetic Exchanges: 2 starch, 1½ fat.

⑤ INGREDIENTS

FROZEN YOGURT FRUIT POPS

My grandson, Patrick, who's now in high school, was "Grammy's helper" for years. We made these frozen pops for company, and everyone, including the adults, loved them. They're delicious and good for you!

—JUNE DICKENSON PHILIPPI, WV

PREP: 15 MIN. + FREEZING
MAKES: 1 DOZEN

- 2¼ cups (18 ounces) raspberry yogurt
- 2 tablespoons lemon juice
- 2 medium ripe bananas, cut into chunks
- 12 freezer pop molds or 12 paper cups (3 ounces each) and wooden pop sticks

1. Place the yogurt, lemon juice and bananas in a blender; cover and process until smooth, stopping to stir mixture if necessary.

2. Pour mixture into molds or paper cups. Top molds with holders. If using cups, top with foil and insert sticks through foil. Freeze until firm.

Per fruit pop: 60 cal., 1g fat (0 sat. fat), 2mg chol., 23mg sod., 13g carb. (10g sugars, 1g fiber), 2g pro.
Diabetic Exchanges: 1 starch.

★★★★★ **READER REVIEW**

"So easy to make and tastes great, too. My toddler and I just love these pops."

LAURAMANNING TASTEOFHOME.COM

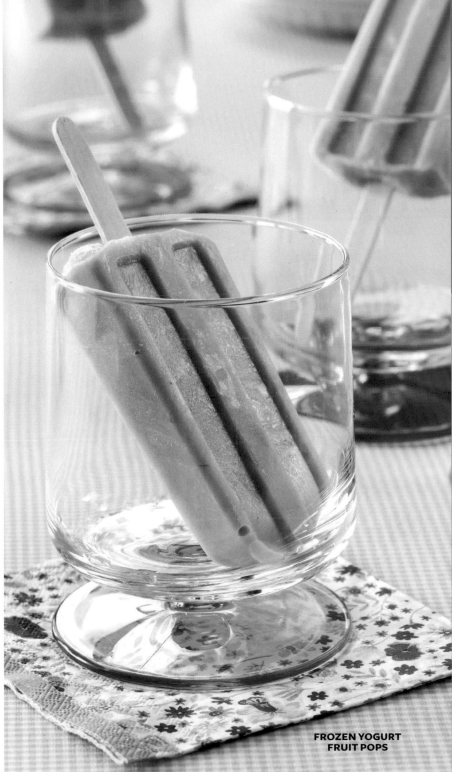

FROZEN YOGURT FRUIT POPS

CHOCOLATE-TOPPED
STRAWBERRY CHEESECAKE

CHOCOLATE-TOPPED STRAWBERRY CHEESECAKE

Creamy and airy, this gorgeous dessert is the perfect special something for a summer dinner party. I love the mix of smooth strawberry cheesecake and crumbly chocolate crust—and how elegant it looks on the table.

—KATHY BERGER DRY RIDGE, KY

PREP: 45 MIN. + CHILLING
MAKES: 12 SERVINGS

- 1-¼ cups chocolate graham cracker crumbs (about 9 whole crackers)
- ¼ cup butter, melted
- 16 ounces fresh or frozen strawberries, thawed
- 2 envelopes unflavored gelatin
- ½ cup cold water
- 2 packages (8 ounces each) fat-free cream cheese, cubed
- 1 cup fat-free cottage cheese
  Sugar substitute equivalent to ¾ cup sugar
- 1 carton (8 ounces) frozen reduced-fat whipped topping, thawed, divided
- ½ cup chocolate ice cream topping
- 1 cup quartered fresh strawberries

1. Preheat oven to 350°. Mix cracker crumbs and butter; press onto bottom and 1 in. up sides of a 9-in. springform pan coated with cooking spray. Place on a baking sheet. Bake until set, about 10 minutes. Cool on a wire rack.

2. Hull strawberries if necessary; puree in a food processor. Remove to a bowl. In a small saucepan, sprinkle gelatin over cold water; let stand 1 minute. Heat over low heat, stirring until gelatin is completely dissolved. In food processor, process cream cheese, cottage cheese and sugar substitute until smooth. While processing, gradually add gelatin mixture. Add strawberries; process until blended.

3. Transfer to a large bowl; fold in 2 cups whipped topping. Pour into crust. Refrigerate, covered, until set, 2-3 hours.

4. Loosen sides of cheesecake with a knife; remove rim from pan. Top with chocolate topping, remaining whipped topping and the quartered strawberries.

Note: This recipe was tested with Splenda no-calorie sweetener.

Per slice: 244 calories, 8g fat (5g saturated fat), 16mg cholesterol, 463mg sod., 29g carbohydrate (17g sugars, 2g fiber), 10g protein.
Diabetic Exchanges: 2 starch, 1½ fat.

GINGER PLUM TART

Sweet cravings, begone! This free-form tart is done in only 35 minutes. Plus, it's super-delicious when served warm.

—TASTE OF HOME TEST KITCHEN

PREP: 15 MIN. • **BAKE:** 20 MIN. + COOLING
MAKES: 8 SERVINGS

- 1 sheet refrigerated pie pastry
- 3½ cups sliced fresh plums (about 10 medium)
- 3 tablespoons plus 1 teaspoon coarse sugar, divided
- 1 tablespoon cornstarch
- 2 teaspoons finely chopped crystallized ginger
- 1 large egg white
- 1 tablespoon water

1. Preheat oven to 400°. On a work surface, unroll pastry sheet. Roll to a 12-in. circle. Transfer to a parchment paper-lined baking sheet.

2. In a large bowl, toss plums with 3 tablespoons sugar and cornstarch. Arrange plums on pastry to within 2 in. of edges; sprinkle with ginger. Fold the pastry edge over plums, pleating as you go.

3. In a small bowl, whisk egg white and water; brush over the folded pastry. Sprinkle with remaining sugar.

4. Bake 20-25 minutes or until the crust is golden brown. Cool in pan on a wire rack. Serve at room temperature.

Per piece: 190 cal., 7g fat (3g sat. fat), 5mg chol., 108mg sod., 30g carb. (14g sugars, 1g fiber), 2g pro.
Diabetic Exchanges: 1½ starch, 1 fat, ½ fruit.

FAST FIX

FRESH FRUIT SAUCE

I used to peel the fruit when making this sauce, but not anymore. The skins help hold the juicy summer fruit together when they are left on.

—KATIE KOZIOLEK HARTLAND, MN

PREP/TOTAL TIME: 10 MIN.
MAKES: 2¼ CUPS

- 1 tablespoon cornstarch
- 1 cup orange juice
- ⅓ cup honey
- 1 cup sliced fresh peaches
- 1 cup sliced fresh plums
  Vanilla ice cream

1. In a small saucepan, mix cornstarch and orange juice until smooth; stir in honey. Bring to a boil over medium heat; cook and stir until thickened, about 1 minute.

2. Remove from heat; stir in fruit. Serve warm over ice cream.

Per ¼ cup sauce: 71 cal., 0 fat (0 sat. fat), 0 chol., 1mg sod., 18g carb. (16g sugars, 1g fiber), 0 pro.
Diabetic Exchanges: 1 starch.

GENERAL RECIPE INDEX
Find every recipe by food category and major ingredient.

APPETIZERS & SNACKS
Artichoke Hummus, 41
Avocado Endive Boats, 45
Baked Pot Stickers with Dipping Sauce, 42
Balsamic-Goat Cheese Grilled Plums, 33
Blueberry Salsa, 38
Cheesy Snack Mix, 38
Chicken, Mango & Blue Cheese Tortillas, 33
Curried Chicken Meatball Wraps, 36
Fresh Fruit Salsa with Cinnamon Chips, 37
Garden-Fresh Wraps, 41
Garlicky Herbed Shrimp, 34
Gorgonzola Polenta Bites, 43
Homemade Guacamole, 40
Mango Avocado Spring Rolls, 34
Meatballs in Cherry Sauce, 38
Mini Feta Pizzas, 35
Mocha Pumpkin Seeds, 37
Pickled Shrimp with Basil, 46
Raisin & Hummus Pita Wedges, 42
Roasted Grape Crostini, 45
Roasted Red Pepper Tapenade, 33
Three-Pepper Guacamole, 47
Tomato-Jalapeno Granita, 45
Wicked Deviled Eggs, 46

APPLES & APPLE JUICE
Apple Spiced Tea, 17
Broccoli & Apple Salad, 81
Chilled Turkey Pasta Salad, 168
Ginger-Kale Smoothies, 19
Gran's Apple Cake, 299
Maple Apple Baked Oatmeal, 22
Waldorf Turkey Salad, 167
Wendy's Apple Pomegranate Salad, 85

APPLESAUCE
Chocolate Chocolate Chip Muffins, 287
Spicy Applesauce Fruit Bread, 287

ARTICHOKES
Artichoke Cod with Sun-Dried
  Tomatoes, 220
Artichoke Hummus, 41
Parmesan Chicken with Artichoke
  Hearts, 143
Spinach & Artichoke Pizza, 232

ARUGULA
Melon Arugula Salad with Ham, 192
Salmon & Spud Salad, 224

ASPARAGUS
Asparagus Beef Stir-Fry on Potatoes, 94
Asparagus-Mushroom Frittata, 23
Asparagus Turkey Stir-Fry, 166

AVOCADOS
Avocado Endive Boats, 45
Baby Kale Salad with Avocado-Lime
  Dressing, 77
Homemade Guacamole, 40
Mango Avocado Spring Rolls, 34
Shrimp Avocado Salad, 210
Three-Pepper Guacamole, 47
Tuna & White Bean Lettuce Wraps, 205

BACON
Bacon & Swiss Chicken Sandwiches, 131
Broccoli with Garlic, Bacon & Parmesan, 259
Brussels Sprouts with Bacon & Garlic, 260
Chard & Bacon Linguine, 190
Cod with Bacon & Balsamic Tomatoes, 214
Hearty Vegetable Lentil Soup, 66
Red, White & Blue Potato Salad, 81
Special Occasion Beef Bourguignon, 113
Spinach Steak Pinwheels, 106

BANANAS
Banana-Pineapple Cream Pies, 304
Banana Wheat Bread, 278
Frozen Chocolate Monkey Treats, 303
Frozen Yogurt Fruit Pops, 305
Raspberry-Banana Soft Serve, 304
Wholesome Banana Bread, 285

BARLEY
Barley Beef Burgers, 121
Comforting Beef Barley Soup, 57
Turkey & Vegetable Barley Soup, 50

BEANS
Artichoke Hummus, 41
Avocado & Garbanzo Bean Quinoa
  Salad, 238

Balsamic Three-Bean Salad, 77
Black Bean-Tomato Chili, 53
Black Beans with Bell Peppers & Rice, 231
Bow Tie & Spinach Salad, 241
Chicken Burrito Skillet, 156
Chili-Rubbed Steak with Black Bean
  Salad, 103
Easy White Chicken Chili, 56
Garlic Tilapia with Spicy Kale, 222
Greek Salad Pitas, 239
Red Beans & Sausage, 170
Sausage & Greens Soup, 66
Slow-Cooked Chicken Chili, 245
Southwest Breakfast Pockets, 24
Tomato & Garlic Butter Bean Dinner, 230
Tuna & White Bean Lettuce Wraps, 205
Turkey Pinto Bean Salad with Southern
  Molasses Dressing, 162

BEEF (also see Ground Beef)
Ancho Garlic Steaks with Summer Salsa, 120
Asparagus Beef Stir-Fry on Potatoes, 94
Balsamic Beef Kabob Sandwiches, 115
Chili-Rubbed Steak with Black Bean
  Salad, 103
Comforting Beef Barley Soup, 57
Easy & Elegant Tenderloin Roast, 118
Easy Marinated Flank Steak, 98
Feta Steak Tacos, 118
Italian Crumb-Crusted Beef Roast, 98
Mediterranean Pot Roast Dinner, 248
Open-Faced Roast Beef Sandwiches, 104
Peppered Beef Tenderloin, 96
Philly Cheesesteak Rolls, 102
Slow Cooker Beef Tostadas, 255
Smoky Espresso Steak, 110
Special Occasion Beef Bourguignon, 113
Spinach & Feta Burgers, 94
Spinach Steak Pinwheels, 106
Sublime Lime Beef, 106
Summer Salad with Citrus Vinaigrette, 110
Teriyaki Beef Stew, 245
Vegetable Steak Kabobs, 110

BEETS
Beet & Sweet Potato Fries, 261
Beet Salad with Lemon Dressing, 84

ALPHABETICAL RECIPE INDEX